Essentials in Hospice and Palliative Care:
A PRACTICAL RESOURCE FOR EVERY NURSE

Essentials in Hospice and Palliative Care:
A PRACTICAL RESOURCE FOR EVERY NURSE

Katherine Murray
RN, BSN, MA, CHPCN(C), FT

Life and Death Matters
Victoria, BC

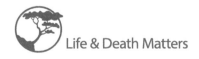

Life & Death Matters

www.lifeanddeathmatters.ca

Published by Life and Death Matters, Victoria, BC, Canada
www.lifeanddeathmatters.ca

Illustrations by Joanne Thomson
Editing by Sarah Weber and Ann-Marie Gilbert
Design by Greg Glover

Library and Archives Canada Cataloguing in Publication

Murray, Katherine, 1957-, author
        Essentials in hospice and palliative care : a practical resource for
every nurse / Katherine Murray, RN, BSN, MA, CHPCN(C), FT.

Includes bibliographical references and index.
ISBN 978-1-926923-11-6 (paperback)

    1. Hospice care. 2. Palliative treatment. 3. Hospice nurses. I. Title.

RT87.T45M85 2016   616.02'9   C2016-906184-1

Disclaimer

DEDICATION

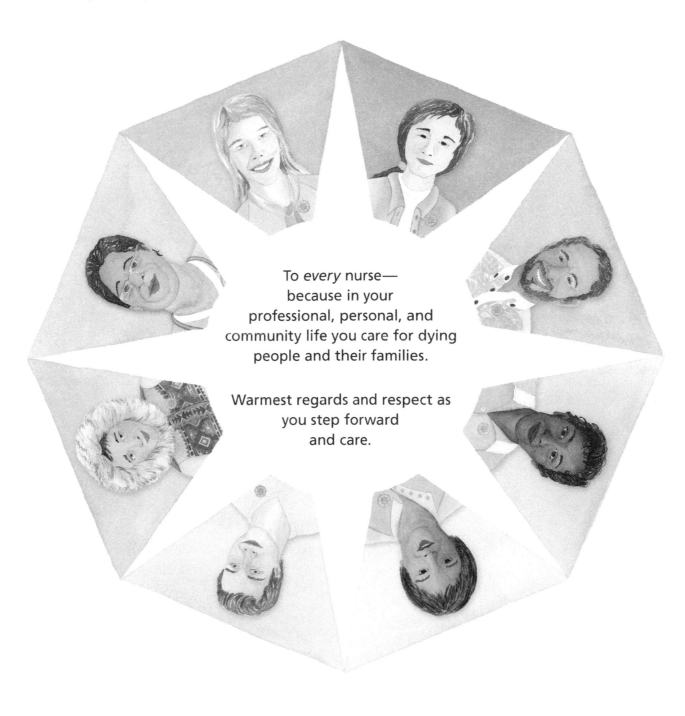

To *every* nurse—
because in your
professional, personal, and
community life you care for dying
people and their families.

Warmest regards and respect as
you step forward
and care.

About the Cover

The arbutus tree shown on the cover of this book is native to southeastern Vancouver Island, the nearby Gulf Islands, the adjacent coast of mainland British Columbia, and some areas along the west coast of the United States. Often rooted in the crevices of rock faces along the shore, this tree, with its gnarled and twisted branches, hangs over the edge and is blown about by the wind. The smooth, papery bark peels off as new bark grows. Each arbutus is unique.

The arbutus inspires me with its ability to grow, survive, and even thrive in such rough and rocky areas. This tree graces the cover of my book because to me the arbutus symbolizes the strength of the human spirit, the amazing ability of human beings to survive, grow, and even thrive in difficult, harsh, and even traumatic situations. Like the tree, we too get gnarled as we age. And like the tree, we are all unique.

The arbutus reminds me of those I care for, those who grew in the midst of dying, who grew as they cared for their loved ones or in the years following.

The arbutus reminds me of you, the many nurses I have worked with over the years. You also struggle with personal and work challenges, you provide excellent care, and you inspire me with your stories.

I wish you well as you continue on your path of caring for others. I hope that you will find great satisfaction and growth in doing this work.

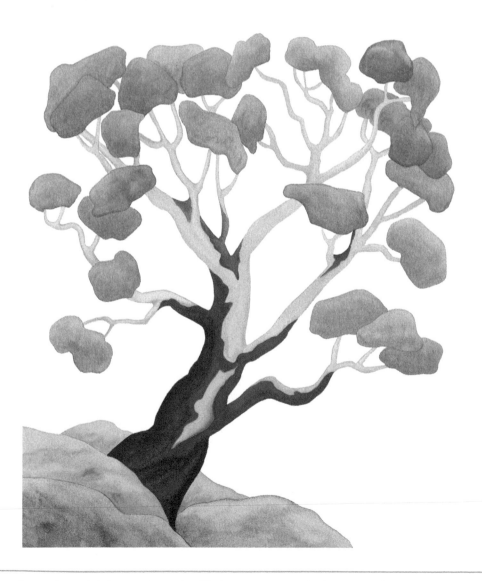

ACKNOWLEDGMENTS

I am extremely grateful to the people who helped me in the development of this book.

I am grateful for the hospice and palliative care nurses who strengthened my practice and who influenced the education I provide. I thank Terry Downing, Coby Tschanz, Della Roberts, Deanna Hutchings, Terry Webber, Jeanne Weis, Dr. Ann Syme, Uta Rach, Krystal Anne Murray Brown, Chelsea Knowles, Maggie Moreton, Sarita Van Dyke, Brenda Hearson, Ann Brignell, and nurse practitioners Camara Van Brennan and Janice Robinson.

Thank you to the educators who have mentored me, provided insight, and shared their passion for nursing and nursing education, teaching, and learning. In particular I thank Jeanne Weis, Coby Tschanz, Joanne Thomson, Dr. Lorelei Newton, Dawn Witherspoon, Andrea Leatherdale, Leanne McKinzey, Dr. Carrie Mines, Laura Bulmer, Zola Goebel, Esther Aguilar, Dr. Gweneth Doane, and Dr. Kathy Kortes-Miller and Patricia Strachan.

I am grateful for the privilege of working with these hospice and palliative care physicians in the clinical setting, with the Palliative Response Team, through educational endeavors and in international projects: Drs. Pippa Hawley, Deb Braithwaite, Joshua Shadd, Daphna Grossman, Sharon Koivu, Doris Barwich, Jim Wilde, Michael Downing, and Fraser Black.

Working with counselors and spiritual care providers helped me to better understand the psychosocial perspective. I am thankful for the time spent with Allyson Whiteman, Elizabeth Causton, Michelle (Misha) Butot, Susan Breiddal, Michelle Dale, Wendy Wainwright, and Dr. Carla Cheatham.

I am grateful for the personal support workers, including Jackie McDonald, who represents the many health care workers, health care assistants, and nursing assistants I have met through the years who have taught me much and who provide phenomenal care for the dying and their families.

I am grateful for all those who assisted in this project through research and contributions, specifically the following people:

⯈ Jeanne Weis, Terry Webber, Allyson Whiteman, and Terri Litfin for their help in searching the literature and identifying treasures of knowledge and best practice.

⯈ Dr. Kelli Stadjuhar and the Initiative for a Palliative Approach in Nursing Leadership and Education (iPANEL) team for their phenomenal work on integrating a palliative approach into care.

⯈ Dr. John Mastrojohn, Dr. Christy Torkildson, Pam Malloy, Dr. Ira Byock, Dr. Terry Martin, Dr. Cheryl Parrott, Lynn Tobin, Marlene Lee, and Sara Collins, who helped me to understand the perspective from the United States.

⯈ Michelle Dale, who shared her guidelines for family conferences and the analogy of the marathon of caregiving.

⯈ Dr. Lorelei Newton, Dr. Janet Storch, Barbara Mason, and Erika Paxman, who helped me to explore ethics in nursing and, in particular, ethics in dying and in caring for the dying person and their family.

⯈ Kelsey Rounds, who contributed knowledge and research about marginalized populations and their experiences with health care.

⯈ Dr. Betty Davies and Dr. Rose Steele for their research on best practices health care professionals, which informed Chapter 3. Betty has been an example to me of excellence in nursing since the 1970s.

⯈ Misha Butot, who helped write "A Personal Creed on Love in Professional Practice" and, with creative support from Coby Tschanz, Allyson Whiteman, and Joanne Thomson, worked with me to summarize the "Ten Principles of Love in Professional Practice" (based on Misha's initial research).

⯈ Dr. Darcy Harris and Dr. Phillip Larkin for their input on compassion.

⯈ Elizabeth Causton, who wrote the metaphor of the "family dance" and provided content on therapeutic boundaries, roadblocks to communication, and responding to questions.

⯈ Jim Mulcahy, who shared "A Story about Care," and who shared his thoughts about care as a recipient and a caregiver.

⯈ Bruce Kennedy, an expert and dedicated hospice palliative care pharmacist and researcher, who provided valuable input to the section on using opioids in hospice and palliative care.

⯈ Cari Hoffman who provided insight and guidance for the section on advance care planning.

⯈ Dr. David K. Wright, who provided the comprehensive content about physician-assisted dying, and worked with me to write this excellent section.

- Andrea Warnick, a fellow student in the thanatology program at Hood College, who wrote the piece on working with children.

- Dr. Ann Syme for sharing her ideas and resources on sexuality and intimacy.

- Dr. Carla Cheatham for her research on spiritual care, and her contributions to the FICA Spiritual Care Assessment tool.

- Dr. Françoise Mathieu, who contributed to the piece on compassion fatigue in the books I wrote for personal support workers and nursing assistants: *Integrating a Palliative Approach: Essentials for Personal Support Workers* (2014) and *Essentials in Hospice and Palliative Care: A Resource for Nursing Assistants* (2015). The materials in those texts were adapted for this text for nurses.

- Carrie Bergman from the Center for Contemplative Mind in Society, who provided insight and shared the illustration of the Tree of Contemplative Practices.

Many organizations and people helped form the foundation of this text. I gratefully acknowledge:

- The two national education providers—Pallium Canada (Learning Essentials Approaches in Palliative Care [LEAP]) and, in the United States, the End-of-Life Nursing Education Consortium (ELNEC).

- Dr. Betty Ferrell and Dr. Nessa Coyle, editors of and contributors to *The Oxford Textbook of Palliative Nursing*. They are leaders in palliative care nursing in the United States and internationally.

- The two national hospice and palliative care associations—the Canadian Hospice Palliative Care Association (CHPCA) and, in the United States, the National Hospice and Palliative Care Organization (NHPCO), and their respective leaders Sharon Baxter (executive director) and John Mastrojohn (chief operating officer).

- Victoria Hospice Society, which provided me with almost 25 years of work experience, on-the-job education, and the opportunity to teach and attend some seminal educational events.

- The College of Licensed Practical Nurses of Alberta, which gifted me with an in-kind donation of work time from Jeanne Weis. She provided her expertise as a strong hospice and palliative care nurse and a former licensed practical nurse. She has a Master of Nursing degree and brought with her to this project her experience in policy writing. This gift was a vote of confidence and support, and included the college's express desire to have a resource that would help students in practical nursing programs achieve the competencies related to hospice and palliative care. Thank you, Linda Stanger, Teresa Bateman, and Glenda Tarnowski.

I need to acknowledge that my involvement with hospice and palliative care nursing started in my childhood. My dear aunt, Frances Montgomery, the master family caregiver, introduced me to caregiving and compassionate communities when I was a teenager, and my mother, Yetta Lees, not only taught me of community, but also asked and allowed me to be part of the community that cared for her when she died.

I have said often that I am very good at gathering together excellent people into a team. The team members that worked directly on this book are:

- Joanne Thomson—How did I ever attempt to provide education without an artist in my life? Creating educational resources with Joanne has thrilled me. Together we wrestled with concepts and explored ways to create "delicious and digestible" resources, and then Joanne would retreat to her studio and later return with illustrations that inspired and strengthened the written materials. Thank you.

- Greg Glover—Thank you for your outstanding work on the complex layout of this book, which helps make it visually delicious and educationally digestible. Your insight and experience have been invaluable to this project.

- Ann-Marie Gilbert—This book would not have been finished if it were not for you. You endured and even enjoyed the process right through to completion. I thank you, Ann-Marie, and appreciate your many, many contributions.

- Sarah Weber and Ann-Marie Gilbert—You are phenomenal editors. Thank you both. Your attention to detail is incredible. Wow! I stand all amazed!

- Kim Garnett— We at Life and Death Matters knew when we first met you that we needed you, your leadership, and your ideas. Thank you for coming on board and for staying on board!

As well I thank Ted, my hubby of over 35 years. Thank you for your help, your encouragement, and your constant belief in me. ¡Gracias, mi amigo!

And to our kids—Jenny, Naomi, Michael, Krystal, and Geordie—thank you for all the lively dinnertime conversations about dying, loss, and grief. Thank you for helping me to live more fully and to love more deeply.

Kath

CONTENTS

PREFACE

A Text for Every Nurse

Every nurse cares for dying people. Whether you nurse in a hospice or a palliative care, medical, intensive care, or long-term care unit, you care for people who are dying, you care for their family members, and you care for people experiencing loss and grief. You care in your professional and your personal life, and you care as a member of the larger community. This text will help every nurse to integrate a palliative approach into care by incorporating the principles and practices of hospice and palliative care across all care settings, early in the disease process, for people with any life-limiting illness.

This text was created to be "delicious and digestible." The colorful, evocative illustrations make it delicious for the eyes, helping you envision the concepts of hospice and palliative care in practice. The stories bring flavor and depth to the concepts and principles, and build your appetite to turn the page and see what is next. The text is digestible, because current best practice, principles, and practical care strategies are provided in bite-sized pieces that you can easily absorb and use in your practice. The ultimate goals are for nurses to learn how to provide excellent physical and psychosocial care for the dying person and their family, and to feel more confident, competent, and compassionate in doing so.

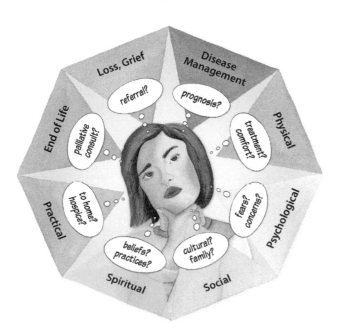

The illustration with the nurse within the star is used in this text as an icon to prompt reflections on what best practice might be for a given situation. The icon will be your cue to consider the care issues presented and reflect on how best to provide care.

I hope that this text will both be an educational tool and inspire you to claim or to reclaim and to celebrate the art and science of hospice and palliative care nursing.

Visit the Life and Death Matters website for learning activities and new companion resources for this text, Essentials in Hospice and Palliative Care: A Resource for Every Nurse.

Essential Reading for Every Nurse

Every nurse provides hospice and palliative care. This text provides knowledge, skills, and strategies for providing excellent hospice and palliative care and, as such, is an essential resource for every nurse.

Use these chapter summaries to decide how you want to approach the book in a way that will best meet your needs.

Chapter 1: The Dying Process

Causes of death have changed in the past 100 years. Read this chapter to learn about the common patterns of dying for people in the 21st century and the impact of these patterns on the dying person, their family, and the health care system.

Chapter 2: Integrating a Palliative Approach

Learn about the first hospice that Dame Cicely Saunders created, the philosophy, principles, and practices of hospice and palliative care, and how they have been shaped, woven together, and reformed into the current practices of integrating a palliative approach.

Chapter 3: Preparing to Care

Strategies for best practice, including compassion and providing love in professional practice, are explained in this chapter. Learn to reflect on how you provide care, and to consider how you can integrate best practice interactions.

Chapter 4: Using Standardized Tools

The screening, assessing, and communication tools referenced in the text are gathered together in this chapter—a hospice and palliative care toolbox. When a tool is mentioned in the text, refer to this chapter to view the full-size tool and read the instructions for use.

Chapter 5: Enhancing Physical Comfort

In Part 1, read the principles and practices for enhancing physical comfort—the heart of providing care—in hospice and palliative care. In Part 2, learn to recognize and assess common symptoms dying people experience and to incorporate strategies for managing symptoms using non-pharmacological comfort measures and pharmacological measures.

Chapter 6: Providing Psychosocial Care

Explore common psychosocial needs of the dying person and their family and learn strategies for supporting them. Examine and reflect on medical assistance in dying, and physician assisted dying and the impact on HCPs. Consider the importance of strengthening the "social" in psychosocial.

Chapter 7: Last Days and Hours

Learn the common changes that a dying person might experience in their last days and hours, and ways to provide comfort and support for the person and their family. Understand the importance of preparation in planning for care at the time of and following death, and the use of rituals.

Chapter 8: Caring for *You*!

Develop your understanding of compassion fatigue and your ability to self-evaluate for early signs of compassion fatigue. Learn ways to minimize your risk of developing compassion fatigue by caring for yourself even as you strive to provide excellent care for others.

Addressing Ethical Issues

The text in "Ethics Touchstone" boxes addresses ethical principles and issues. The term "touchstone" is commonly used to mean a standard against which to evaluate quality or genuineness. In this text, the ethics touchstones draw upon the following codes of ethics:
- The International Council of Nurses (ICN) (Appendix 1)
- The Canadian Nurses Association (Appendix 2)
- The Canadian Council for Practical Nurse Regulators (CCPNR) (Appendix 3)
- The American Nurses Association (ANA) (Appendix 4)

The ethics touchstones also include thought-providing reflective questions designed to unearth previously unnoticed or overlooked ethical dimensions of practice. As you read, use the ethics touchstones to assess the value of your new understandings in terms of relationships, responsibilities, behaviors, and decision making, as well as for self-reflection and peer feedback. Return to these touchstones as your nursing practice develops, and reconsider your earlier responses to the reflective questions.

The icon for the ethics touchstones consists of a box to represent the framework in which every nurse provides care, a heart to remind you to provide care from the heart, and an "e" signifying ethical questions for reflection.

The 2012 code of ethics of the ICN states, very simply, that "nurses have four fundamental responsibilities: to promote health, to prevent illness, to restore health, and to alleviate suffering" (International Council of Nurses, 2012). This text will help you to fulfill the responsibilities the ICN has identified as you work to prevent or manage common symptoms, support healthy grieving, prevent or respond to complicated grief, and decrease suffering associated with dying, death, loss, and grief.

Developing Cultural Competence and Cultural Humility

The text incorporates stories to help nurses develop cultural competence and cultural humility. The stories provide nurses with the opportunity to reflect on their ethnocentric view, to develop awareness of other people's cultural beliefs and values, and to develop cultural skills for communicating with, interpreting, and engaging with people of different cultures. With these practices the nurse can mindfully respect and support the person and family and their cultural wishes.

Incorporating Leadership and Advocacy

As a nurse you are in a unique position to lead and advocate for the dying person and the family. You witness suffering, and you assess physical and psychosocial issues. Throughout the text you will be encouraged to consider your role as a leader and advocate in your day-to-day work as you strive to integrate hospice and palliative care across the continuum of care.

I wish you well, and mostly I wish that this text helps you increase your competence, confidence, and compassion in caring for the dying person and their family.

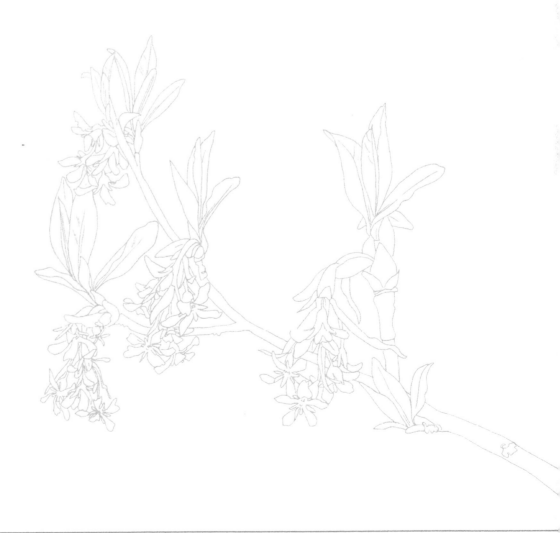

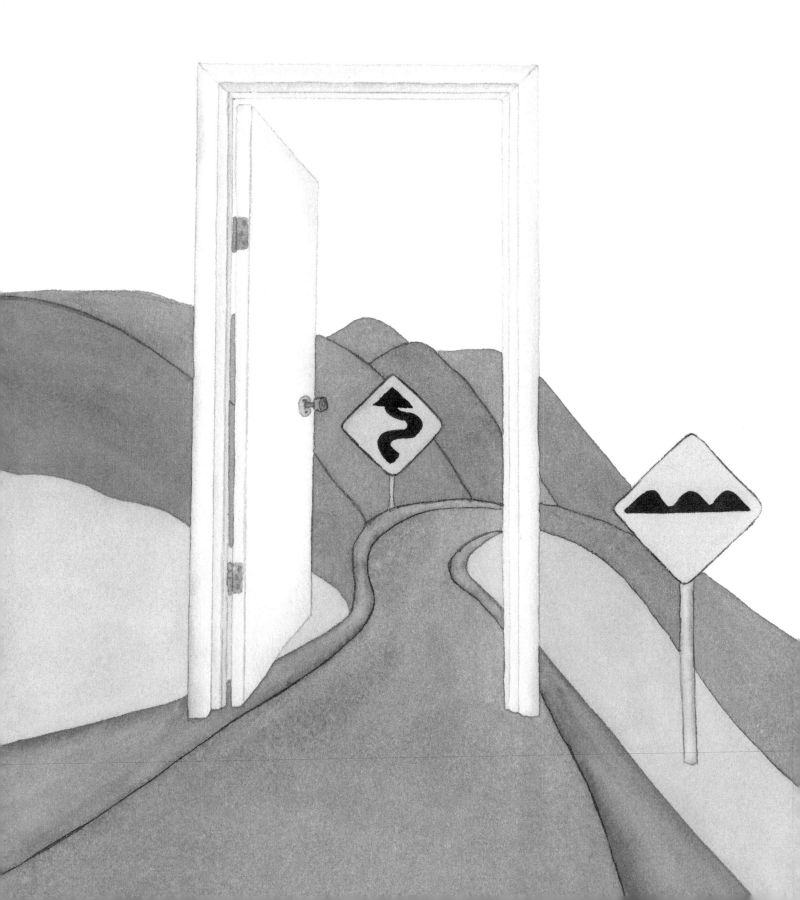

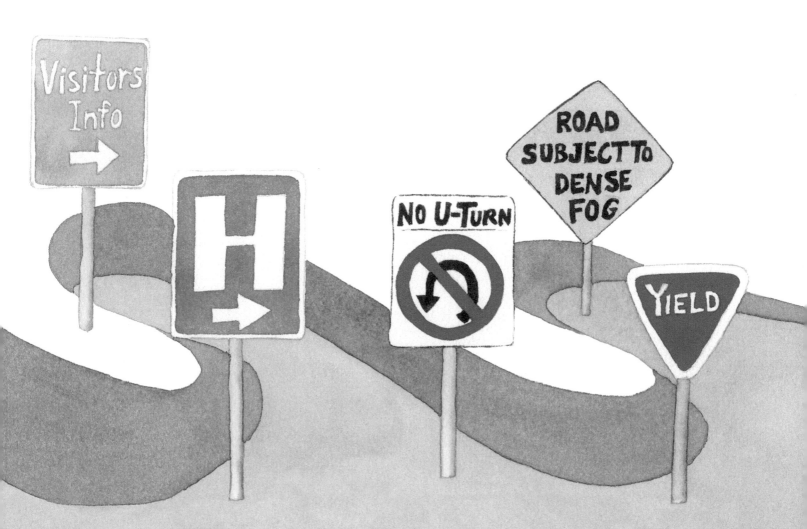

Understanding the Dying Process

Common Patterns of Dying

When I studied thanatology (the study of death, dying, and bereavement), one of the questions students considered was, "When does dying begin?" The answers, of course, ranged from birth to the visible onset of illness, to last days and hours. The answer I always liked best was, "At 40, when the dog dies and the kids leave home!" (At this point I am 60ish and still hoping to get a dog. The kids have come back home!) In fact, dying begins differently for each person, depending on the illness and the person's own health.

What does dying look like? To answer this question, you might observe the physical changes the person experiences in their last days and hours. However, understanding what dying looks like in this century requires that you look further back than the last days, back to the weeks, months, and perhaps years prior to death.

To answer the question "What does dying look like?" you need to understand the changes in the way people are dying in the 21st century.

This chapter explores common patterns of dying and discusses the reality that a dying person is still very much a living person.

Palliative care is now seen as a valuable service from time of diagnosis. Why? Because the dying person may have many needs for holistic care early on.

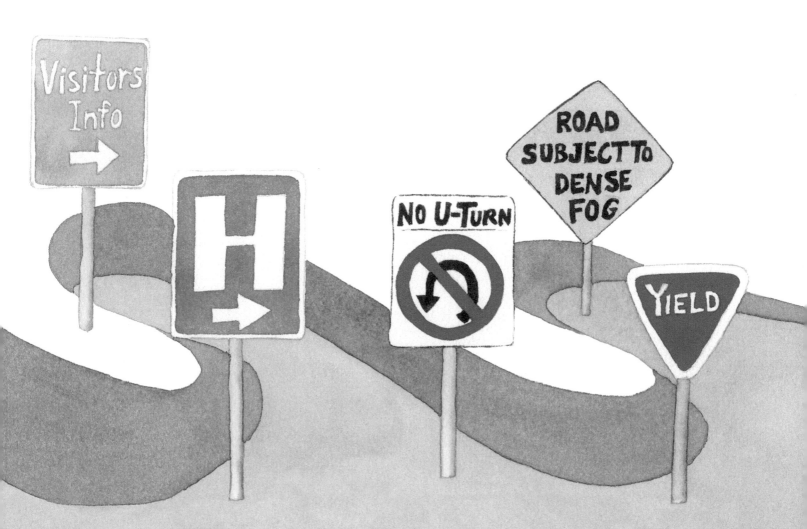

Defining People Referred to in This Text

Dying person: I use this term (or simply "person") because I cannot bear to use the word "client" to describe someone who is so vulnerable and so unable to be a "consumer." I also cannot use the word "patient" to describe someone who probably feels anything but patient, and I cannot use the word "resident," as it is not applicable in all settings.

Family: This term means anyone that the person defines as family, as well as anyone significant to the person. For simplicity, I use "family" rather than using "family and significant others" repeatedly.

Health care provider (HCP): This term means trained people who are paid to provide care (e.g., nurses, physicians, nursing assistants, personal support workers, medical assistants, counselors, and spiritual care providers), including health care workers.

Health care worker: This term means any paid frontline worker. In Canada they may be called personal support workers or health care assistants, as well as other titles, while in the United States they may be called nursing assistants, nurse's aides, medical assistants, patient care technicians, or a variety of other titles.

Caregiver: This term means any unpaid caregiver, such as a friend or family member, who provides care for the dying person.

Nurse: This term means "every nurse," that is, anyone trained in the nursing profession, including, but not limited to, practical nurses, vocational nurses, registered nurses, psychiatric nurses, and retired nurses.

Physician/nurse practitioner: This term is used to identify a person responsible for diagnosing, treating, and managing the dying person's symptoms.

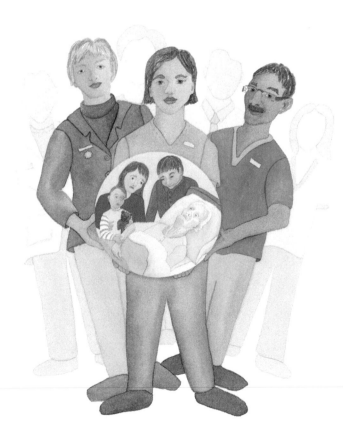

People Have Never Died Like This

> *My grandfather was a farmer. One morning he was sick. He worked in the fields all day. At night he was worse. His pain was excruciating. My grandmother sent for the doctor. The doctor came in the morning, laid him on the kitchen table, and cut open his abdomen. He was full of gangrene. He died three days later.*

 Ethics Touchstone
How might you respond to this death as a professional? How might your response differ if the person who died was an elderly member of your family?

A hundred or a thousand years ago, people did not die as they die today. In fact, never in known human history have people died as they are dying today in the developed world.

A hundred years ago, when a farmer developed a serious illness, a week later the farmer was either back working in the field or buried in it. Death was mostly due to infections and occurred over days, sometimes weeks. The advent of the sanitary techniques and the medical treatments of public health now help people survive illnesses that previously would have killed them (Gawande, 2014). In industrialized nations, the vast majority of the population now survives childhood illnesses and lives to a greater age than ever before.

As people live longer, aging and dying will include developing one or more life-limiting, serious, progressive illnesses such as cardiac and respiratory diseases and cancers in their senior years. While 70% of Canadian deaths result from chronic diseases, among seniors aged 65 years and older, 74% suffer with pain and discomfort of one or more chronic life-limiting illnesses (CHPCA, 2015). As the last of the baby boomers reach age 65, seniors may comprise up to 25% of the population by the year 2036 (Statistics Canada, 2011). People suffering with chronic, progressive illnesses will require care over many years, substantially increasing the care burden. Given the changes in demographics, however, fewer HCPs and caregivers will be available to provide care.

To be prepared to meet the needs of the dying person and their family, it is important to understand the common patterns of dying and acknowledge that the dying process entails more than the physical changes occurring in the last days and hours of life. It is equally important to recognize that while people are dying, they also continue to live. HCPs need to support people to live while dying.

> The term "life-limiting illness" refers to any illness, acute or chronic, that is likely to shorten or "limit" a person's life. "Life-limiting illness" is a gentler term than "terminal illness" and may be more easily accepted by the dying person and their family. People with life-limiting illnesses can benefit from a palliative approach early in the disease process.

Common Trajectories of Dying

Dying is a unique process for each person but usually occurs in one of four patterns: sudden death, steady decline, stuttering decline (the "roller coaster"), and slow decline. Each decline reflects changes in the person's function and abilities, specifically changes in:

- Ambulation—the ability to move around
- Participation in activities
- Personal care
- Eating and drinking
- Cognitive functioning

A person's decline in function over time can be illustrated as a line on a graph. The line—the progression of the decline—is known as the "trajectory" or pattern. Each trajectory has different challenges for the dying person, their family, and HCPs. HCPs can observe changes in a dying person's abilities as a way to understand their declining condition. This section defines the parameters of these trajectories, the illnesses that are often involved, and the challenges for the person and their family.

Sudden Death

Approximately 10% of people in developed nations will die suddenly. A heart attack, major stroke, or car accident are common causes of sudden death. In most cases of sudden death (Figure 1), the dying person and the family do not know that death is imminent.

As a nurse you may witness a sudden death or arrive just after a sudden death. Chapter 7, "Providing Psychosocial Care," includes information on what to do after a sudden, unexpected death has occurred in the home setting.

Figure 1. The sudden death trajectory

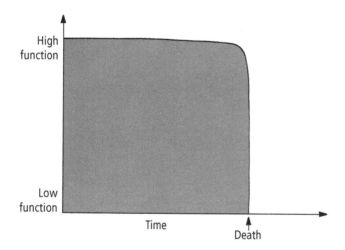

> **Sudden Death**
>
> *I was playing baseball when my brother called to tell me that our mom had had a heart attack. I went straight to the hospital but was too late. It is hard to believe. I wish we had been prepared. It would have been easier if she had been sick for a while so that I could have said good-bye and told her that I loved her. I feel like I was hit by a truck!*

 Ethics Touchstone
Have you, or anyone you know, been affected by the sudden death of a loved one? Were there advantages to this trajectory? Were there disadvantages?

When I ask people how they want to die, there are always some who say they would prefer a sudden death. They often state that they do not want to be a burden on their loved ones. However, grieving people whose loved one has died suddenly often express regret that they did not have time to say good-bye or to prepare for or anticipate the death, and may say that they wish they could have provided care. These people may say,

> *Well it might have been a good death for her, but it was not a good death for me.*

Steady Decline

The steady decline pattern of dying (Figure 2) is often observed in people dying from cancer. They may be relatively strong for a long period of time, even for years, after their diagnosis and treatment. At some time they experience a significant steady decline in function and strength, signifying the last six months of life. They may be confined to bed only in the last weeks before death.

Figure 2. The steady decline trajectory

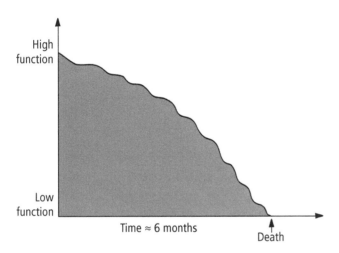

The following story of Yetta Lee's dying illustrates this steady decline. Because her death was anticipated, Yetta (my mother) and our family had opportunities to prepare, share, and care. Yetta was grateful to have the knowledge that she was dying. The family gathered, cared for her, and prepared for her death. She chose what she wanted to do with her limited energy and time. She registered with the provincial palliative care program. People offered assistance, expressed gratitude, and reminisced.

The steady decline can have a few benefits, but there are times when it may feel too fast. People may feel they have no time to prepare, that they are constantly racing to catch up to a "new normal." The decline may feel especially fast when a person is not ready or able to process information when it is shared, when there are significant differences in how individual family members hear and act on the information received, or when the health care team does not share, early in the process, information about the seriousness of the illness and what to anticipate.

Most people believe that a steady decline is how most people die. In fact, less than 20% of people die in this way.

Steady Decline

On September 12th, Yetta walked 12 kilometers—not bad for an 82-year-old. However, 10 weeks later she felt quite fatigued and visited the doctor.

"Fatigue," she said. "Oh, and my right side is sore."

On November 8th she was told that the ultrasound and CT showed a tumor. The surgeon very gently and kindly told her, "You have an inoperable tumor ... How long? ... Hmm ... maybe 6 to 12 months."

She got as busy as her energy would allow her. She organized papers, resigned from committees, checked on a few people she was concerned about. She connected with her closest friends.

Within six weeks we, her four kids, gathered and celebrated Christmas. She talked about the light in a season of darkness. She ate whipping cream and decided life was too short for cheap wine. She nibbled small bits of anything she felt like eating and nothing else.

"What do you want? What is important to you in dying?" I asked. She was very clear, "I do not want any pain." Repeatedly she described her last months as "the richest period of my life."

As weeks passed, Yetta slept more. She became unstable on her feet. She came close to death a number of times, but then she would perk up again.

And then, on the 16th of January in the quiet of the night, she breathed her last breaths and was gone.

Ethics Touchstone
A steady decline is commonly thought to be how most people die, but is the trajectory for only 20% of people. What are the advantages and disadvantages of the steady decline trajectory?

Stuttering Decline—the Roller Coaster

The stuttering decline trajectory (Figure 3) describes people who alternate between periods of decline and periods of recovery. A period of decline may result from the exacerbation of an illness or be caused by a fall, a fracture, a new illness, or a combination of these events. At times, the person may require hospitalization and treatment, or an adjustment of medications to help them stabilize. Following stabilization, the person may recover some of their previous functioning and may again enjoy the activities they used to do. The person may be stable for weeks or months, and then decline again when their chronic illness changes or they experience another infection, fall, or illness. Eventually, the repeated declines lead to death. In approximately 70% of dying people, the pattern of decline follows a stuttering or slow trajectory to death.

Figure 3. The stuttering decline trajectory

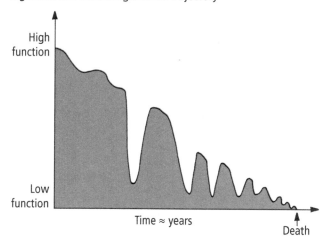

The stuttering decline is likely to be experienced by people with life-limiting illnesses such as organ failure, congestive heart failure, and kidney disease, as well as people with illnesses such as Parkinson's disease or dementia-related illnesses.

Sarah's story (see box at right) illustrates her experiences caring for Tom through a stuttering decline. She talks of her fatigue and the challenge of not knowing the future. When Tom improves, she wonders if he is getting better. Each time he declines, she wonders if he is dying. Sarah may consider the downs and ups as part of the ongoing illness and not realize the overall decline. She may not notice that the number of episodes and exacerbations is increasing.

Estimating the time remaining until death for people in stuttering decline is difficult. Research indicates that half of the people with advanced progressive illnesses will not know the week before they die that the next week will be their last. Even the day before they die, many of these people will be thought to have up to six months to live.

Caring for a person experiencing a stuttering or slow decline has its unique challenges. Reflecting on her own caregiving experiences, Michelle Dale, a hospice counselor, expresses the challenges beautifully in her story "Caring for the Dying—It's Like Running a Race" (see page 8).

Stuttering Decline—the Roller Coaster

My name is Sarah. I am Tom's wife and caregiver. Tom has chronic obstructive pulmonary disease. He was diagnosed 15 years ago, but the last 8 years have been the hardest, with repeat hospital admissions, decreased abilities, and increased needs. I have heard it said that the typical patient with this disease goes to death's door a number of times before dying. At least five times the children have gathered to say good-bye.

June 9: Last week the doctor came in and, squatting to make eye contact with Tom, asked us what we wanted. Tom said that he was tired—tired of hospitals, emergencies, tests, and more treatments. I very carefully suggested hospice. Tom and the doctor agreed.

June 15: We came home by transport ambulance. The kids came home to help. In the night, I wept. I am exhausted. I wonder if he will die soon.

July 16: How long will this go on? The nurses and health care workers come daily. I willingly let them help.

July 18: Tom is eating so little even with me trying to help him eat.

August 9: Tom has been restless for the last three nights. We sit with him constantly. He has more difficulty breathing. He is confused, sometimes talking to people who aren't there.

August 17: We celebrated our 60th anniversary two months early. He is very weak. He is confused again.

August 20: Tom died this morning.

Slow Decline

Figure 4. The slow decline trajectory

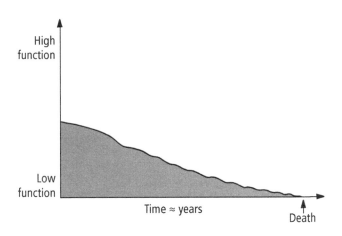

The slow decline trajectory (Figure 4) happens over a period of years. There may be periods of decline and improvement similar to those in the stuttering decline trajectory, but the ups and downs in a slow decline are more subtle. In contrast to the stuttering decline trajectory, the highs are not as high and the lows are not as low, making the slow decline trajectory seem gradual and sometimes unnoticeable. However, the people who are providing direct care or are involved daily with the dying person may notice the small changes. When the person has a good day, the family may wonder whether the person is getting better, and when the person has a bad day, whether death is near.

Parkinson's disease, dementia-related illnesses, and frailties cause this type of slow decline in a person's abilities. With the slow trajectory, people often lose the ability to care for themselves long before they are imminently dying. Unless they develop a significant infection or other medical crisis, people may linger for years. In these cases, the time until death is very difficult to estimate.

Usually, dying people who suffer from Alzheimer's disease first lose their ability to do tasks that require higher levels of thinking, such as balancing a checkbook. Then they lose basic-level functioning, such as being able to do their own personal care, or walk or eat independently. If the person lives long enough, they will lose the most basic abilities, including the ability to swallow.

People with other types of dementia may experience a differently shaped decline. People with vascular dementia may experience a small stroke that results in a decline in functioning (a step down) and then stabilize (remain at a plateau) until the next stroke occurs. Death may occur following a stroke.

Slow Decline

Mom was diagnosed with Parkinson's disease nine years ago, and with Alzheimer's disease five years ago. She did pretty well for the first years, with only a few visits to the doctor. But over the years it got more difficult to care for her. First, she would leave the house and go walking. Then she would get lost, so I had to go with her. Then she would just wander and not really go anywhere, but there was the possibility that she would get lost. Then she did not want to go anywhere or do anything. She started to resist care. She got restless and sometimes agitated and stopped finding pleasure in the cat, stopped watching TV, and did not like to be read to anymore.

At some point, the nurses assessed her and followed up by sending nursing assistants to help her with bathing and meals. Volunteers from the local dementia care program provided some respite care. I appreciated this help, but it was not enough. Nights were long; I slept poorly and got up too frequently. Then she fell, cut herself, and bruised her hip. She went by ambulance to emergency and then into a care home.

It was absolutely the most difficult thing I have ever done, leaving her there. I came home and wept. I was so tired of caregiving, but it was still hard to give the caregiving to someone else. And the staff, well, they seem fine, but there are so many of them.

Now, she does not know me. It is as if she is dead—but her body is still here. When I sing to her she becomes agitated. She does not participate in any activities.

She has bladder infections regularly. She hardly eats anything. She has difficulty swallowing, and sometimes does not eat at all. Last month they thought she was dying, but they have thought that before … I sometimes wonder if she will outlive me.

Caring for the Dying—It's Like Running a Race

I've often said to families that caring for the dying is like running a race in which the distance keeps changing. For example, at the time of diagnosis my aunt and my family were all shocked, convinced (due to the words of the doctor) that she had a very short prognosis. We were in a 100-meter sprint.

Everyone came, everyone called and sent letters and flowers, and made declarations of love.

Nobody was thinking about pacing.

And then things changed. It became clear that we were in, maybe, a 10-kilometer race. She had a treatment plan. There was hope being offered by her oncologist. We needed to slow down. We wished we had trained.

Then she had the surgery and it was awfully hard and everyone moved in again. We were back in a short-distance mentality—maybe not a 100-meter dash, maybe an 800-meter race. We needed to give everything, but we had to save a little for the finish.

Now she is doing well again. The prognosis is uncertain. There is talk of survival. Everyone realizes that we are in a marathon. Nobody trained. Someone needs to take responsibility for the water and food stations. We need volunteers to stand at the tricky corners to make sure we don't get lost.

As hospice workers we are the ones at the tricky corners.

We don't need to run the race, but we need to know how hard it is. We need to know how confusing and exhausting it is when the finish line keeps getting moved. Imagine being in a marathon and having 2 miles to go and then seeing a new sign that says, "Only 10 miles to go." How does one continue?

Michelle Dale

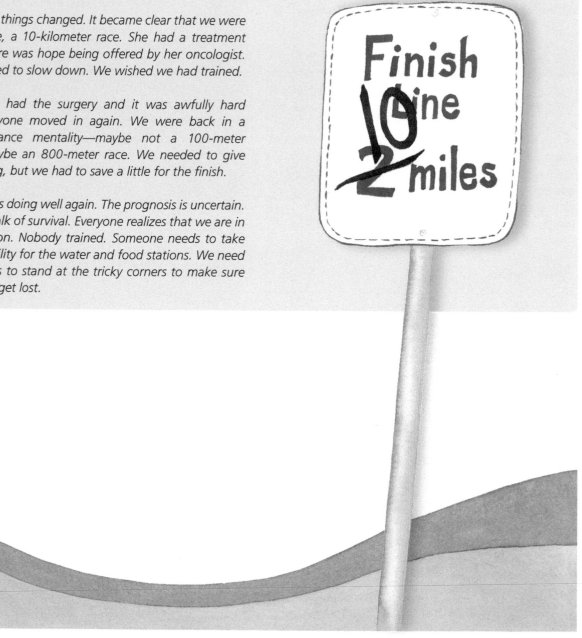

Reflections

People may experience common trajectories of dying but will have unique experiences. Dying is a deeply personal experience that also affects the dying person's family and community. Dying is not easy, and there are no rehearsals. As one woman said, "Dying ain't for wimps." However, in the midst of dying there can be room for living. This brings me to think of Gary Quinton.

Gary was diagnosed two years before we met. He was at a table, at the edge of a large auditorium where I delivered a talk titled "Alzheimer's is a terminal illness." I noticed him as I spoke because he was smiling and nodding. I wondered, "Who is he? Is he a family member? Does he have Alzheimer's disease? Why does he appear to understand? What am I saying that resonates with him?" After the presentation I turned, and there he was. "Who are you?" I asked. "My name is Gary Quinton" he replied. "But who are you?" I asked again, "Why do you 'get it'"?

Then Gary told me his story. He told me of being diagnosed with Alzheimer's a few years before. He told me how some people do not want to talk about dementia or acknowledge dementia as being a terminal illness, just like they did not want to talk about cancer many years ago. Gary and his wife, Judy, have continued to share some of their adventures since we first met. Gary still rides his bike around the city where they live, but takes the bus when the roads are too icy and it's snowing too hard. He prefers to live at risk rather than to stay home. He travels each summer to a Tai Chi conference, alone, by airplane, through a large international airport. Over the last few summers the couple has joined walking tours, hiking through rural prairie lands and European cities. I am not sure how Gary's memory is these days. I wonder if he remembers our time together. Regardless, I am sure that he enjoys the moments.

Gary and Judy remind me that dying is also about living, and living fully. Caring for those who are dying is about learning to live well and being reminded to live life fully in the face of challenges, changes, and uncertainty.

As I reflect on the experience of dying and of caregiving, I am struck by what I have witnessed and what I have learned. I am impressed by people who seem to live and die with grace, compassion, and courage. I am equally amazed at those who fight against death through to their last breath. All these stories are stored in my heart and my memory. The stories come to me when I ponder and when I am at a crossroad. They inspire me when I am deciding how to face challenges, changes, and uncertainty.

Ethics Touchstone
Think about the four different patterns of decline (trajectories) and place them in order of your most preferred (good death) to least preferred (bad death) way of dying. What are the reasons that prompted you to assign the most and least preferred methods of decline?

Would you want a different trajectory for a loved one?

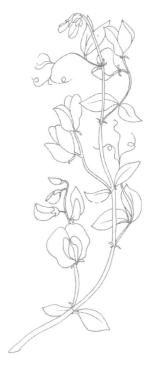

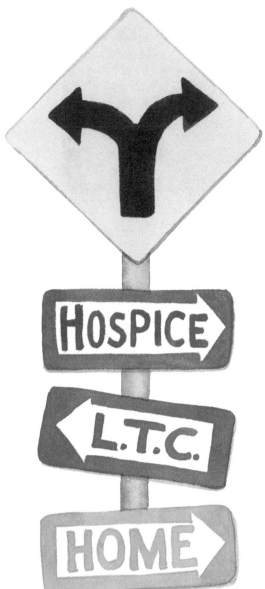
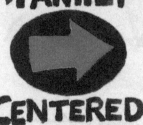
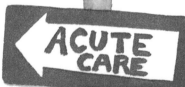

Integrating a Palliative Approach

A Dream of Better Care for the Dying

Historically, care of the dying was the responsibility of the family and the community. People died in their own homes. In the mid-1900s, with medical advances and the building of acute care hospitals, care of the dying was moved to the hospitals. People lived their last months, weeks, or days under the care of physicians, nurses, and other health care providers (HCPs).

It was in a busy acute care hospital that Cicely Saunders, a social worker and former nurse, met David Tasma. Tasma was living alone in London, England. He was dying. They talked for hours about the challenges that dying in an acute care hospital presented, and envisioned a place and philosophy of care designed specifically to address the needs of the dying person and their family—care that would relieve suffering and improve quality of life.

Following Tasma's death, Saunders spoke with a surgeon colleague about her dream. He suggested that she would be better able to make changes to care of the dying if she was a physician. Saunders then returned to study and earned a medical degree. With the holistic perspective of a nurse, a social worker, and now a medical doctor, she saw and understood the "total pain" that people experienced. In fact, she coined that term to describe the various types of pain—emotional, spiritual, physical, bureaucratic, and so on—that people might experience in the dying process.

In 1967, Saunders opened St Christopher's Hospice outside of London, England. In 1979, Queen Elizabeth II honored her with the title "Dame Commander of the Order of the British Empire" for her contributions to hospice and palliative care. Thereafter she was known as Dame Cicely Saunders.

Ethics Touchstone
Provision 6
The nurse, through individual and collective effort, establishes, maintains, and improves the ethical environment of the work setting and conditions of employment that are conducive to safe, quality health care.

Code of Ethics for Nurses (ANA, 2015a)

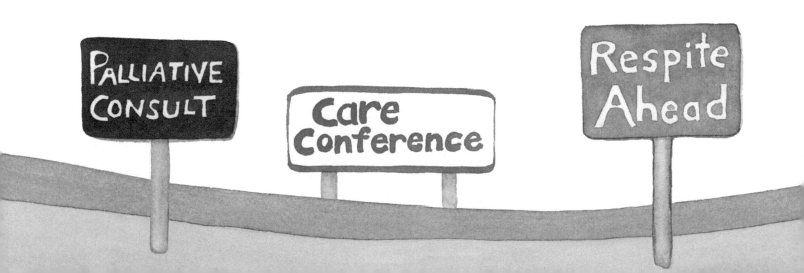

Hospice Care Begins

Saunders introduced the idea of specialized care for the dying to the United States in 1963, during a visit to Yale University. Her lecture about the concept of holistic hospice care to an audience of medical students, nurses, social workers, and chaplains included photos of terminally ill people, and their families. The photos showed the dramatic differences before and after symptoms were controlled. This lecture resulted in the development of hospice care in the United States (NHPCO, 2016a).

Dr. Balfour Mount, a physician in Quebec, Canada, studied in England with Cicely Saunders so that he could better understand the needs of people in his hospital who were dying. He coined the term "palliative care" because the word "hospice" did not translate well into French, which is commonly spoken in Quebec. He opened the palliative care unit at the Royal Victoria Hospital in Montreal in 1974.

Since those early days, hospice care and palliative care throughout the world has become an area of specialization in medicine, nursing, social work, and chaplaincy. Specialists and researchers have developed a great body of knowledge and skills that support holistic, person-centered care for the dying person and the family.

The values of hospice that Saunders identified continue today in modern hospice and palliative care. She said this of the dying person:

> You matter because you are you, and you matter to the end of your life. We will do all we can not only to help you die peacefully, but also to live until you die.

(Saunders, 2010)

Ethics Touchstone

Dame Cicely Saunders found her calling in nursing but left due to back pain. She trained in social work and, in this role, talked with David Tasma about a way to better meet the needs of the dying person. Why do you think she was encouraged to become a physician to realize her dream of care for the dying?

Do you think that her experience would be different in today's sociopolitical environment?

Would you be able to make the changes to caregiving that she made today in your role as a nurse?

Global Definition of Palliative Care

The World Health Organization (WHO) defines palliative care as "an approach that improves the quality of life of patients and their families facing the problems associated with life-threatening illness, through the prevention and relief of suffering by means of early identification and impeccable assessment and treatment of pain and other problems, physical, psychosocial and spiritual" (WHO, 2012).

Goals of Hospice and Palliative Care

The goals of hospice and palliative care unite the care philosophies and goals of the WHO (WHO, 2012), the Canadian Hospice Palliative Care Association (CHPCA) (CHPCA, 2013), and the (US) National Hospice Palliative Care Organization (NHPCO, 2016b), and identify for all HCPs common ground from which to provide care for the dying. Hospice and palliative care is care that:

- Affirms life and supports the person to live as actively as possible until death
- Regards dying as a normal process
- Considers the dying person and their family to be the unit of care
- Is offered early in the course of illness, with other therapies and investigations
- May influence the course of illness
- Provides support through death and bereavement

Hospice and palliative care promotes care that:
- Does not speed or delay dying or death
- Improves the dying person's quality of life
- Provides pain relief, manages distressing symptoms, and prevents new issues
- Attends to the holistic needs of the person

Hospice and palliative care is best when provided by an interprofessional team, which may include nurses, doc-tors, social workers, volunteers, chaplains, health care workers, psychiatrists, physiotherapy and palliative specialists, and others. The robust scope of the interprofessional team helps to address the dying person's physical, spiritual, social, psychological, ethical, and cultural needs. The size and composition of the interprofessional team will depend on the needs and preferences of the person, the availability of the resources, and the location of care.

Principles of Hospice and Palliative Care

Hospice and palliative care is based on these principles:
- Care is of high quality, ethical, and centered on the person and their family.
- Practices are safe, beneficial, and without undue risk, and are based in evidence and knowledge.
- Care is equally accessible to all people who need it.
- Care is best when provided by an interprofessional team.

(CHPCA, 2012; NHPCO, 2016b; WHO, 2012)

Evolving Models of Hospice and Palliative Care

To increase understanding of hospice and palliative care and the evolution of it over the past decades, three models of hospice and palliative care are provided in Figure 1.

The model in Figure 1a illustrates that the dying person received active life-prolonging treatments until hospice services were provided. In the United States and some places in Canada, the dying person was required to forgo any further curative or life-prolonging treatments before registering with hospice.

Often the criteria for registration with a hospice program or admission to a hospice unit required that the person have a prognosis of six months or less. People may have arrived at hospice after hearing the specialist, often an oncologist, say, "There is nothing more that we can do for you … you should go to hospice."

Providing hospice care in this model did not work well for people who were not ready to forgo active treatment. With this model of care, hospice was more available to people who were dying in a steady decline pattern and had a clear prognosis than to people who were dying with chronic life-limiting illnesses and for whom the time until death was uncertain.

Beginning Palliative Care Earlier

Figure 1b shows how palliative care programs evolved to address people's needs beginning at the time of diagnosis through until admission to the hospice program and the time of death. Hospice was provided in the last six months of life. Bereavement care started at the time of death and decreased over the following months and years.

The first two models in particular represent hospice and palliative care programs that required the development of specialists in hospice and palliative care, for example, a palliative consult team, a palliative care unit, or a free-standing hospice residence.

People who received the palliative care and then the hospice services benefitted from excellent pain and symptom management, as well as psychosocial and bereavement support.

However, people with chronic life-limiting illnesses still had difficulty accessing hospice and palliative care.

Expanding Hospice and Palliative Care

In the 1980s hospice doors were opened to people dying with AIDs, and later to those dying with end-stage cardiac, respiratory, or kidney disease, ALS, and other chronic life-limiting illnesses.

Figure 1. Models of hospice and palliative care

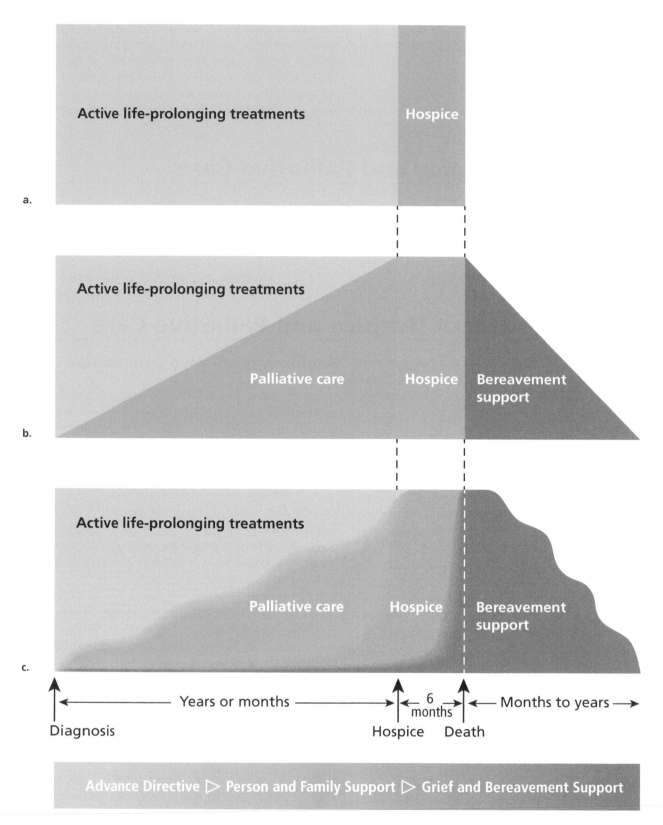

In hospice and palliative care communities, the understanding grew that people dying from any life-limiting illness could benefit from hospice and palliative care.

At the 2006 International Congress on Care of the Terminally Ill, a nephrologist, respirologist, neurologist, and cardiologist each spoke about the struggle to address the needs of the dying people for whom they care. The message of these professionals was clear: people with non-cancer diagnoses experience a significant symptom burden in the dying process and have psychosocial needs; hospice and palliative care programs are needed to serve people who have a non-cancer diagnosis!

A More Responsive Model of Hospice and Palliative Care

Figure 1c represents a more responsive approach to address the needs of people who can benefit from acute life-prolonging treatments while also receiving palliative care support.

This model builds on the strengths of the model shown in Figure 1b. Responding to the needs of the person from the time of diagnosis is referred to as "moving upstream" or "front loading" (Coyle, 2015). As the person moves closer to death, disease-modifying treatments usually decrease and the focus on hospice and palliative care increases.

In both the United States and Canada, more and more people with non-cancer diagnoses are served by hospice and palliative care programs.

In Canada, "hospice palliative care" programs provide palliative consultations, access to benefits, and hospice services all in one service. In such programs, the person may be involved in "hospice" for much longer than six months.

In the United States, people can register for hospice six months before death. However, physicians tend to overestimate the prognosis and delay discussing death, resulting in people being admitted to hospice programs only days or weeks before death.

In Figure 1c, the wavy line representing bereavement support illustrates that the need for it may not decrease in a steady decline but instead may fluctuate in the months or years following a death.

In the United States, palliative care is still funded separately from hospice care. Depending on the health care plan and the resources available at each hospital, people can access palliative care consultants or specialists early in the disease process. However, they may not be able to access palliative care services after registering for hospice services.

Improving Quality of Life with Hospice and Palliative Care

In a landmark study published in 2010, people who received palliative care in addition to oncological treatment reported better quality of life and improved mood states, and as a group experienced a longer survival rate (Temel et al., 2010). This study confirmed that hospice and palliative care does improve quality of life for people who are dying.

Another study of 160 people found that early, multidisciplinary hospice care was associated with better pain relief and quality of life, reduced costs, and less aggressive care at the end of life, as well as less psychiatric morbidity (Diamond et al., 2016).

These studies support the essential role of hospice and palliative care in ensuring that dying people have better quality of life, fewer symptoms, and greater satisfaction with their care. According to the CHPCA, dying people who received hospice and palliative care also had fewer emergency room visits and fewer hospitalizations than people who did not receive such care (CHPCA, 2013; Coyle, 2015).

Ethics Touchstone
Provision 7
The nurse, in all roles and settings, advances the profession through research and scholarly inquiry, professional standards development, and the generation of both nursing and health policy.
Code of Ethics for Nurses (ANA, 2015a)

How can nursing students advance the nursing profession? How do the nurses that you work with help to generate nursing and health policies?

Once upon a time I thought that hospice and palliative care meant "doing nothing." When my dad died, I found out that the palliative care team did everything possible to help my dad live a full life right up to the day he died.

Dad had access to a team of people, depending on his needs. When he was in severe pain, he was seen by a palliative care physician and an oncologist. He was offered radiation therapy, not to treat his disease, but to decrease his pain. It was hard for him to get to the treatments, but they decreased his pain and he was able to attend and enjoy my sister's graduation, which meant so much to him.

When he was no longer able to get out of bed, the counselor and nurse talked with him and offered home support help. The health care workers provided daily personal care. Their care helped him to preserve his energy for the things that mattered to him the most.

When Dad's breathing became uncomfortable, the doctor ordered medications to help him breathe easier. The nurses taught us how to give him the medications. They supported us when we realized that he would not get better, and helped to prepare us for when he died. They told us what to expect, what he might do, and what we could do. They gave us phone numbers to call if we needed anything in the middle of the night. They changed what could have been an awful experience into a positive time of being together.

Common Issues in the Process of Providing Care

When a person is dying, the person and their family face uncertainty, multiple losses, and changes in their physical, psychological, and social spheres. Hospice and palliative care seeks to identify and address all these complex and often interconnected issues. The CHPCA identifies eight "Common Issues," and the National Consensus Project for Quality Palliative Care in the United States identifies eight "Domains of Care" (Figure 2) (CHPCA, 2013; Dahlin, 2013; Ferrell et al., 2007). By considering the Common Issues or the Domains of Care, HCPs can ensure that they address the holistic needs of the person and family. In this text, the term "Common Issues" rather than "Domains of Care" is used because it may be more easily understood by the dying person and their family. The CHPCA Common Issues and the US Domains of Care are provided in full in Appendices 5 and 8, respectively.

CHPCA Process of Providing Care

The CHPCA developed a national model of hospice palliative care—the "Square of Care"—to help ensure a consistent, quality approach to care that addressed all needs. Figure 3 shows two sides of the Square of Care, with the steps in the process of providing care appearing horizontally across the top (CHPCA, 2013). While the traditional nursing process has four steps—assessment, care planning, care implementation, and evaluation—the CHPCA process of providing care has two additional steps: information sharing and decision making. Appendix 6 contains the CHPCA chart "Six Steps for Providing Excellent Hospice and Palliative Care" and Appendix 7 presents the diagram of the "CHPCA Process of Providing Care."

Figure 2. Congruence of Common Issues in Canada and Domains of Care in the United States

CHPCA Common Issues	US Domains of Care
Disease Management	Structure and Processes of Care
Physical	Physical Aspects of Care
Psychological	Psychological and Psychiatric Aspects of Care
Social	Social Aspects of Care Cultural Aspects of Care Ethical and Legal Aspects of Care
Spiritual	Spiritual, Religious, and Existential Aspects of Care
Practical	Social Aspects of Care
End-of-Life Care / Death Management	Care of the Imminently Dying Patient
Loss and Grief	Psychological and Psychiatric Aspects of Care

Figure 3. The Square of Care (CHPCA, 2013)

PROCESS OF PROVIDING CARE					
Assessment	**Information Sharing**	**Decision-making**	**Care Planning**	**Care Delivery**	**Confirmation**
History of issues, opportunities, associated expectations, needs, hopes, fears Examination— assessment scales, physical exam, laboratory, radiology, procedures	Confidentiality limits Desire and readiness for information Process for sharing information Translation Reactions to information Understanding Desire for additional information	Capacity Goals of care Requests for withholding/withdrawing therapy with no potential for benefit, hastened death Issue prioritization Therapeutic priorities, options Treatment choices, consent Surrogate decision-making Advance directives Conflict resolution	Setting of care Process to negotiate/ develop plan of care—address issues/ opportunities, delivery of chosen therapies, dependents, backup coverage, respite, bereavement care, discharge planning, emergencies	Care team composition, leadership, education, support Consultation Setting of care Essential services Patient, family support Therapy delivery Errors	Understanding Satisfaction Complexity Stress Concerns, issues, questions

COMMON ISSUES / DOMAINS OF CARE						
Disease Management	Primary diagnosis, prognosis, evidence Secondary diagnoses—dementia, substance use, trauma Co-morbidities—delirium, seizures Adverse events—side effects, toxicity Allergies					
Physical	Pain, other symptoms Cognition, level of consciousness Function, safety, aids Fluids, nutrition Wounds Habits—alcohol, smoking					
Psychological	Personality, behaviour Depression, anxiety Emotions, fears Control, dignity, independence Conflict, guilt, stress, coping responses Self image, self esteem					
Social	Cultural values, beliefs, practices Relationships, roles Isolation, abandonment, reconciliation Safe, comforting environment Privacy, intimacy Routines, rituals, recreation, vocation Financial, legal Family caregiver protection Guardianship, custody issues					
Spiritual	Meaning, value Existential, transcendental Values, beliefs, practices, affiliations Spiritual advisors, rites, rituals Symbols, icons					
Practical	Activities of daily living Dependents, pets Telephone access, transportation					
End-of-Life Care / Death Management	Life closure, gift giving, legacy creation Preparation for expected death Management of physiological changes in last hours of living Rites, rituals Death pronouncement, certification Perideath care of family, handling of body Funerals, memorial services, celebrations					
Loss and Grief	Loss Grief—acute, chronic, anticipatory Bereavement planning Mourning					

The Square of Care model identifies the Common Issues, specifically disease management, physical, psychological, social, spiritual, practical, end-of-life care/death management, and loss and grief. For the purposes of this text, the term "psychosocial" refers to psychological, social, and spiritual issues.

The dying person, their family, and the HCPs are at the center of the Square of Care, where each step in the process of providing care intersects with each of the Common Issues. This is where caregiving occurs. HCPs go through each step of the process for each of the Common Issues the person is experiencing. At any given time, the person, their family, and the HCP may be involved in assessing one issue, sharing information about a second issue, and confirming the management of a third issue. The process of providing care is not linear. It is ongoing and dynamic, responding to changes in the person's Common Issues as disease progresses.

Nurses can use the Square of Care as a visual reminder to follow each step in the process of providing care, and to address or consider each of the Common Issues. The complete model is available online at the CHPCA website (CHPCA.net) and is well worth exploring.

Creating Common Language in Hospice and Palliative Care

Clear definitions of terms and how they are used are key to good communication. It is helpful to use terms that are equally understood by members of the health care team, the person, the family, and the public. This is a challenge, because the language used in hospice and palliative care continues to evolve locally and globally. When working in this field, identifying how these related terms are used in the communities where you live and work will be helpful. You might also want to ask people to clarify what a term means to them.

Sharon Baxter, executive director of the CHPCA, addresses concerns about the variability in the understanding of terms across Canada and in different countries, cities, or even facilities where hospice and palliative care is provided. In a keynote address at the CHPCA annual conference in 2015, she stressed that "the lack of unified definitions should not in any way diminish the provision of compassionate, timely care and education for the dying and their family."

"Palliative" Is a Type of Care

Sometimes people incorrectly label a person in their last days as "palliative" or say, "He's palliative." Consider using these phrases instead:

He is in his last days and hours.

He is actively dying.

Use the term "palliative" only when referring to a type of care, a philosophy of care, or an approach to care.

"People are not palliative. Care is palliative."

Chris Sherwood, hospice and palliative care nurse

Hospice and Palliative Care Programs and Benefits in Canada

In Canada, both provincial and national programs are available to people receiving hospice and palliative care. Most provincial palliative care benefit programs provide medication support, while the local health programs lend equipment and provide other supplies needed to help the person remain in the home. Current information is available on each provincial health care website. The national Compassionate Care Benefit program in Canada provides employment insurance benefits for a family caregiver who must take time away from work to care for their loved one at the end of life (Government of Canada, 2016a).

Hospice and Palliative Care Programs and Benefits in the United States

In the United States, people may receive the Medicare Hospice Benefit, a specialized benefit for people if they are eligible for Medicare Part A (hospital insurance), have a terminal illness, and, according to their doctor, have a prognosis of six months or less (if the disease runs its normal course). Ideally a person registers with hospice in the six months before death; however, difficulties with prognosticating often mean that the person does not register with hospice until weeks or days before death (US Medicare, 2016). More information on this coverage and how a person can apply is available on the Medicare website (medicare.gov).

The Next Steps for Hospice and Palliative Care

Despite all the positive benefits of hospice and palliative care, and the move to address the needs of people with a non-cancer diagnosis, less than 30% of dying people in Canada receive specialty hospice and palliative care services (CHPCA, 2015), and referrals often occur in the last few weeks of life. In the United States, in 2014 approximately 46% of all people who died were under the care of a hospice program; however, half of those received hospice services for less than 17 days (NHPCO, 2015). Late referrals result in dying people and their families not receiving the full benefits of the program (NCHS, 2015). Given the benefits of hospice and palliative care, why do more people not access hospice and palliative care programs?

Current Barriers to Accessing Hospice and Palliative Care

While hospice and palliative care is founded on the principle of equal accessibility, there are barriers that prevent people from accessing such care.

Belief of Ineligibility

The belief persists that hospice and palliative care is only for people dying with cancer or people who are expected to die soon. In 2014, 34% of Canadians were not aware that hospice and palliative care services were available for people with non-cancer diagnoses, and that palliative care programs could serve dying people and their family from the time of diagnosis right through to and following death (CHPCA, 2015).

This false belief that palliative care is for the imminently dying person was supported recently when news reports announced that a prominent politician was "now receiving palliative care" only to be followed by another announcement a few hours later that he had died. Additionally, countries, provinces, states, and communities differ in terms of the criteria people must meet before they can access hospice and palliative care services. This adds to the confusion and lack of understanding about such care.

Insufficient Training for HCPs

Research indicates that only 3% of physicians or nurses in the United States receive training in palliative or end-of-life care in their core curriculum (Diamond et al., 2016; Temel et al., 2010). (There is no current data on nursing education in Canada.) Without this education, an HCP may not fully understand the needs of the dying person and their family, or the value of talking about disease progression, goals of care, and the benefits of hospice and palliative care. The result is that an HCP who is not taught the philosophy, principles, and practices of hospice and palliative care will not be able to integrate them into caring for the dying.

Taboos and Fear of Talking about Death and Dying

HCPs may not talk about dying or death because they are not comfortable with the topic, they do not want to cause the dying person or their family to lose hope, or they sense that the dying person and family may not be receptive to such a discussion (Beernaught et al., 2014; Synder et al., 2012). HCPs may struggle to say "You're dying," opting instead to use vague euphemisms. This can result in a miscommunication of the diagnosis or prognosis.

The dying person and family may also be uncomfortable talking about death and dying, and often believe that the "specialist" will talk about death and about hospice or palliative care at the appropriate time (Friedman, Harwood, and Shields, 2002; Temel et al., 2010).

Lack of Clear Prognosis, Especially with a Non-Cancer Diagnosis

In the United States in particular, and in many programs in Canada, the dying person needs to have a prognosis of less than six months in order to qualify for hospice care. As mentioned in Chapter 1, "Understanding the Dying Process," the trajectory of a person dying with chronic illness has many ups and downs. The person with chronic illness may be "on death's doorstep" and recover several times before actually dying. Geriatrician, hospice physician, and author Joanne Lynn suggests that 50% of people suffering with chronic illness will not know they are in their last week of life a week before they die (Lynn, 2004). She says, "If you are waiting for a drum roll to announce that you are going to die, it is not going to happen in most cases." The family and HCPs also may not know that death is near.

Ethics Touchstone
What are some ways that every nurse can help reduce barriers to providing excellent care of the dying?

Underserved Groups

Certain groups of people are at increased risk of not accessing or receiving hospice and palliative care services. According to research, people in some age, racial, socioeconomic, ethnic, or religious groups and people who have certain gender or sexual orientations are less likely than other people to receive adequate hospice and palliative care. Compared with people who access hospice and palliative care services, members of some minority groups differ in their understanding of or affinity for hospice and palliative care services and their desire to continue with life-prolonging treatments. Other groups are less likely to have the opportunity for care, or their care needs are not recognized as being unique (Hughes, 2015; Kirolos et al., 2014).

Elderly: Historically, hospice and palliative care services were provided to adults who were dying from cancer but not to the frail elderly. Older people living in their homes or in residential care facilities often do not receive hospice and palliative care.

Children: The number of children surviving with life-limiting illnesses continues to increase due to advances in medical technology. In the United States, the majority of children (75–80%) receive their health care coverage through Medicaid, which may or may not include hospice

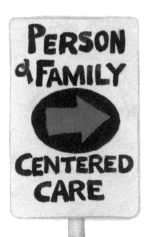

and palliative care services. Additionally, children comprise only 2.8% of people who benefit from hospice and palliative care services, with the result that few resources are allocated to meet the needs of dying children (Kaiser Commission on Medicaid and the Underinsured, 2009; NCHS, 2012). For the same reason, community resources are often insufficient to meet the needs of dying children discharged from hospital. Given the low numbers of children who would benefit from hospice and palliative care services, maintaining providers' skills and competencies and allaying their fears are also significant barriers to access to such care. HCPs who usually care for adults may not have experience managing the more diverse and complicated conditions children have. The ethnic and cultural challenges noted above, the fear of death, especially the death of a child, and inexperience among clinicians are significant barriers to accessing palliative and hospice services for children and their families.

People with physical or developmental disabilities: People who have physical or developmental disabilities are often prevented from accessing hospice and palliative care because of poverty and lack of resources (Stienstra and Chochinov, 2006). Unfortunately, compared with people who do not have such disabilities, people who do are also at higher risk for developing chronic illnesses earlier in life due to the lifelong impact their disabilities have on their physical health (NHPCO, 2009). Additionally, some people with physical or developmental disabilities feel more vulnerable because of the negative attitudes of HCPs who are not educated about the different experiences and abilities of a person who is disabled (VP-NET, 2006).

> *Martin, a 64-year-old male with Down syndrome who lives in a group home, is experiencing increasing complications due to diabetes, dementia, and heart failure. Martin is also experiencing a delirium and is increasingly unresponsive. His intake and urinary output have decreased. The HCPs are concerned that Martin is imminenetly dying. The physician recommends transfer to the hospital for assessment, because a hospice and palliative care consult is not available for residents of the group home.*

People who identify as LGBTQ: Even today, the stigma attached to people who identify as being lesbian, gay, bisexual, transgendered, or queer still exists, and such people may fear being judged or labeled by HCPs whose values and beliefs are different from theirs. People in this group who are now seniors may have experienced significant rejection, isolation, and criticism in past decades when homosexuality was considered a mental disorder, a criminal offence, and a justifiable reason for being fired from a job. Until recently, in some places it may have been acceptable to force LGBTQ people into medical treatments, such as electroshock therapy. These experiences may have shaped the LGBTQ person's perception of the health care system. It is therefore understandable when LGBTQ seniors such as Gladys (see the story that follows) are uncomfortable with the medical system and fearful about how HCPs will receive them (American Geriatrics Society Ethics Committee, 2015).

Gladys is a 70-year-old woman with ALS. She is very independent. She cared for herself and lived alone with occasional support from health care workers until her recent and rapid decline. She was admitted to the hospice for her last months. Gladys has requested no visitors. She also has requested not to be cared for by males.

When I look at Gladys, I see a small, frail, gray-haired woman. She has no photographs and no memorabilia in her room. I wonder why she is not allowing family or friends to visit. As I build my relationship with her, I ask her about family and friends. After a while, she confides that her partner of 20 years died from breast cancer 4 years ago. They never had kids but were part of a local lesbian group and had a large family of choice.

I wonder if she is afraid to allow people to visit because the staff will recognize that she is a lesbian, and if she is worried about being treated poorly if people know that she is a lesbian. I ask her if this is why she has refused visitors. She starts to talk about her experience of "coming out" and her experiences with the health care system decades ago. It is obvious that she was deeply wounded by those experiences.

As we talk, I wonder what we as a team can do to build trust so that she feels comfortable inviting her family to visit and sharing herself more openly with us.

Together we explore this topic.

People with mental illnesses: People with mental illnesses are recognized as a vulnerable population, but very little is known about the specific needs of such people with respect to hospice and palliative care (iPANEL, 2016;

Tuffrey-Wijne, Hogg, and Curfs, 2007; Woods et al., 2008). In the story about Sam that follows, the challenges that a homeless person with mental health issues confronts are evident.

Homeless people: People who are homeless may not qualify for hospice and palliative care services simply because they lack a fixed address or home. Many homeless people will not seek out hospice and palliative care services, whether due to cost, lack of referral, or lack of understanding of benefits or needs. This population is largely underserved. Providing hospice and palliative care to homeless people is challenging for many HCPs, because of cultural differences between the HCP and the person receiving care. Suspending judgment and working with compassion are cited as important factors when providing hospice and palliative care for the homeless (Collier, 2011). Recently hospice and palliative care has been introduced into homeless shelters so as to enable symptom management for the person in their own environment of comfort (Podymow, Turnbull, and Coyle, 2006).

Sam is a 56-year-old male with esophageal cancer, HIV, and schizophrenia who has been living on the streets and in homeless shelters for the past 25 years. He is sometimes aggressive, uses a lot of foul language, is restless, and often refuses offers of help. He has pain in his neck, shoulders, and chest. He is not able to access a palliative care consult or a visiting hospice program because he has no fixed address. He sleeps at the shelter sometimes.

Mariel is a single parent with two children. She also has stage 4 lung cancer and cannot afford treatment. She has lost her job because of illness and is now living out of her car.

People who live in rural or remote areas: For dying people who live in rural or remote areas, hospice and palliative care specialty services may not be available. Accessing such services may require traveling to where they are provided, which can be expensive and cause discomfort for the dying person and the family (Johnson et al., 2011; Lynn, 2004).

> *Trent lives in a rural community that is two hours from the nearest city. His health has been declining lately, and he now must travel to the city twice a week for dialysis and treatments to manage his emphysema. There are no hospice services available in his community, and he does not want to die alone in the city.*

Future Challenges for Hospice and Palliative Care

In addition to the barriers noted above, the following constitute challenges that will become salient in future decades:
- An increasing number of people dying
- An increasing number of people aging with chronic life-limiting illnesses who will require care for longer periods of time
- Fewer family caregivers, given that the baby boom generation had fewer children than previous generations

It is unlikely that the specialist model of hospice and palliative care will be able to meet future needs of the dying.

Shifting Gears: Integrating a Palliative Approach

In 2003, Palliative Care Australia (PCA) used a population-based approach to evaluate the overall needs of dying people and the barriers they encountered to receiving hospice and palliative care. The organization estimated that 65% of the dying could receive good care from their primary care providers alone. Of the remaining 35%, some would require episodic access to hospice and palliative care consultations and services, while others would require ongoing care by specialty hospice or palliative care services. This information enabled PCA to determine, on the basis of estimated numbers of people dying, the type and quantity of services to provide for different communities (Palliative Care Australia, 2005).

The PCA research emphasizes the important role of the primary care provider in caring for the dying. It also directs the primary care provider to access specialty services when needed.

Primary care providers, according to PCA, are general practitioners, physicians, community care nurses, acute care staff, and residential care home staff. A specialist whose primary area of specialty is not hospice or palliative care—for example, a cardiologist—might also be part of the primary care team and may want to call on the palliative care consultant for help in managing dyspnea or for ideas on how to support family members.

Integrating a Palliative Approach into Care

When the primary care team integrates hospice and palliative care into care, this is known as "integrating a palliative approach."

> **To integrate a palliative approach is to integrate the principles, practices, and philosophy of hospice and palliative care into the care of people with any life-limiting illness, early in the illness trajectory, across all care settings.**
>
> *Kath Murray*

Care is no longer focused only on end-of-life care and can include disease-modifying treatments, as well as a focus on providing comfort care and reducing suffering. Anyone who is aging and/or has a chronic life-limiting illness can benefit from a palliative approach being integrated into their care (CHPCA and QELCCC, 2015). Life-limiting illnesses include COPD, end-stage cardiac or kidney disease, dementia-related illnesses, Parkinson's disease, and ALS (CHPCA and QELCCC, 2015).

According to research by the Initiative for a Palliative Approach in Nursing: Evidence and Leadership (iPANEL), a palliative approach involves the following:
- Adopting the foundational principles of palliative care
- Adapting the knowledge and expertise in palliative care to meet the needs of people living the trajectories of chronic life-limiting illnesses
- Embedding and contextualizing this adapted knowledge and expertise "upstream" into the delivery of person-centered care across different health care sectors and professions

(Sawatzky et al., 2016)

In practice, integrating a palliative approach involves:
- Acknowledging that dying well includes living well until the time of death

- Opening conversations about the physical changes that are part of the dying process
- Sharing information
- Initiating discussions about advance care planning, goals of care, the illness trajectory, the benefits and burdens of treatment options, substitute decision makers, and so on
- Providing holistic care by addressing physical symptoms as well as emotional and spiritual suffering

---

Care of the dying is not just the responsibility of specialist providers. Care of the dying and their families is the responsibility of all HCPs, including nurses. There will never be enough specialist palliative care providers to provide good end-of-life care for all.

In the acute care setting in particular, nurses tend to consider dying people as not "belonging" in that setting and therefore tend to want to call the palliative consult team or have dying people admitted to a hospice or palliative care unit. Nurses do not know that care of the dying is their responsibility, and that they can provide excellent care.

Dr. Kelli Stadjuhar, principal investigator,
iPANEL research

What can you do to integrate a palliative approach into the care that you provide? Ask yourself these questions:
- How could this person benefit from a palliative approach?
- Is there anything that I need to understand about palliative care that would help me to provide better care?

At times the dying person will require more expertise than is available on a particular unit. When this is the case, it is appropriate to ask, "Would this person benefit from a referral to a specialty hospice and palliative care consult team?" It is helpful to know when and how to access a consult team. You may find that, as you access consult services, your ability to integrate palliative care in your setting will increase. Collaboration not only strengthens care in the moment, but also can strengthen your ability to care in the future.

Integrating a Palliative Approach into Residential Care

In Canada, the average length of stay in long-term care is now less than 18 months. Given this short time frame to death, integrating a palliative approach into care from the first contact with the person and their family is more than appropriate.

Asking the "Surprise Question" to Identify Who Might Especially Benefit from a Palliative Approach

From time of diagnosis through to death, anyone diagnosed with a life-limiting illness might benefit from a palliative approach. Supporting the person and family through diagnosis, decision making, and care planning is integral to a palliative approach.

In Canada and the United States, one of the first steps in identifying people who are declining and approaching death is to ask the Surprise Question:

Would you be surprised if this person were to die in the next year?

It is difficult to know the best timing for asking the Surprise Question, because of variables such as the person's illness, co-morbidities, and different policies governing when to integrate a palliative approach. A person who is expected to die within the next months or year may present with any, some, or all of the following characteristics:
- Frequent hospital admissions for the same symptom
- Difficult-to-manage symptoms
- Increasingly complex care requirements (e.g., the person has difficulty functioning independently)
- Added specialty needs, such as requiring a ventilator or assistance with feeding
- Decreasing appetite and/or involuntary weight loss (anorexia or cachexia)

Asking the Surprise Question

Asking and answering just one Surprise Question helped HCPs identify people who were likely to die in the coming year/months/weeks and facilitated advance care planning. The Surprise Question for nurses was,

Would you be surprised if this patient died within the next year? Months?

By considering this question, HCPs working with cancer patients were able to accurately predict 60% of people who would die within the coming year (Green, 2015). In fact, according to a new study, the Surprise Question was more predictive than other clinical factors, such as the cancer stage, the patient's age, and the time from diagnosis (Vick et al., 2015).

The Surprise Question identified only 60% of the people who died within one year. Therefore, nurses are advised to also evaluate general and clinical indicators of decline.

In Great Britain, the Gold Standards Framework Prognostic Indicator Guidance (GSF PIG), shown in Figure 4, has three steps to identify a person who might benefit from a palliative approach being integrated into their care. This tool was developed to help identify and support people who might be in their last year of life (Thomas, 2011). Step 1 is a variation of the Surprise Question, while in Steps 2 and 3, general and specific clinical indicators of decline are assessed for the person. The recurring assessment of these indicators is key to understanding the person's needs and knowing when a palliative approach might be beneficial.

Figure 4. The Gold Standards Framework Prognostic Indicator Guidance

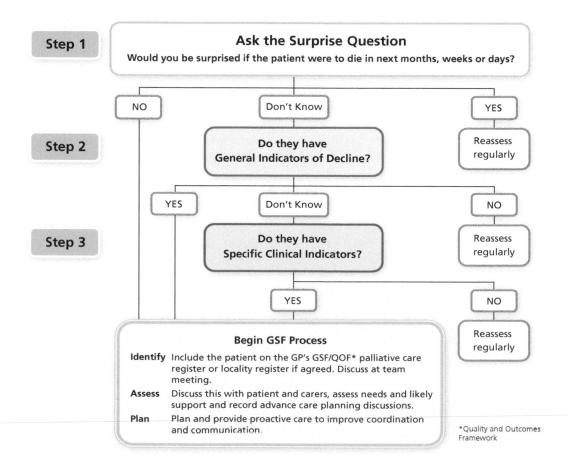

When the answer to the Surprise Question is "No," it triggers nurses and the health care team to begin the GSF process of identifying, assessing, and planning care. When the answer to the Surprise Question is "Yes," the health care team assesses the person for general and specific indicators of decline. Answering "Yes" for any indicators of decline will also trigger the GSF process. Tools to help answer the Surprise Question and to assess general and specific decline are available in Chapter 4, "Using Standardized Tools."

For nurses beginning to integrate a palliative approach, it will be essential to educate the public about the benefits to the person and family of integrating a palliative approach early in the disease process, including how such an approach may more effectively support the needs of people living with a progressive life-limiting illness.

When to Consult with a Hospice and Palliative Care Specialist

Sometimes, despite the excellent care provided by the primary care team, symptoms may persist and remain unrelieved, or the dying person's goals are unmet. Hospice and palliative care consult teams are specialist teams, often consisting of a physician, a nurse, a social worker, and others such as a pharmacist and spiritual counselor, who can assist primary care teams as needed with:
- Complex pain and symptom management issues
- Complex psychosocial or spiritual needs of the person or family
- End-of-life discussions that the primary care team does not feel able to address or for which the person and family need more support

If the dying person's symptoms are not being managed and/or their goals are not being met, then consider a referral to a hospice or palliative care team.

Case Study: Integrating a Palliative Approach on a Medical Unit

In this case study, Pritam has been transferred from the coronary care unit to the medical unit.

Pritam is a 73-year-old male with a history of cardiac disease. He was admitted one week ago to the coronary care unit following a myocardial infarction while shopping. CPR was performed immediately by a bystander. Pritam's PPS (score on the Palliative Performance Scale) is 20%, he is sleeping most of the time, and he can answer questions but has periods of delirium. He has pulmonary and peripheral edema, his breathing is labored, and he is receiving oxygen at 5 L/min. The urinary catheter is draining clear urine. Pritam is not a candidate for surgery or rehabilitation. At a family meeting held in the coronary care unit, the decision was made to keep him comfortable. He was transferred to the medical unit.

The nurse on the medical unit receives him and considers the Common Issues that Pritam and his family may be experiencing, and how she might best assess and address their needs. The illustration indicates a few of her thoughts.

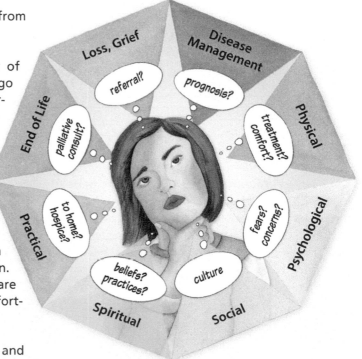

Summary

Modern hospice and palliative care began almost 50 years ago with the work of Cicely Saunders. She founded the first hospice and continued to work to provide better care for the dying. Through her leadership, hospice care and palliative care became specialty fields within health care. Specialist physicians, social workers, chaplains, nurses, and others on the interprofessional team met the needs primarily of people dying with cancer. Over the past 30 years, however, hospice and palliative care has been extended to people dying with chronic life-limiting illnesses (e.g., AIDS, COPD, CVD).

Yet still, less than 30% of dying people access hospice and palliative care in Canada, and less than half of the dying receive hospice care in the United States. Referrals to hospice often occur in the last weeks of life, and therefore dying people miss many of the benefits of the services. Barriers to access include lack of knowledge about eligibility; lack of training for the health care team; fears that professionals, the dying person, and their family have about discussing death and dying; and lack of services for underserved populations. Added to these barriers are the predictions that, over the next decades, the number of people dying will increase while the number of family caregivers and number of HCPs will decrease. The current model does not have the capacity to meet the needs of the dying.

Ethics Touchstone
Part I:D. Preserving Dignity, 7
Nurses maintain appropriate professional boundaries and ensure their relationships are always for the benefit of the persons they serve.
Code of Ethics for Registered Nurses (CNA, 2008)

Shifting gears to integrating a palliative approach will help to meet the needs of the future dying, who are cared for by the primary care team, with assistance from specialists as needed. Educating HCPs to integrate a palliative approach will help remove barriers that prevent people from accessing hospice and palliative care. As this occurs, the elderly, ethnic minorities, and other marginalized populations will have greater access to the benefits of hospice and palliative care.

Integrating a palliative approach can result in the philosophy of hospice and palliative care permeating a busy medical unit and becoming part of the fiber of care in residential care. This also means that you, as a nurse, can recognize the strength and importance of your role in providing excellent care for the dying person and their family, and advocating for specialist services when needed.

Ethics Touchstone
Provision 7 states that the nurse advances the profession through research and scholarly inquiry.
Code of Ethics for Nurses (ANA, 2015a)

Explore the contributions of a nurse you have met, or read or heard about, who has helped advance the nursing profession by engaging in research, scholarly inquiry, teaching, or workplace improvements.

What do you think are current barriers to nursing leadership in the workplace?

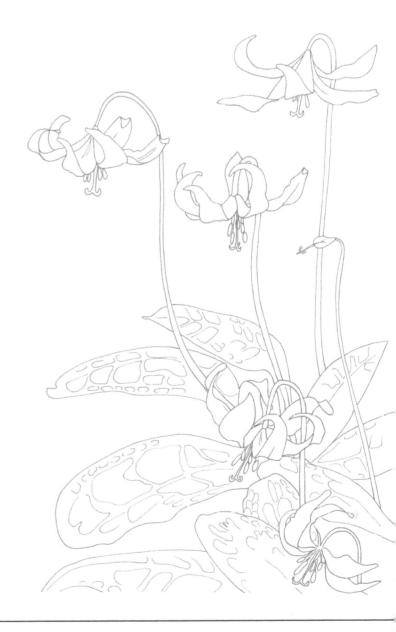

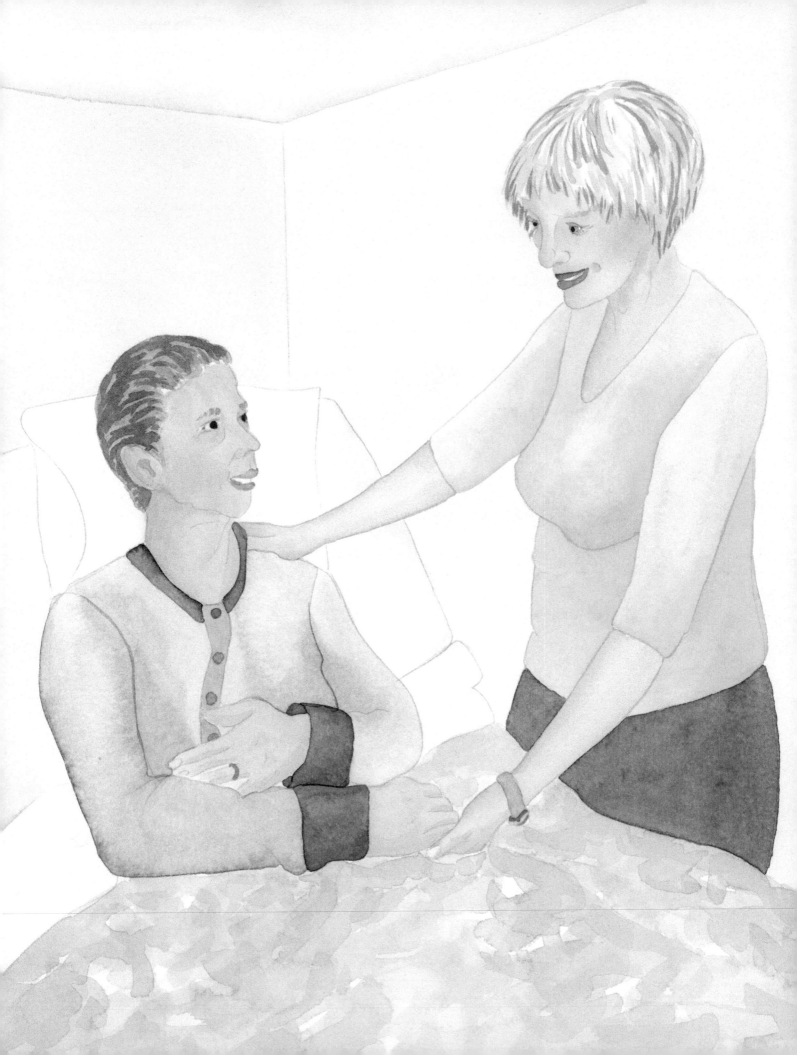

Preparing to Care

Preparing to Care—a Personal Journey

I came to hospice and palliative care nursing as a curious child. My earliest recollections of death include a dead rat and a lovely transparent leaf. I tried to nurse both back to life, with no success. When my siblings and I found a dead bird, we opted for burial. As a teenager I lived with my Aunt Frankie. Frankie, a nurse, was the master family caregiver. She cared for many family members and friends through aging, illness, and dying. I learned that death is part of life.

During high school and university, I encountered death and learned that even the young die. I learned that people die from cancer, accidents, and suicide. When I was in my 20s my father, uncle, and a few dear friends died. I saw severe pain that went untreated and respiratory congestion that led to distress and anguish. My compassion for the dying grew.

While the hospice movement spread globally, I completed my nursing degree. In 1988 I began working at Victoria Hospice, on the west coast of Canada. As a nurse working on the inpatient unit and then as a member of the Palliative Response Team, I worked with health care providers who showed me their incredible skills and compassion. I cared for people who died in the hospice and palliative care unit and those who died at home. I learned to prepare to care as I also learned

more about diseases, disease progression, symptom management, and the dying process.

I also learned from the dying and their families. They taught me how to be more comfortable talking about death, as well as the importance of sharing information, responding to questions, and having difficult conversations. And in walking with dying people on their journey, I learned to put aside my agenda and to try instead to address their concerns and their needs. I learned that I could not fix, but I could companion and I could "be with" suffering. They taught me how to prepare for dying.

From my colleagues, in particular the nurses, counselors, and physicians, I learned about best practices in symptom management, ways of being, communication skills, and humor. I was fortunate to have colleagues who debriefed after visits and were happy to reflect together to fine-tune and improve care. These interactions continue to help me as I prepare to provide care.

From early childhood and on through my nursing years, I have been passionate about learning and curious about people, and yearn to provide excellent and compassionate care—in particular, excellent care for the dying person and their family. Through my practice I have learned the importance of preparing to care.

Preparing to Care—an Essential Practice

The "journey of the dying" is a metaphor frequently used to describe the path a person follows as they die. Nurses are often companions for people on their journey of dying. As the companion, nurses need to prepare for the journey—to prepare to care.

Consider what you need to know, to be, and to have for this particular journey, with this particular person. You might ask yourself, "What will be supportive? Helpful? Needed?" You might wonder, "How do I need to be within myself so that I am able to support this person in their journey and do not try to take them on my journey?"

To be a companion on someone's journey you will need to gather information, acquire skills, and learn ways of being that together will develop into best practice. This chapter will help prepare you to be a companion on someone else's journey, by providing the knowledge to develop these skills and ways of being.

While this preparation may feel simple, it can profoundly enhance your capacity to provide hospice and palliative care with compassion, confidence, and competence. When health care providers (HCPs) prepare to provide hospice and palliative care, the dying person and family receive excellent care, and the professional minimizes stress and avoids burnout (Causton, 2016; Davies et al., 2016).

Striving for Best Practice

Preparing to care is, in part, about developing knowledge and skills for providing the best care possible. Over the past 20 years, hospice and palliative care has improved the quality of life of the dying, as HCPs have learned about best practice. Research by Dr. Betty Davies and Dr. Rose Steele identifies beliefs and attitudes of health care professionals[1] that provide the best care possible for parents and their dying child (Davies et al., 2016). Their research is similar to themes found in compassionate caregiving and the principles of "incorporating love in professional practice." Discussed below are three aspects to consider when developing your best practice in providing hospice and palliative care.

Best Practice Is What You Bring

Davies and Steele asked the question, "What makes for excellence [defined as best practice] in health care professional/parent interactions?" They asked parents to identify health care professionals who provided the best care, and then observed their practices. Their analysis identified common behaviors that these health care professionals demonstrated at all times and in all interactions. The researchers suggest best practice and best practice interactions that they believe all health care professionals can adopt when providing care (Davies et al., 2016).

As you strive to increase your competencies, consider the following behaviors and how you might integrate them into your practice.

At the core of best practice was honoring and valuing the intrinsic worth of people from all cultural groups and providing the person with autonomy and control, clearly echoing the Code of Ethics for Nurses, Provision 1: "The nurse practices with compassion and respect for the inherent dignity, worth, and unique attributes of every person"(ANA, 2015a). Davies and Steele's research also identified that best practice health care professionals:

- Are curious about the world and, in particular, desire to understand the experiences of the dying person and their family
- Are committed to learning about their field of work
- Withhold judgment and refrain from labeling people
- Understand that the person, family, disease, and health care professionals are all connected

Ethics Touchstone

Ethical practice is the underpinning of best practice HCPs. Integral to weaving a palliative approach into nursing practice and your way of being with the dying person and family is the examination of your beliefs and values regarding how people experience chronic illness, dying, and death. To provide best care, it is essential to reflect on what you believe excellent care is, and challenge yourself to discover what constitutes excellence.

The goal of hospice and palliative care is to provide care that honors the person and family. The context in which care is provided changes constantly as do the needs, experiences, beliefs, and values of the person receiving care. The many changes in the setting, the situation, and the people involved will require changes in how care is provided. In order to provide best care, it will be essential to consider the ethical dimensions of nursing practice.

---

1. The term "health care professionals" is used in this book to refer to Davies and Steele's research subjects. That term should not be confused with the more general term "health care providers (HCPs)."

Best Practice Is Compassion in Caregiving

Cicely Saunders saw dying people suffering in hospital and was empathetic to their experience; she felt their pain. She wanted to find better ways to care for the dying. This ability to be with suffering, along with the desire to transform it, is called compassion.

The root of the word "compassion" means "to suffer together" (UC Berkeley, 2016). Compassion is the feeling that arises when you witness a person's suffering and have the desire to help relieve it. Joan Halifax, an eminent instructor in medical schools who teaches about compassion, states: "The intention to transform suffering is one of the features that distinguishes compassion from empathy" (Halifax, 2013). Learning to be compassionate means being willing to go to difficult and painful places with another person. Theologian Henri Nouwen writes,

Let us not underestimate how hard it is to be compassionate. Compassion is hard because it requires the inner disposition to go with others to the places where they are weak, vulnerable, lonely and broken. Compassion is not our spontaneous response to suffering. What we desire most is to do away with suffering by fleeing from it or finding a quick cure for it … And so we ignore our greatest gift, which is our ability to enter into solidarity with those who suffer. When we provide care with compassion and love in our practice, we are willing to go to the places where we ourselves, and those we care for, feel vulnerable, uncertain or uncomfortable.

(Nouwen, McNeill, and Morrison, 1981)

Ethics Touchstone
Principle 1: Responsibility to the Public Licensed Practical Nurses, as self-regulating professionals, commit to provide safe, effective, compassionate and ethical care to members of the public.
Code of Ethics for Licensed and Registered Practical Nurses (CCPNR, 2013)

GRACE Model of Compassionate Response

Joan Halifax developed the GRACE Model of Compassionate Response, which organizes compassion into core domains and provides guidance on how to use these core domains when caring for dying people and their families (Halifax, 2014).

G: Gathering Attention. Get grounded within yourself, using whatever strategies work for you. You might find it helpful to purposefully slow down and take a deep breath, pause, touch something physical, then focus on the person, the situation, and interaction.

R: Recalling Intention. Recall what brought you to this work in the first place. Reflect on the reasons that you do this work. What was your deepest desire in becoming a nurse? Your hope? What keeps you motivated? Recalling these intentions can help to ground and connect you with the dying person and the family from a place of your highest values.

A: Attuning to Self and Others. There are two parts to this section of the model. First, check in with yourself. Notice what is going on for you in your own mind and body. Identify and set aside any biases, burdens, or barriers you may have that could shift you away from your intention.

Second, tune in to the other person and family or to team members. Sense what they may be experiencing in this situation and how they may be experiencing you. Allow yourself to notice and experience empathy or a deep intuitive connection, and, finally, allow the encounter to unfold without preplanned goals or expectations. Encourage mutual exchange between all who are present.

C: Considering What Will Serve. As the exchange continues, check in with yourself and ask, "What will best serve here?" Draw on your knowledge, expertise, and experience, but do not allow them to dictate what will happen. Stay open to the possibility that this encounter might be completely different from any you have experienced before.

E: Engaging and Ending. Hopefully what arises is compassion that is mutually respectful and practical. Such compassionate interaction requires a clear ending for the dying person, family, or team member. Ending involves releasing, letting go, and recognizing that this particular encounter is now over. Clear endings create space and the ability to focus on the next encounter or task.

Nurses are encouraged to use the GRACE Model to help focus and be open to what each unique dying person and their family bring to their particular circumstances.

Reflections on Compassion

Dr. Philip Larkin is a practitioner and educator whose warmth and wisdom seem to embody hospice and palliative care. He is a nurse, an educator, and the president of the European Association of Palliative Care. This is his summary of compassion:

- Compassion is not just a worthy endeavor. It is a clinical imperative.
- Compassion is more than a feeling or aspiration. It is an action.
- Compassion is only compassion when you do something about it.
- Compassion works alongside many attributes like empathy, sympathy, presence, silence, care, love, power, and altruism.
- To be a compassionate practitioner means practicing both the art and the science of hospice and palliative care.
- To provide compassionate care is to understand that presence is often far more valuable than practice.
- To provide compassionate care is to be able to care for self, to acknowledge our weaknesses as well as our strengths, and to be aware of how much we can achieve together as opposed to alone.

(Larkin, 2016)

Best Practice Is Incorporating Love in Professional Practice

Michelle (Misha) Butot, a counselor and clinical social worker, was curious about the ways that self-reflective and social-justice-oriented HCPs thought and practiced "love" in their work with dying people. It is important to clarify that love in professional practice is *not* about love in a romantic sense. Butot's research looked at HCPs of different ages, genders, and cultural and spiritual backgrounds, and identified behaviors and attitudes that were best practice for them and that also illustrated compassion in practice. Despite the diversity of participants, many of the perspectives HCPs expressed about the key role of love in their work were remarkably similar (Butot, 2005). This research about love in professional practice shares many of the attributes and ways of being that Davies and Steele identified as best practice interactions (Davies et al., 2016). It also shares

characteristics of cultural humility and providing care with compassion (Austerlic, 2009; Mazanec and Panke, 2015).

This past year I worked with Misha Butot and three other colleagues to rewrite her findings in language that is easily accessible. They are summarized in "Ten Principles of Love in Professional Practice" below.

As you read these principles, reflect on what you consider to be a "loving" way and a "compassionate" way of engaging in providing holistic care through the life trajectory and specifically in the last months, weeks, and days of a person's life.

"A Personal Creed on Love in Professional Practice" (see page 34) embodies my reflections on the Ten Principles of Love in Professional Practice and is included as a way to help you consider what love in professional practice might look like for you.

Ten Principles of Love in Professional Practice

Incorporating love in professional practice means:

- Acknowledging all human beings as whole and interconnected
- Acknowledging all human beings to be worthy of value and deserving of rights and respect
- Coming to the dying person open-minded, open-hearted, and deeply curious about who they are, what is true for them, and how best to provide their care
- Coming to the dying person fully engaged in one's own life, relationships, and community
- Committing to personal growth, including self-reflection, and to ongoing professional growth
- Committing to creating an accepting atmosphere that is devoid of judgment and includes the possibility of mutual honesty
- Caring with compassion and mindfulness
- Engaging with the dying person even when one of us is vulnerable, uncomfortable, or uncertain
- Being open to be changed by the dying person and by this work
- Being willing to support, recognize, and bear loving witness to your changing

Ethics Touchstone
Reflect on the Ten Principles of Love in Professional Practice, and be open to discovering and hearing within yourself where your values and beliefs currently lie.

Understanding Love in the Context of Professional Practice

Love is not without boundaries. In fact, love needs boundaries that touch both parties and that separate people to provide space and distance. Love is not about fixing things or trying to fix things. Love is about being with, desiring to help, and not being invested in a certain outcome.

Tom Kitwood, a pioneer in the field of dementia care, writes about love in dementia care:

Love within the context of dementia care includes comfort in the original sense of tenderness, closeness, the calming of anxiety, and bonding.

(Kitwood, 2003)

Stephen Post, a researcher on the health benefits of helping others, writes about altruistic love:

Altruistic love involves both a judgment of worth, and a related affirmative affection. Love is manifest in care, which is love in response to the other in need; it is manifest in compassion, which is love in response to the other in suffering; it is manifest in companionship, which is love attentively present with the other in ordinary moments.

(Post, 2003)

Kitwood's and Post's words have been an inspiration to HCPs and others providing compassionate care in dementia care. Davies and Steele, Larkin, Butot, Kitwood, and Post are only a few of the authors who have written about best practice, and compassion and love in practice.

A Story about Care

I am 63 years old and was diagnosed five years ago with an aggressive type of lymphoma. I was treated with chemotherapy. After a relapse I received a stem cell transplant. During that time, my wife and three of our four children were diagnosed with Huntington's disease.

During my first hospitalization, the more they studied me and looked at me, the more I felt myself getting smaller and smaller as a person. But there were some individuals whose caring encouraged recovery of "me."

... The bone marrow biopsy was upsetting. I was upset. I did not understand what was happening. There was a young nurse there, and she held my hand. It was the first time in three or four weeks of medical appointments that someone had done that, that someone had touched me in a way that was not entirely clinical in nature. At the end of the procedure and after the doctor left the room, she uttered a sigh and said, "I hate that procedure."

I thanked her and told her how "cared for" that made me feel.

And she said, "Thank you for holding my hand, because it was difficult for me to watch this and to witness you in that process."

I was a person to her. I was not a pathology.

Another time, in the hollow of the night, which was a scary time for me, a nurse sat down by my bed. She said, "I am just going to talk with you if that is all right." She talked about her kids and she let me talk about my kids, what I did as a profession, and she asked me about those things. She was addressing me, as a person, a complex individual, not just asking about my medical history, but my personal history. I loved her for that. I just loved her for that.

Often late at night when I am alone, the nurse comes in, and I share the depth of my soul with the nurse. I share with the nurse because the visits with the doctors are during the day and are only a few minutes long, and because I can't share with my family. I do not want to add to their grief. Think about it, if you are "caring for me," do you care for me?

(Mulcahy, 2014)

A Personal Creed on Love in Professional Practice

To you, for whom I will care—when I love in professional practice:

I want to care for you with love in my professional practice. I want to live an ethos of love in professional practice.

I recognize that dying is a blessed and bewildering path of personal growth. I acknowledge that in caring for you, I have the opportunity to learn with you, and I thank you for teaching me.

When I love in professional practice, I will see you as whole and dignified, with strengths and challenges that may be unfamiliar to me. I will respect you. I will honor your hopes and concerns for yourself and others. And I will care for you with tenderness. And, I will realize that we are connected, we breathe the same air, and we need each other.

When I love you in professional practice, although your face, your body, your thoughts are shifted with disease, I will remember that you have rights to justice, equity, care, and warmth.

When I love you in professional practice, I will honor that you know your needs and the needs of your loved ones better than I do. I will open my eyes, my ears, and my heart to try to understand what is important to you and how you would have me care for you. I will feel for you in your suffering, empathize and care deeply about you. I will adapt the care plan to best meet your desires and concerns. Your desires and concerns will mean more to me than efficiency and the tasks that I have. I am here to help you live as you are and to contribute to the well-being of your family and community. I will wait with you.

When I love you in professional practice, I will know that I cannot change or fix what is happening, but I can be with you. I will know that I cannot tell you how to die, what to do, what to talk about or think about, or what to believe. However, I will also take the risk at times to share my truth with you, to share my observations and understanding with you, and I will also support you to act on your insights as you will. Even so, I will respect that you may not want to talk, that you may want to step back. I will respect that sometimes you may hope for what seems impossible, and I can be present with you all the same.

When I love you in professional practice, I will come fully immersed in my life, living my life fully, engaged in my relationships and in my community. I will not expect you to fill that part of my life for me. I will engage with you, support your desire and ability to engage fully in your life, relationships, and community. And I will stay engaged with you, even if there is conflict or if doing so is not comfortable. I will build my stamina and ability to be with you in times of uncertainty, vulnerability, and fear.

When I love you in professional practice, I will understand that while you are dying, you are also living, and I so want to support you fully.

When I love you in professional practice, I am willing to know and to not know, to make mistakes and to do things "right." I will know that I can read about you in your chart and think that I know you, but I am willing to find that you are different than I thought.

When I love you in professional practice, I am open-hearted and open-minded. I am willing to meet you where you are, to be open to you as you define yourself and to your experience of life. I will withhold judgment. May my eyes behold you as someone who is loving and beloved.

When I love you in professional practice, I am willing to be changed by you and willing to be changed by this work. Yes, when I love you in professional practice, I can join you on the path of personal growth, in living–dying. Always I will celebrate and remember the opportunities to provide loving care to someone who is beloved.

When I love you in professional practice, I am willing and I want to take action to support you in your suffering.

With love in professional practice,
Kath Murray and Misha Butot

If you were the nurse caring for the dying person in "A Story about Care" (see page 33), how comfortable would you be in holding his hand?

How might that person's experience have been different if you had stood back and observed the procedure?

Preparing by Striving for Best Practice Interactions

The research by Davies and Steele also emphasizes the importance and value of the relationship and interactions between the health care professionals and the dying person (often called the nurse–client or the nurse–patient relationship) (Davies et al., 2016). "A Story about Care" (see page 33) illustrates best practices when the person discusses the care nurses provided him when he was sick and in hospital. This section discusses best practice interactions in providing care and as aspects of relating to people and families, highlighting how these interactions pertain to hospice and palliative care, to compassion, and to cultural humility.

Best Practice Interactions—How You Provide Care

Davies and Steele's research identified these ways of relating in all health care professionals who provided the best care:

- Being flexible and willing to respond to the changing needs of the people they care for, and putting aside their own agendas and tasks to best meet the needs of the dying person in the moment
- Developing and adapting priorities, responding to changing needs, and following up and evaluating care plans
- Engaging authentically by listening, empathizing, observing for strengths, being kind, maintaining hope, and developing trust in therapeutic relationships
- Engaging in reflective practices to learn about themselves and the families they are working with, and constantly seeking ways to improve their practice
- Incorporating their own life experiences into relating to the dying person and family, while focusing on the person and understanding boundaries
- Being aware of their strengths and limitations, and the impact of their behavior on others

If you are a nursing student or new graduate, focus on developing one behavior at a time, and work toward integrating all the behaviors into practice over time.

Best Practice Interaction Strategies

The way that HCPs relate to the person is vital to the perception of excellent care. These interactions are opportunities to value the person, to validate their experiences, and to understand their care needs. Strive for best practice interactions, and consider using the Psychosocial Assessment Form (see Chapter 4, "Using Standardized Tools") to record valuable information learned about the person and family.

The following behaviors may help develop best practice interactions.

Being Curious

Meeting people and being curious about their life—their stories, strengths, and history—are among the joys of nursing and support best practice interactions. Learning about the person—exploring who the person is and who the family members are—is essential to providing person-centered and culturally sensitive care.

Many tools are available to help you learn about the person and the family. Dr. Harvey Chochinov, a world-renowned palliative care psychiatrist and researcher who investigates the emotional and psychological needs of the dying, developed the "Dignity Question" with the Dignity Therapy Team (Chochinov et al., 2016, Chochinov, 2010). It is a profound question:

What do I need to know about you as a person to give you the best care possible?

The person's answer can help you fine-tune the care plan to best meet their needs. For example, you might ask about the person's culture and traditions.

Many hospices use a psychosocial assessment tool as part of their ongoing assessment to ensure that vital information about the person's life is shared with HCPs. The psychosocial assessment includes a review of the person's life, beliefs, practices, and fears, and questions about family and support. A psychosocial assessment tool, adapted from the Victoria Hospice tool, is included in Chapter 4, "Using Standardized Tools."

Ethics Touchstone
Reflect on the difference between curiosity that enriches professional relationships and curiosity that is self-serving. How can you ensure that you provide care that is respectful to the person in a culturally sensitive way?

In addition to helping you personalize the care plan for the dying person, exploring these topics will help you connect and establish common ground with the person and their family.

As you ask questions, remember that it is appropriate to explore topics that will enhance the therapeutic relationship. It is inappropriate to ask questions simply to satisfy your own curiosity. Be aware that observing may be more appropriate than asking questions.

Doing What Is Possible to Meet the Person's Needs

Barnard, Hollingum, and Hartfiel (2006) cite "doing what is possible" to meet the needs of the person as an important component of palliative care nursing. They express this by saying,

Let's make this day the best day that we can for you so if there is something we can do for you, we will.

The essence of doing what is possible is being open to the needs of the person. As Davies and Steele indicate, putting aside your agenda and being flexible so that the person's needs are the priority are ways to ensure best practice interactions (Davies et al., 2016). One way I express this when I am providing personal care is by saying,

This may not be a day at the spa, but if it were, what would you want?

Connecting

Connecting is a relational skill that builds and maintains trust, and communicates value and respect. Connecting occurs in many ways—with laughter, tears, the holding of hands, and being with the person in moments of silence and grief. At times it is important to connect visibly with the person and their family, while at other times it may be more appropriate to move into the background and support the person and family as they connect. It is not always possible to know the person before connecting. In the story below, a nurse connects with a person without the benefit of knowing the person in advance.

I went for a colonoscopy. The nurse and physician performing the task were clinical, hard, and driven. They paid little attention to me as they carried out the procedure. They interacted with me only to tell me what to do.

Then another nurse entered the room. She came and sat by my head. She introduced herself, called me by name, took my head in her hands, and spoke gently to me.

She cradled my head in her hands and talked quietly to me about me while the "others" finished the procedure. Her words were more than comforting; they were transformative.

Focusing on Strengths

Discovering a person's and family's strengths is another relational skill. The role of the nurse, like the role of the therapist, is to discover both the problems and the strengths in the person and the family you provide care for. Consider using the Psychosocial Assessment Form in Chapter 4, "Using Standardarized Tools," to help discover the strengths of the person and their family.

In the following story, the HCP focuses on the strengths and withholds judgment.

One day I had the good fortune to meet an elderly woman who had been homeless and lived on the street for most of her life. I found myself quick to judge and pity her for her lack of worldly possessions and stable lifestyle. Then she spoke of her freedom to be fully present in and open to life, to the experiences and people she met without the distraction of "things." She said that she traveled light in life and that her legacy was in the memories of the generous gifts of time and attention that she left with those she loved. She didn't judge others for their choices and chose not to be defined by those who felt the need to judge her.

The strengths noticed by the HCP were essential content for a review of the woman's rich life in her last weeks.

A positive approach can help you, as a nurse, understand the person's strengths, integrate them into the care plan, and remind the person of their strengths if they have forgotten them.

Being Flexible and Responsive

Being flexible and responsive is essential when the person and the family are the focus of care. In the story below, the nurse exemplifies one aspect of best practice interactions by responding to the person's and family's needs as they change.

There was so much that we needed to understand. We were overwhelmed. The nurse somehow understood that, and he knew what we needed to understand before each procedure.

He would return after the procedure, check in, see what was needed next, and then share a bit more information. He did that regularly. It seemed as if he was adapting his messages to meet us where we were each time. He walked us step by step through the maze of investigations and diagnoses, and he made it possible for us to understand what was happening ... just one bit at a time.

In this situation the nurse tailored the education and communication to meet the needs of the person and family at a very stressful time, always ensuring that he was meeting their needs as they defined them. Strong relational skills helped the nurse be supportive by knowing when to step in and when to step out.

Seeking to Understand by Asking Open-ended Questions

One aspect of best practice interactions is seeking to understand. In conversations, the relational skill of asking open-ended questions can help you learn about the person, their history, and their experiences with the health care system. This aspect can help inform the care team of ethnic, cultural, or religious concerns or values.

Asking open-ended questions in a gentle, timely manner can help create a space where the dying person feels safe to explore difficult topics. Sharing their story may help the person develop a greater understanding of self and of what he or she is experiencing.

Here are some examples of open-ended questions:

Mmm ... can you tell me more?

What do you think?

What do you think is happening now?

Can you give me an example?

What do you need right now in order to feel safe?

What do we need to know about you as a person to provide the best care possible?

When providing care for people with serious illnesses, it may be helpful to ask about the person's experience of being sick, accessing the health care system, and perhaps the story of their diagnosis or treatments. You might hear people talk of misdiagnosis, long waits for treatment, or poor communication among members of the health care team. In hearing these stories, you might identify ways of being that are especially important to this particular person and family.

"Can you tell us about your diagnosis and treatment?" I asked.

Without hesitation she shared stories of misdiagnosis and miscommunication. We realized very quickly the importance of clear communication and accurate information.

Listening

Learn to listen to a person with the sole intention of hearing them. Often when people listen, their eagerness to be next to speak can prevent them from hearing what is said and what is intended. In a busy work environment, when time feels limited, you may find that you are half-listening while also thinking about your other work responsibilities (Doane and Varcoe, 2016). This can be a disservice to the person as well as the health care team. Listening is essential to learning about the person and their understanding of their health. It can also be a useful intervention that enables the person to share their story, ask questions, consider their options, and confirm their choices.

Listening is a whole body experience. As you may have learned in a basic communication course, lean forward and attend to what the person says, how they say it, and what their body is saying. Let them know with your body language that you are present and listening, that you do not have an agenda, and that you are prepared to be with them until they finish speaking. Respond in ways that let the person know they are being heard. Bear witness, be with, and companion.

The next time you are in conversation—a minute from now, an hour from now, tomorrow—monitor your own listening habits. See if you can catch yourself waiting to speak. See if you can force yourself to stop and listen more actively. First, count the number of seconds you allow between when one person finishes speaking and you begin. Then try to double your pause time and see what happens.

(Doane and Varcoe, 2016)

Responding

A relational skill that strengthens relationships and supports the dying person and their family includes responding to what they say in ways that encourage conversation. Refrain from minimizing the problem and offering false reassurance, excessive praise, or platitudes. Avoiding these and other "roadblocks" to communication is an important relational skill that facilitates communication; conversations flow more easily without roadblocks.

Avoid Responding with Roadblocks

Minimizing the problem
When you get a parking ticket, it may make you smile when someone reminds you that it could have been worse: "My friend got a parking ticket and a speeding ticket on the same day." But when a person is dying, efforts to minimize the person's problems are likely to leave the person feeling unheard and misunderstood.

Offering false reassurance
When a person is constipated, it may be helpful for a nurse to assure them that the medication will resolve the problem. But when a person is dying, offering false reassurance such as "Everything is going to be just fine" does not address the deep worries and anxieties the person is experiencing.

Offering excessive praise
If you repeatedly praise the person for being strong, resilient, and resourceful, they may not want to share or acknowledge their feelings of loss, hopelessness, or fear, or to ask for help when they feel weak, fragile, or lost.

Offering platitudes
Platitudes are statements such as "Time heals all wounds" or "The grief will pass." These statements are not true—time does not heal, and grief does not simply pass. Sharing the truth compassionately with the person is more helpful.

Maintaining Hope

HCPs need to understand that receiving hospice and palliative care does not mean that the person no longer has hope. Hope is transitional and changes through different life experiences. When a person is facing death, that does not mean there is no hope, but it may mean that the person's hopes have changed.

At the time of initial diagnosis, the person may hope for a cure. As the illness progresses and cure is no longer an option, the person may hope to have control over symptoms and to live to experience specific events. As you can imagine, people are unique in their hopes. While one person hopes for the reassuring presence of family, someone else may hope for reconciliation with an estranged child, and another person may hope for spiritual guidance.

Some people find hope easily throughout their experience, while others struggle to maintain or find hope. As a nurse you can foster hope by being open to discussing the hopes, fears, and struggles that the person is experiencing. You can support hope by allowing the person to freely express their hopes and their thoughts as you avoid judging or questioning them. You can support hope by discussing the person's experiences in a way that allows hope to have a place (Olsson et al., 2010).

When I was first diagnosed with breast cancer, I hoped for cure, to be free of the disease and to go on with my life as it had been. I proceeded with surgery and treatments (chemo and radiation) filled with hope that the disease would be removed from my body once and for all. It was that way for about four years. Then I noticed I was having difficulty with my breathing. Testing showed that the cancer was back and now in my lungs. This time cure was not being offered, only time. My hope shifted to having enough time to see all the people I cared about both near and far, to ensuring that my family would be okay with the care decisions I was making, and that I would have enough time for organizing all my paperwork. As I became weaker and less able to do things, my hope shrank along with my world. Now I was hoping for a peaceful, pain-free death. I was hoping that I would be able to die without fear and that everyone knew how much I loved them. And now, my world is tiny and I hope that I will be able to let go with ease.

Ethics Touchstone
How might the experience of hope of the person in the preceding story be different if they were supported to see how curative treatments and palliative care treatments can be provided simultaneously?

Witnessing changes in hope as a person's death nears can help you understand and be comfortable with the changing face of hope. Chapter 6, "Providing Psychosocial Care," examines interventions to support hope.

Being with Suffering without Trying to Fix It

Elizabeth Causton, palliative care counselor and social worker, has researched effective ways of communicating when providing hospice and palliative care. She knows, after years of work on a palliative response team, that when you work with people who are dying, every day you work in the face of unfixable pain and suffering. The issues are often complex when cure is not an option and death is on the horizon. Some things can be fixed, for example, constipation or physical discomfort. Emotional pain and grief, however, cannot be fixed. It is inappropriate to attempt to cover or mask emotional pain and grief in the same way that one tries to cover or mask physical pain. It is inappropriate to try to fix the unfixable; it cannot be fixed (Causton, 2016).

The Fix-It Trap
Thinking that it is your job to fix the unfixable will change what you see and hear and focus on. You may be in the Fix-It Trap if you:
- Listen for and respond only to those problems that you can fix
- Ask to be assigned to people with "simple" problems and avoid people whose issues are complex
- Focus on tasks that are familiar and comfortable, and turn away from more complex issues without obvious solutions
- Do not distinguish between palliating physical pain and responding to grief

Instead of trying to fix a problem, strive to be with the person, bearing witness to their pain, hearing what they say about it, and validating it.

Remember that the purpose of listening is to bear witness, and to discover how to support, be with, and companion the person and family. If, on the other hand, you listen with the intention of fixing, you may not hear any of the problems that cannot be fixed and may be unable to support the person in their suffering of "unfixable" pains. However, when you listen, companion, and support, the person will feel cared for, and moments of healing can happen.

The Fix-it Trap is based on the belief that it is your job to "fix" everything, that something needs fixing in the first place and the delusion that we can actually do that.

(Causton, 2016)

Offering Silence

The most important thing that nurses can learn to say is *nothing*. People are human beings, not "human do-ings." Being quiet and still is often as effective as or more effective than doing or saying something. Sitting still and breathing may be one of the most effective ways to listen and support.

I saw her standing, alone and crying. I did not know her. I did not know why she was crying. I did not know what to do. I went to her side, stood next to her, and after a bit I put my arm around her shoulder. I wanted to be supportive, but I had no idea what she might find helpful.

I stood silently, and eventually I thought to breathe. Slow and deep—deep enough that she could feel my breathing through our physical contact.

After a while she stopped crying. She turned to me, opened her phone, and showed me the word she had programed to come to the screen each time she opened the phone: "BREATHE."

Ethics Touchstone
Reflect on how you feel being silent with someone when you want to be supportive. Think about how you are with silence. What is it like for you?

You can be a compassionate presence without having to do or say something to fill up the space. When you are present and real, you invite the person to be present as well. In this gentle, safe place the person may experience their suffering, fear, pain, and confusion in a different way.

To "be there" for someone who is in a difficult situation, stop for a moment. Pay attention to the natural rhythm of your breathing. Notice that you inhale, exhale, pause, inhale, exhale, *and pause*. The silent pause is as much a part of the natural breathing pattern as the inhaling and exhaling. If you skip the pause, you will hyperventilate, a practice that cannot be sustained indefinitely.

In a similar way, natural communication patterns include times of pausing and moments of silence. Yet people are often uncomfortable in shared silent moments and, as a result, either avoid or interrupt them. Many people asso-ciate silence with emptiness or absence, when in fact si-lence is full of presence; there is always something going on in the spaces between one's words and actions. Embra-cing silence is a conscious clearing of space, making room for whatever needs to happen. Silence requires some de-gree of trust—in yourself, in the other person, and in the situation itself. Silence requires that you give up control of the space long enough to allow something to happen. Silence allows you to consider what you might do next to support the person and family. Silence allows you to clean your slate and be open to respond to what happens next.

He was in his last weeks. He was quiet and with-drawn. I cared for him each day, and I struggled to know how I could connect with this man who did not talk. I knew that he liked to be quiet, so I put a "stop-per on my talker." I talked very little as I provided care.

When it was quiet on the unit, I would go and sit with him. I would ask, "Do you want me to read, or do you just want me to sit with you?" Often I just sat quietly.

One day he said, "I am glad you are here. The nurse yesterday did not stop talking!" I realized that my silence was helpful. When he died, his daughter thanked me and said how he had appreciated the quiet care that I had provided.

Ethics Touchstone
What purpose does ongoing talking (chatter) serve for the nurse?

Silence can be a gift that gives people who are dying and people who are grieving the time to collect their thoughts, to ponder, to face challenges, to prepare, and to regroup. Silence can be a gift for those who are fatigued; the space may provide them time to gather the energy to speak. As a nurse, you do not need to fill this silent space with words—fill it with quiet presence.

Good communication is often seen as a skill, but com-munication that includes silence is an art.

When I was a child, I was taught that in order to be safe when crossing the street I needed to stop, look, and listen. Stop, look both ways, and listen for oncoming cars.

As a young hospice nurse, I realized this wisdom applied when caring for a dying person and their family. When I stop, I put my agenda and needs on hold. When I look, I look at the person, their physical presence, their surroundings, their family. When I listen, I listen to what is being said and consider what might be felt but not said. If I stop, look, and listen, then sometimes I am invited to cross the street and journey with the dying person. At some point, the person moves forward alone on their journey, and I remain behind. My life is changed. And sometimes I feel that I have been taught by "the masters."

Ethics Touchstone
Think about how this approach (stop, look, and listen) may promote the person's dignity and sense of control over their own health.

Offering Empathy

Empathy is our very human ability to see the perspective of and feel the emotions of another person. Teresa Wiseman, a nursing scholar in England, identifies four characteristics of empathetic behavior (Wiseman, 1996):
- Seeing the world as others see it
  It sounds like this is really hard for you. I want to understand ... can you tell me more?
- Staying out of judgment—so hard to do in a society that judges so often
- Understanding another person's feeling—connecting with one's own feelings and being able to connect with the other person's feelings
- Communicating your understanding of that person's feelings
  I hear that you are frustrated and angry about the miscommunication within the team. Tell me how you are feeling.

Empathy is different from sympathy. Sympathy is feeling bad for someone in their current circumstance or situation, whereas empathy is putting yourself in that person's place by trying to see and understand the situation as they experience it. Sympathy can close a conversation, whereas being empathetic opens the door to connection and communication.

A video by Dr. Brené Brown, a researcher, author, and storyteller, illustrates the difference between sympathy and empathy. See "Brené Brown on Empathy" at the Life and Death Matters website (lifeanddeathmatters.ca /brenebrown).

Empathy is about listening:

It sounds like this is really hard for you. I want to understand how this is for you. Can you tell me more?

Empathy is about being with:

I am here for you. Please tell me what would be helpful.

Empathy is about acknowledging uncertainties:

It sounds like you are living with much uncertainty. How is this for you?

Empathy is about being present in the face of unfixable pain:

I can see the pain in your eyes and hear the pain and worry in your voice. I am here with you.

Building Cultural Competence and Cultural Humility

Culture helps shape people's behaviors and their interactions with other people. People from a shared culture can more easily understand and work with one another because their ideas and beliefs are similar. Cultural competence in HCPs is important for communicating and providing care for people from other cultures, and helps to prevent miscommunications, misunderstandings, and false assumptions.

Nurses can better strive for cultural competence by first being curious about and seeking cultural knowledge from the dying person and family, and second by developing their own cultural self-awareness (California Health Advocates, 2007; McGee and Johnson, 2014; Mazanec and Panke, 2015). The goal is to acknowledge and respect the person's culture, including their beliefs and values.

Cultural competence is not a goal per se; instead it is a lifelong commitment to honoring and respecting the people you care for. It may best be described as cultural humility, because humility is central to cultural competence. A person must be humble to continually engage in self-reflection and be committed to lifelong learning and a reflective practice. HCPs must be humble to openly admit that they do not have all the answers, and to acknowledge that answers the dying person and their family have are as valid as those of the medical team. HCPs must be humble so as to avoid stereotyping that comes with awareness of other cultures and, instead, view each person as a truly unique and valuable being (Tervalon and Murray-Garcia, 1998). Cultural humility requires HCPs to be curious, open, and willing to be in uncomfortable situations, and to put aside their own agenda in caregiving. These characteristics of cultural competence and cultural humility dovetail smoothly with Davies and Steele's work, where curiosity, openness, willingness to be with the person in diverse situations, and letting go of agendas are just a few of the characteristics that identify best practice interactions.

Cultural humility is the essence of providing compassion in caregiving. Cultural humility empowers the dying person and family as participants and contributors in a bilateral therapeutic relationship (Austerlic, 2009).

Ethics Touchstone

Reflect on your cultural biases and beliefs regarding the health of Aboriginal people. Read the following statement, explore the topics identified, and then reflect on your biases and beliefs in the context of the call to action.

Call to Action Number 24

"We call upon medical and nursing schools in Canada to require all students to take a course dealing with Aboriginal health issues, including the history and legacy of residential schools, the *United Nations Declaration on the Rights of Indigenous Peoples*, Treaties and Aboriginal rights, and Indigenous teachings and practices. This will require skills-based training in intercultural competency, conflict resolution, human rights, and anti-racism."

(Truth and Reconciliation Commission of Canada, 2012)

Ethics Touchstone

Part I:A. Providing Safe, Compassionate, Competent and Ethical Care, 3
Nurses build trustworthy relationships as the foundation of meaningful communication, recognizing that building these relationships involves a conscious effort. Such relationships are critical to understanding people's needs and concerns.

Code of Ethics for Registered Nurses (CNA, 2008)

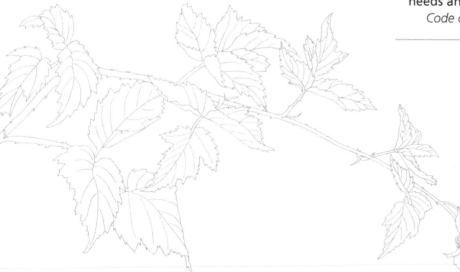

Personal Strategies for Preparing to Care

This section discusses the following strategies for preparing yourself to provide care for the dying and their family:

- Developing a reflective practice
- Establishing and maintaining therapeutic boundaries
- Establishing and maintaining self-care practice

These preparations can enhance your capacity to provide hospice and palliative care with compassion, confidence, and competence. When health care professionals provided care following best practice, the dying person and their family reported receiving excellent care, and the health care professionals minimized their personal stress and avoided burnout (Davies et al., 2016).

Developing a Reflective Practice

Developing a reflective practice can help prepare you to provide care (Barnard, Hollingum, and Hartfiel, 2006; Causton, 2016; Davies et al., 2016). The term "reflective practice" is commonly used to refer to the process of considering your values, judgments, beliefs, opinions, culture, stereotypes, experiences, and so on—informally called "your baggage"—and learning to understand their influence on your behavior. All people have baggage. It is neither good nor bad—it is a part of being human.

Reflecting on the Baggage You Bring

The "journey of the dying" has already been mentioned as being a common metaphor for the path a person follows as they die. Nurses are often companions for people on their journey. When companioning someone, it is im-

portant to be clear that it is *their* journey, not your journey. When you consider what to bring on this journey, it is important to reflect on what would help make this the best possible journey for the dying person, rather than taking what you would want if the journey were yours. There are benefits to traveling light and bringing only what you will need.

Nurses can prepare to care for the dying by developing a reflective practice and making conscious decisions about what to bring with them in terms of their beliefs, values, and biases. In the series of images below, a nurse is carrying all the baggage from her life. Next, she sorts her baggage to decide what is appropriate to take with her when providing care. She does not want her baggage to hinder her or weigh her down when caregiving. In the final image, she has much less baggage. She knows what is in the bags and how to work with it, and is not burdened by the weight of carrying too much.

Engaging in a reflective practice and becoming aware of your baggage allows you to decide what to take with you when providing care and what to leave behind. With this self-awareness, you are wholly available to support and assist the dying person and family in their journey. With your excess baggage identified and placed to the side, the path forward is clear, and you will be less likely to trip on your baggage and confuse your personal issues with what is happening professionally.

Davies and Steele's definition of a reflective practice included health care professionals' thinking about their

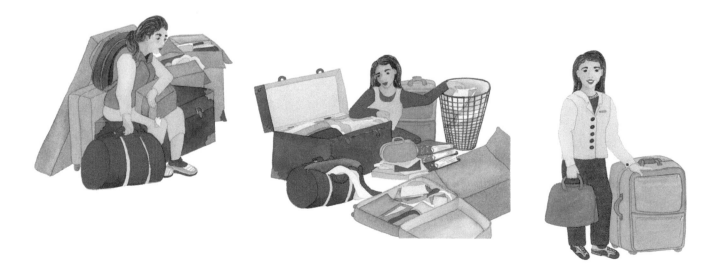

interactions with the parents of a dying child. The health care professionals reflected on their own behavior and what they might want to repeat in other situations and what they might want to change. According to Davies and Steele, developing your reflective practice helps you to hear, listen, and respond best when working with the dying (Davies et al., 2016).

Stephen Levine, a poet, an author, and a teacher best known for his books on dying, once said that "working with people in crisis is similar to reading Braille: you need to feel your way moment by moment" (Levine, 1989). Carrying less baggage makes it easier to be flexible and attend to the needs of the dying person in the moment and to "feel your way," moment by moment.

Activities for Developing a Reflective Practice

Davies and Steele identified curiosity as being integral to best practice for health care professionals—being curious, open-minded, and self-aware. Being curious about yourself will help you develop your reflective practice. Reflective activities—for example, meditation, pondering, praying, journaling, receiving counseling—can be excellent tools for exploring your thoughts and feelings, biases, needs, wants, hopes, dreams, and beliefs.

You will be more comfortable with someone who is dying when you are aware of your fears and biases. The knowledge you gain from your reflective practice will help you to provide better care, as fear and other personal issues can block your ability to see and hear others and communicate openly with them. It is significant that in Davies and Steele's research, best practice health care professionals engaging in reflective practices reported less burnout than their peers. Thus, reflective practice benefits the dying person, their family, *and* you as the nurse.

Reflective activities can also be used to "pause and prepare" in the moment before providing care. They can provide the inner space allowing you to put your baggage aside, right in the moment, and be open to the dying person's care needs. If you are unfamiliar with the practice of preparing to care, follow the instructions in the "Guided Reflective Activity for Preparing to Care" section that follows. Try using this activity before entering a dying person's room, knocking on the door, or making a difficult phone call.

Guided Reflective Activity for Preparing to Care

Take a few deep slow breaths in and out. Feel your feet on the ground. Feel the breath enter and leave your lungs. You may want to touch a wall as well to enhance your connection to the earth. Focus briefly on these physical connections.

Now remember that you are here to companion someone on their journey. Consider the person and their family. Reflect on your desire to care. Notice what is happening inside your mind and body. What biases and beliefs do you hold about the person, their family, their situation? Will your beliefs assist you in this relationship or will they stand in the way? Do you need to put them aside, question them, or seek help from a colleague to challenge your beliefs?

Refresh yourself with a few slow breaths, in and out.

Consider the person you are caring for and what will be of assistance to this person and family. What are their concerns? What are their needs?

Refresh with a few slow breaths, in and out. In the quiet of the breath, allow yourself to feel the person's journey, their needs. Consider how you might engage with the person in a way that is supportive.

Take another breath, slowly in and out, and remind yourself of your connection to the earth. When you are ready, proceed with your visit, introduce yourself, and engage.

Establishing and Maintaining Therapeutic Boundaries

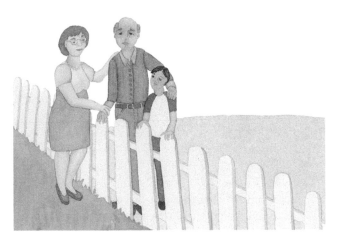

Therapeutic boundaries are invisible lines or edges in relationships, similar to the fence in the illustration above, that help you to know where your values and beliefs end, and where the other person's begin (Causton, 2016). Establishing therapeutic boundaries is a component of self-care, which is also integral to Davies and Steele's best practice interactions between health care professionals and the people for whom they provide care (Davies et al., 2016). Therapeutic boundaries help you to remember that you are a companion on someone else's journey. When you have healthy therapeutic boundaries, you can be present and feel deeply but still think clearly and act wisely in your work, and are less likely experience compassion fatigue.

Caring for the dying is difficult—it means saying hello, knowing that one day you will disconnect. Thinking about boundaries may remind you that while you care deeply about some families, you need to acknowledge that you are an "intimate stranger" who entered their lives in a moment of need. Thinking about boundaries may remind you that although you may feel like family, you are not family; you have not shared the family history, nor have you known this family except during their experience of illness and loss. You are there to provide care as part of a job. Maintaining boundaries helps you remember your role and provides you the space in which to remember whose needs you are trying to meet and whose emotions you are feeling.

Maintaining clear boundaries can be particularly difficult when you are caring for a dying person in their home and supporting their family. The family may expect more from you than is realistic. The person may start thinking of you as a close friend rather than as an HCP. They may ask your opinions on treatments or ask you to sign documents.

You may want to give them your home phone number and visit outside of work hours. When you maintain clear boundaries, you will be able to remember your role as an HCP and know how to respond to these requests or expectations.

When you provide care for a dying person and their family, you do so in moments that are heart-warming, life affirming and sacred. You also provide care in difficult, painful situations. Boundaries may help you to separate yourself from the suffering, pain, and sorrow.

Signs That Therapeutic Boundaries Are Not Clear

When you are not clear about therapeutic boundaries, you may lose your ability to think clearly and act wisely and ethically, especially when you are in a situation characterized by strong emotions, difficult family dynamics, or challenging issues related to care of the person who is dying. If you can relate to any of the following experiences, your boundaries may not be clear.

You experience extreme emotions

Experiencing extreme emotions may indicate that something about the situation or the people in it is resonating with something important, perhaps even unresolved, in your own life, as this example shows:

> *I cry at everything. I feel like I have no skin. I feel out of control. I feel like I'm giving so much of myself at work I don't have anything left to enjoy or be part of my life at home. My daughter said to me, "Mom, you don't laugh anymore."*

The emphasis here is on an extremely strong gut reaction that may even catch you by surprise. This is not the same as the appropriate, shared grief that you experience in the course of your work.

You feel ownership of the dying people you are caring for

Ownership issues arise when you feel unwilling to "share" the person for whom you are caring with other nurses. For example, you may think,

> *I am the one they like the best, and I am the best one to care for them ... no one else can do it as well as I can.*

You may lack therapeutic boundaries if you find yourself phoning on your days off to check on a person in whose care you are involved, or you lack trust in your colleagues' ability to provide excellent care.

You try to take control

Feeling the need to control a dying person's or their family's decisions about care or treatment is an indication that you may be struggling with boundary issues. Putting pressure on a dying person or their family to behave in a certain way, or insisting that they accomplish certain things before death, are other signs of blurred boundaries.

Signs That Therapeutic Boundaries Are Established

When therapeutic boundaries are in place, you may cry with those you care for, but you will know why you are crying. You will share personal information only if it will benefit the person you are caring for. You observe and assess rather than judge and label. You work with your team and communicate about care strategies that work well for the dying person. You help people know that they will be well cared for even when you are not on duty. You listen to the dying person and their family, but you do not try to influence their decisions, and you let them make decisions that feel right to them.

Strategies for Establishing Therapeutic Boundaries

Paying attention to and valuing personal and work-related boundaries are crucial factors in building healthy relationships and preventing fatigue related to the stress of over-involvement. Developing a reflective practice—knowing your own needs, feelings, and beliefs—will assist you in establishing and maintaining therapeutic boundaries.

The following ideas may help you become better at maintaining therapeutic boundaries:

- Identify your boundaries
  - As established by scope of practice by the nursing college/regulatory body
  - As established by your job description and policies in the work setting
  - As related to legal and ethical principles.
- Write reflectively about your boundaries.
- Collect images of boundaries and use them to make a collage.
- When you are in a situation where boundaries seem blurred, talk with a supervisor, colleague, or counselor to explore what may be happening.
- Engage in self-care, because when you take care of yourself and know your own needs, you will be better able to recognize the need for good boundaries and maintain them.
- Do things you love. Find ways to set work aside and enjoy life. You are worth it! (See Chapter 8, "Caring for *You*!")
- Consider the metaphor of the "family dance" (see next page) as a way to understand the benefits of boundaries.

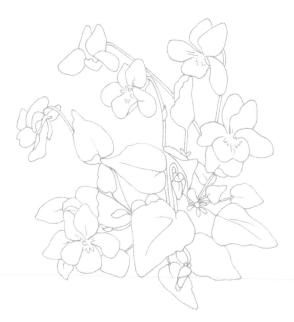

Working from a Therapeutic Distance—the Metaphor of the Family Dance

A "family dance" is one way to describe the different ways that family members interact with one another. A family dance—the music, the steps, and the rhythm—is unique to a family. The family dance evolves over generations as family members respond to joy, sorrow, change, and loss. Every step of the dance has a reason and a history. Do not assume, however, that the family understands what they are doing and why they are doing it.

When one participant in the dance sits or lies down on the dance floor because of illness or death, the family has to change its dance to accommodate the loss. The dance must change instantly, which creates confusion and chaos.

As the family struggles, it is tempting to get onto their dance floor and teach them your family dance steps! However, your dance steps may not work on their dance floor. You also lose the unique and valuable perspective that staying at the edge of the dance floor provides.

When you stay at the edge of the dance floor, you maintain your therapeutic boundaries, thereby decreasing the risk of becoming overinvolved and lost in your work. When you stay on the edge of the dance floor, you can:

- Observe from a neutral place, without judgment
- Explore—consider what you know and need to know to understand this person or the situation
- Imagine what a helping, healing, and validating response might look like
- Preserve the integrity of the family dance

But, staying on the edge of the dance floor is difficult, as the border is often fluid and not easy to identify. In addition, everyone has "hooks"—people or situations that touch them in some deep, unconscious place. For example, when you care for someone who is your age, or whose father reminds you of your father, or whose child is the same age as your child, it is easy to be "hooked." Before you even know what's happening, you may find yourself hooked onto someone else's dance floor, wondering how on earth you got there.

People who care for the dying have an obligation to do this work with awareness. It is important that you do your "homework" by identifying your own hooks and paying attention to signs that you may have stepped onto someone else's dance floor. It is also important to acknowledge that, at some time, all HCPs are likely to become overinvolved with a person or family in their care. Knowing the signs of overinvolvement is crucial.

Work hard to maintain your boundaries and stay off the dance floor of the dying person. Being aware of your own hooks can help you work from a therapeutic distance.

(Causton, 2016)

Establishing and Maintaining Self-Care Practice

Self-care is an essential best practice for nurses and all other members of the health care team who provide care for the dying. Burnout can occur and is a reality for HCPs who connect and disconnect from people and families time and time again in their work. It is worth repeating that Davies and Steele identify self-care as integral to best practice (Davies et al., 2016) and Butot identifies self-care as part of love in professional practice (Butot, 2005). In addition, it is significant and worth restating that Davies and Steele found that health care professionals who engaged in best practice experienced no or little burnout.

Strategies for self-care are the focus of Chapter 8, "Caring for *You!*"

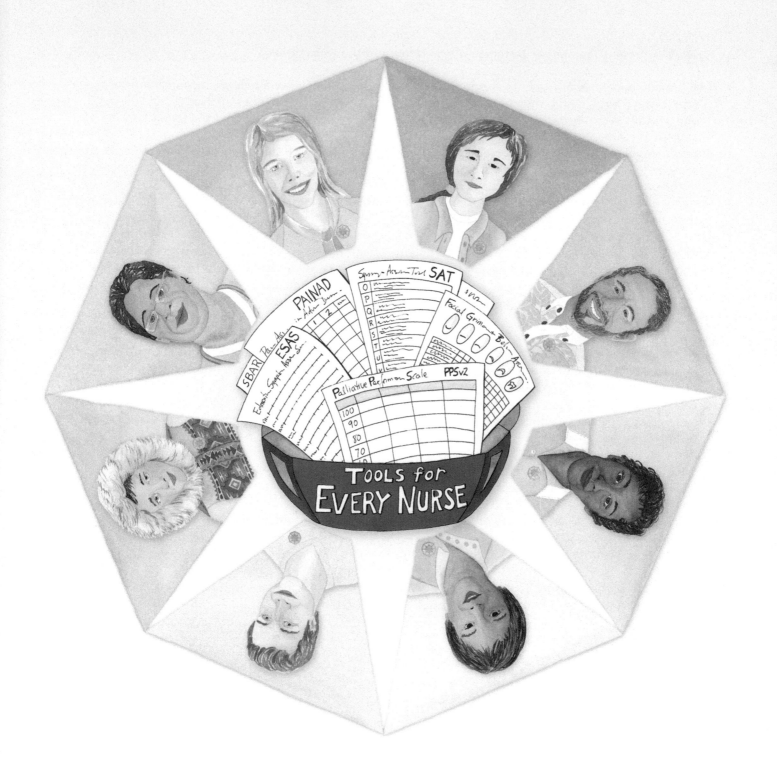

Using Standardized Tools

The Rationale for Using Standardized Tools

The focus of this chapter is to provide health care providers (HCPs) with standardized tools for gathering information and for screening and assessing symptoms as you strive to provide excellent hospice and palliative care. Standardized tools have been validated by multiple researchers and are known to gather consistent information.

The standardized tools presented here are widely used across Canada and the United States; however, this collection of tools is not exhaustive. In your practice, you might encounter other standardized tools commonly used in your location, community, hospital, or hospice. Follow your employer's policies and procedures when determining which tool to use.

It will be helpful to familiarize yourself with these tools so that when the need for a tool arises you know where to find it. As with any tool kit, you will want to choose when and how to use the tools.

Do not feel that you need to read this chapter from beginning to end. Rather, become familiar with the tools, and refer to them as they are mentioned throughout the text.

Note the following:
- Certain assessment tools, such as the Palliative Performance Scale (PPS), can be completed on the basis of observation; others require input from the dying person and/or the family.
- People may experience "assessment fatigue" when presented with too many questions. It may be helpful to clarify with the person and the family when and how to best complete the assessment.

Tools Described in This Chapter

Best Practice for Assessments and Information Sharing

Being curious and asking questions about the dying person and their family are behaviors of best practice HCPs (Davies et al., 2016). Assessment, sharing information, supporting informed decision making, and planning, implementing, and evaluating care are integral to the process of providing care. Just as you would ask a person how they prefer their eggs to be cooked, it is helpful to ask how to best assess, share information, support informed decision making, and include the person and family in care planning, implementation, and evaluation. This does not need to occur in the initial interview. The art is in realizing that some of this is intuitive and you see it, sense it, and will be able to know what questions to ask. The important thing is to make sure that people understand and are supported to make decisions.

Some examples of questions and conversations that you might adapt to the needs of the person and family follow:

Many people are asking you many questions as we strive to get to know you, your needs, and how best to help you. The questions can be overwhelming at times, and answering them can be exhausting. Do you have any suggestions for us on how to best collect the information that we need, and yet not exhaust you in the process?

Sometimes people like to answer all the questions themselves, whereas other people like to have family members help with the assessment. What is your preference?

You are receiving a lot of information, and you will continue to get more information in the coming weeks and months. Can you tell me how you like to receive information [brochures? Internet? videos?]? As your disease/illness changes/progresses you will be asked to make many decisions. Do you like to make decisions with your family present, or do you like to decide on your own?

In some families, there is one person who makes decisions. In other families, the family members make decisions together. What are your preferences for making decisions? How can we best support you to make decisions? If there is anything that we can do to support you in making decisions, please let us know.

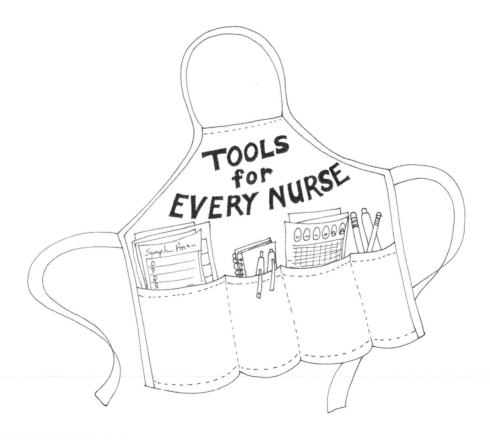

Screening Tools for Identifying When to Integrate a Palliative Approach

Hospice and palliative care are moving upstream, closer to the time of diagnosis. Identifying people who will benefit from having a palliative approach integrated into their care in the months and years before dying is essential to this upstream movement. Four tools are discussed in this section: the Gold Standards Framework Prognostic Indicator Guidance (GSF PIG); the Supportive and Palliative Care Indicators Tool (SPICT); a tool for prognosticating one-year mortality; and a tool for prognosticating one-year mortality after hospital admission. Use these tools, or the tools used in your community or facility, to address needs and inform goals-of-care conversations.

Gold Standards Framework Prognostic Indicator Guidance (GSF PIG)

The GSF PIG tool (Figure 1) (Thomas, 2011), developed in Britain, is used to determine whether a person might benefit from a palliative approach being integrated into their care.

Instructions: Use this tool to assess any person who is aging, living with a progressive life-limiting illness, or entering residential care, or whose health is suspected to be declining.

Follow the three steps in the process to determine whether a person might benefit from the integration of a palliative approach into their care. The following pages present criteria for Step 2, assessing General Indicators of Decline (see purple box in Figure 1) and Step 3, assessing Specific Clinical Indicators of decline (see red box in Figure 1). Chapter 2, "Integrating a Palliative Approach," contains more information about this tool.

A person showing any general or specific clinical indicators of decline would benefit from the integration into their care of a palliative approach. This person would need to be reassessed regularly to evaluate changing needs. The GSF process, shown in the green box in Figure 1, would also begin.

Figure 1. Gold Standards Framework Prognostic Indicator Guidance

(continued on next page)

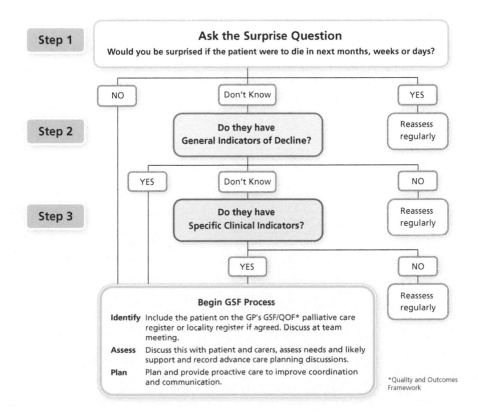

Step 1: The Surprise Question

For patients with advanced disease of progressive life limiting conditions—Would you be surprised if the patient were to die in the next few months, weeks, days?

- The answer to this question should be an intuitive one, pulling together a range of clinical, co-morbid, social and other factors that give a whole picture of deterioration. If you would not be surprised, then what measures might be taken to improve the patient's quality of life now and in preparation for possible further decline?

Step 2: General Indicators

Are there general indicators of decline and increasing needs?

- Decreasing activity—functional performance status declining (e.g. Barthel score) limited self-care, in bed or chair 50% of day) and increasing dependence in most activities of daily living
- Co-morbidity—regarded as the biggest predictive indicator of mortality and morbidity
- General physical decline and increasing need for support
- Advanced disease—unstable, deteriorating complex symptom burden
- Decreasing response to treatments, decreasing reversibility
- Choice of no further active treatment
- Progressive weight loss (>10%) in past six months
- Repeated unplanned/crisis admissions
- Sentinel event e.g. serious fall, bereavement, transfer to nursing home
- Serum albumen <25g/l

Functional Assessments

- **Barthel Index** describes basic Activities of Daily Living (ADL) as 'core' to the functional assessment. E.g. feeding, bathing, grooming, dressing, urinary continence, fecal continence, toileting, transfers, walking, climbing stairs
- **PULSE** 'screening' assessment
  P (physical condition)
  U (upper limb function)
  L (lower limb function)
  S (sensory)
  E (environment)
- **Karnofksy Performance Status Score**
  0–100 ADL scale
- **WHO/ECOG Performance Status**
  0–5 scale of activity

Step 3: Specific Clinical Indicators

Flexible criteria with some overlaps, especially with those with frailty and other co-morbidities.

a. Cancer—rapid or predictable decline

- Metastatic cancer
- More exact predictors for cancer patients are available e.g. PPS. 'Prognosis tools can help but should not be applied blindly'

b. Organ Failure—erratic decline

Chronic Obstructive Pulmonary Disease (COPD)

At least two of the indicators below:

- Disease assessed to be severe (e.g. FEV1 <30% predicted)
- Recurrent hospital admissions (at least 3 in last 12 months due to COPD)
- Fulfils long term oxygen therapy criteria
- MRC breathlessness scale, Grade 4/5—shortness of breath after 100 metres on the level or confined to house
- Signs and symptoms of right heart failure
- Combination of other factors—i.e. anorexia, previous ITU/NIV resistant organisms
- More than 6 weeks of systemic steroids for COPD in preceding 6 months

Heart Disease

At least two of the indicators below:

- CHF NYHA Stage 3 or 4—shortness of breath at rest on minimal exertion
- Patient thought to be in the last year of life by the care team—The 'surprise question'
- Repeated hospital admissions with heart failure symptoms
- Difficult physical or psychological symptoms despite optimal tolerated therapy

Renal Disease

Stage 4 or 5 Chronic Kidney Disease (CKD) whose condition is deteriorating with at least 2 of the indicators below:

- Patient for whom the surprise question is applicable
- Patients choosing the 'no dialysis' option, discontinuing dialysis or not opting for dialysis if their transplant has failed
- Patients with difficult physical symptoms or psychological symptoms despite optimal tolerated renal replacement therapy
- Symptomatic Renal Failure—nausea and vomiting, anorexia, pruritus, reduced functional status, intractable fluid overload.

- 'The single most important predictive factor in cancer is performance status and functional ability'—if patients are spending more than 50% of their time in bed/lying down, prognosis is estimated to be about 3 months or less.

General Neurological Diseases

- Progressive deterioration in physical and/ or cognitive function despite optimal therapy
- Symptoms which are complex and too difficult to control
- Swallowing problems (dysphagia) leading to recurrent aspiration pneumonia, sepsis, breathlessness or respiratory failure
- Speech problems: increasing difficulty in communications and progressive dysphasia. Plus the following:

  Motor Neurone Disease
  - Marked rapid decline in physical status
  - First episode of aspirational pneumonia
  - Increased cognitive difficulties
  - Weight loss
  - Significantly complex symptoms and medical complications
  - Low vital capacity (below 70% of predicted using standard spirometry)
  - Dyskinesia, mobility problems and falls
  - Communication difficulties

  Parkinson's Disease
  - Drug treatment are less effective or increasingly complex regime of drug treatments required
  - Reduced independence, needs ADL help
  - The condition is less well controlled with increasing "off" periods
  - Dyskinesia, mobility problems and falls
  - Psychiatric signs e.g., depression, anxiety, hallucinations, psychosis
  - Similar pattern to frailty—see below

  Multiple Sclerosis
  - Significantly complex symptoms and medical complications
  - Dysphagia + poor nutritional status
  - Communication difficulties e.g., dysarthria + fatigue
  - Cognitive impairment, notably the onset of dementia

Figure 1. Gold Standards Framework Prognostic Indicator Guidance

c. Frailty/Stroke/Dementia—gradual decline

Frailty

Individuals who present with Multiple co morbidities with significant impairment in day to day living and:
- Deteriorating functional score e.g. performance status—Barthel/ECOG/Karnofksy
- Combination of at least three of the following symptoms:
  - weakness
  - slow walking speed
  - significant weight loss
  - exhaustion
  - low physical activity
  - depression

Stroke
- Persistent vegetative or minimal conscious state or dense paralysis
- Medical complications
- Lack of improvement within 3 months of onset
- Cognitive impairment / Post-stroke dementia

Dementia

There are many underlying conditions which may lead to degrees of dementia and these should be taken into account. Triggers to consider that indicate that someone is entering a later stage are:
- Unable to walk without assistance and
- Urinary and faecal incontinence, and
- No consistently meaningful conversation and
- Unable to do Activities of Daily Living (ADL)
- Barthel score <3.

Plus any of the following:
- Weight loss
- Urinary tract Infection
- Severe pressures sores—stage three or four
- Recurrent fever
- Reduced oral intake
- Aspiration pneumonia

It is vital that discussions with individuals living with dementia are started at an early to ensure that whilst they have mental capacity they can discuss how they would like the later stages managed.

Supportive and Palliative Care Indicators Tool (SPICT™)

The SPICT (Figure 2) (NHS Lothian, 2016) is a screening tool developed at the University of Edinburgh to help identify people at risk of deteriorating or dying in the near future, and to determine whether they might have supportive or palliative care needs that should be addressed. This tool is especially helpful for identifying such people who do not have cancer, and can help identify people early in their decline so that advance care planning and treatment goals and options can be discussed before their health is in crisis.

Instructions: Use this tool to assess any person who is living with a progressive life-limiting illness, is entering residential care, or whose health is suspected to be declining.

Figure 2. Supportive and Palliative Care Indicators Tool (SPICT™)

Supportive and Palliative Care Indicators Tool (SPICT™)

THE UNIVERSITY
of EDINBURGH

NHS
Lothian

The SPICT™ is a guide to identifying people at risk of deteriorating and dying. Assess these people for unmet supportive and palliative care needs.

Look for general indicators of deteriorating health.

- Unplanned hospital admissions.
- Performance status is poor or deteriorating, with limited reversibility; (person is in bed or a chair for 50% or more of the day).
- Dependent on others for care due to physical and/or mental health problems.
- More support for the person's carer is needed.
- Significant weight loss over the past 3-6 months, and/ or a low body mass index.
- Persistent symptoms despite optimal treatment of underlying condition(s).
- Person or family ask for palliative care, treatment withdrawal/limitation or a focus on quality of life.

Look for clinical indicators of one or more advanced conditions.

Cancer

Functional ability deteriorating due to progressive cancer.

Too frail for cancer treatment or treatment is for symptom control.

Dementia/ frailty

Unable to dress, walk or eat without help.

Eating and drinking less; swallowing difficulties.

Urinary and faecal incontinence.

No longer able to communicate using verbal language; little social interaction.

Fractured femur; multiple falls.

Recurrent febrile episodes or infections; aspiration pneumonia.

Neurological disease

Progressive deterioration in physical and/or cognitive function despite optimal therapy.

Speech problems with increasing difficulty communicating and/ or progressive swallowing difficulties.

Recurrent aspiration pneumonia; breathless or respiratory failure.

Heart/ vascular disease

NYHA Class III/IV heart failure, or extensive, untreatable coronary artery disease with:
- breathlessness or chest pain at rest or on minimal exertion.

Severe, inoperable peripheral vascular disease.

Respiratory disease

Severe chronic lung disease with:
- breathlessness at rest or on minimal exertion between exacerbations.

Needs long term oxygen therapy.

Has needed ventilation for respiratory failure or ventilation is contraindicated.

Deteriorating and at risk of dying with any other condition or complication that is not reversible.

Kidney disease

Stage 4 or 5 chronic kidney disease (eGFR < 30ml/min) with deteriorating health.

Kidney failure complicating other life limiting conditions or treatments.

Stopping dialysis.

Liver disease

Advanced cirrhosis with one or more complications in past year:
- diuretic resistant ascites
- hepatic encephalopathy
- hepatorenal syndrome
- bacterial peritonitis
- recurrent variceal bleeds

Liver transplant is contraindicated.

Review current care and care planning.

- Review current treatment and medication so the person receives optimal care.
- Consider referral for specialist assessment if symptoms or needs are complex and difficult to manage.
- Agree current and future care goals, and a care plan with the person and their family.
- Plan ahead if the person is at risk of loss of capacity.
- Record, communicate and coordinate the care plan.

Please register on the SPICT website (www.spict.org.uk) for information and updates.

SPICT™, April 2016

Using the tools described here for prognosticating one-year mortality will enable HCPs to identify people who are at high risk of dying within the coming year, and to confidently engage them in discussions about advance care planning, goals of care, and integrating a palliative approach into care.

Choose the appropriate tool, depending on whether the person is living in their home or community care, or has recently been admitted to hospital.

Three-Criteria Tool for Predicting One-Year Mortality

You and Fowler developed a tool (Figure 3) (You and Fowler, 2014) that provides three criteria for predicting mortality within one year for a person living in the community or a facility.

Instructions: Evaluate a person using the three numbered criteria below. Any person that meets criterion 1, 2, or 3 is at high risk of dying in the coming year, and therefore would benefit from conversations about advance care planning, goals of care, and integrating a palliative approach into their care. This tool can be used to assess any person who is aging, living with a progressive life-limiting illness, or entering residential care, or whose health is suspected to be declining.

Figure 3. Three-Criteria Tool for Predicting One-Year Mortality

1. Age ≥ 55 years and 1 or more of the following advanced chronic illnesses:
- Chronic obstructive pulmonary disease (2 of the following: baseline arterial partial pressure of carbon dioxide > 45 mm Hg, cor pulmonale, episode of respiratory failure within the preceding year, forced expiratory volume in 1 s < 0.5 L)
- Congestive heart failure (New York Heart Association class IV symptoms and left ventricular ejection fraction < 25%)
- Cirrhosis (confirmed by imaging studies or documentation of esophageal varices) and 1 of the following: hepatic coma, Child class C liver disease, Child class B liver disease with gastrointestinal bleeding

- Cancer (metastatic cancer or stage IV lymphoma)
- End-stage dementia (inability to perform all activities of daily living, mutism or minimal verbal output secondary to dementia, bed-bound state prior to acute illness

Or

2. Any patient ≥ 80 years of age admitted to hospital from the community because of an acute medical or surgical condition.

Or

3. You answer "no" to the following question: Would I be surprised if this patient died within the next year?

Prognostic Index for Mortality within One Year of Hospital Admission

Walter and colleagues developed the risk scoring system shown in Figure 4 (Walter et al., 2001) to help identify the risk of dying for a person being discharged from hospital. While this index cannot predict who will die, it can indicate how many people with similar risk factors lived and died in the year following hospitalization. This prognostic index can help identify who might benefit from the integration of a palliative approach into their care.

The scoring system can be used to assess any person who is aging, living with a progressive life-limiting illness, or entering residential care, or whose health is suspected to be declining.

The Walter Index is also available online at the ePrognosis website (eprognosis.ucsf.edu/walter.php), and provides an interactive method for calculating a person's risk of dying after hospital admission.

Instructions: Assess the person's risk factors in Step 1 (ADLs means "activities of daily living"). Total their score and go to Step 2.

Locate the row in Step 2 that corresponds to the person's total score, and read across to the value in the 1-year mortality column. This value indicates the percentage of people having the same total score who died in the first year after hospital admission. For example, among people with a total score of 2 to 3, 19% died and 81% lived through the next year following hospitalization.

It will be helpful to discuss with the health care team when a person's score indicates that they are at high risk of dying within a year. This information can be used in addition to the other tools to help determine when a person might benefit from a palliative approach, including advance care planning and goals-of-care discussions.

Figure 4. Prognostic Index for Mortality within One Year of Hospital Admission

Step 1: Determine score using risk factors		
Variable	**Score**	**Tally**
Male sex	1	
Needs assistance with 1–4 ADLs at discharge	2	
Needs assistance with all ADLs	5	
Congestive heart failure	2	
Cancer*	3	
Metastatic cancer	8	
Creatinine > 265 µmol/L	2	
Serum albumin 30–34 g/L	1	
Serum albumin < 30 g/L	2	
	Total Score	

Step 2: Use patient's Total Score to identify their estimated risk of dying within 1 year	
Total score	**1-year mortality (%)**
0–1 points	4
2–3 points	19
4–6 points	34
> 6 points	64

Symptom Screening Tools

Screening tools that help identify the presence or absence of symptoms are usually quick to use and provide information on which symptoms need to be addressed. Such tools do not provide in-depth assessment of the symptom.

Edmonton Symptom Assessment System (ESAS)

The ESAS (Figure 5) (Bruera et al., 1991) is a numerical scale used to gather information on the person's perception of nine symptoms they may be experiencing, and other problems. It is a practical tool that enables a rapid self-evaluation of the nine symptoms, using a horizontal visual scale from 0 to 10, in which 0 means the symptom is absent, 1 means the symptom causes minimal distress, and 10 means the symptom is the worst possible. The tool was developed for use with cancer patients originally and is now used across Canada and the United States for people receiving hospice and palliative care (Cancer Care Ontario, 2010; Richardson and Jones, 2009). The tool provides a "snapshot" of the person's status.

Instructions: Provide the person with a copy of the ESAS to fill out on a regular basis. Clearly identify the time frame (e.g., the present moment, the last 8 hours, the last 24 hours) for the person to consider when completing their self-evaluation. If the goal is to assess for changes in symptoms, ensure that the time between evaluations is consistent. Only the person can provide the answers to the questions in this tool, but the family or an HCP can record them. The tool cannot be used when a person is no longer able to self-evaluate.

When the person indicates that a symptom has become worse since the previous evaluation or that it is a new symptom, follow up by assessing the symptom with the Symptom Assessment Tool (see page 65).

Please circle the number that best describes how you feel NOW. Use the body map on the next page to identify the location of each symptom in your body.

No Pain	0	1	2	3	4	5	6	7	8	9	10	Worst Possible Pain

No Tiredness (Tiredness = lack of energy)	0	1	2	3	4	5	6	7	8	9	10	Worst Possible Tiredness

No Drowsiness (Drowsiness = feeling sleepy)	0	1	2	3	4	5	6	7	8	9	10	Worst Possible Drowsiness

No Nausea	0	1	2	3	4	5	6	7	8	9	10	Worst Possible Nausea

No Lack of Appetite	0	1	2	3	4	5	6	7	8	9	10	Worst Possible Lack of Appetite

No Shortness of Breath	0	1	2	3	4	5	6	7	8	9	10	Worst Possible Shortness of Breath

No Depression (Depression = feeling sad)	0	1	2	3	4	5	6	7	8	9	10	Worst Possible Depression

No Anxiety (Anxiety = feeling nervous)	0	1	2	3	4	5	6	7	8	9	10	Worst Possible Anxiety

Best Wellbeing (Wellbeing = how you feel overall)	0	1	2	3	4	5	6	7	8	9	10	Worst Possible Wellbeing

Other Problem (for example constipation) No _____	0	1	2	3	4	5	6	7	8	9	10	Worst Possible _____ (identify the symptom)

Person's Name _____

Date _____ Time _____

Figure 5. Edmonton Symptom Assessment System (revised version, ESAS-R)

**Please mark on these body images where you experience a symptom. If more than one symptom is iden-
tified, please label each symptom.**

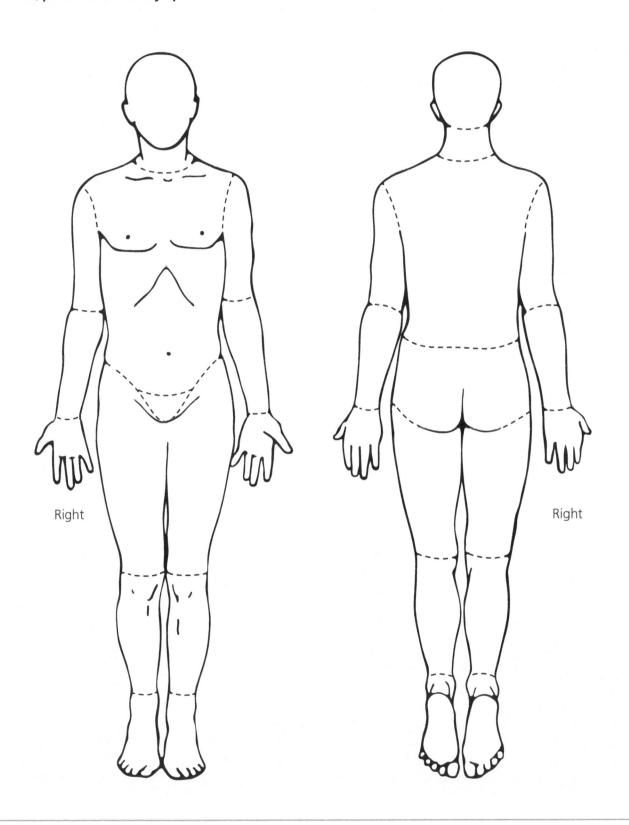

Right   Right

The PPS (Figure 6) (Victoria Hospice Society, 2011) is used to assess a person's ability to perform activities of daily living (ADLs). It assesses a person's performance and distills it into an easily understood value from 0% to 100% on the basis of the person's functioning in five areas: mobility (ambulation), activity and evidence of disease, ability for self-care, intake, and level of consciousness.

The PPS is a widely used in community and hospice and palliative care settings worldwide. As well, it is increasingly being used in long-term care and acute care settings to assess a person's overall functioning, as well as to identify changes in a person's abilities.

You may use the PPS as a guide to observe daily changes in a person's abilities or behaviors, thereby identifying a person's decline and enabling prognosticating. The PPS can provide a quick summary and update, facilitating knowledge sharing and communication about changes in the person's needs.

You are assigned to care for Mr. K. today. He was 60% last week, 40% yesterday, and is 20% today. The family is very upset and has questions and concerns about his condition and his care.

Figure 6. Palliative Performance Scale

(continued on next page)

Palliative Performance Scale (PPS) version 2

Victoria Hospice

PPS Level	Ambulation	Activity & Evidence of Disease	Self-Care	Intake	Conscious Level
100%	Full	Normal activity & work No evidence of disease	Full	Normal	Full
90%	Full	Normal activity & work Some evidence of disease	Full	Normal	Full
80%	Full	Normal activity with effort Some evidence of disease	Full	Normal or reduced	Full
70%	Reduced	Unable normal job/work Significant disease	Full	Normal or reduced	Full
60%	Reduced	Unable hobby/house work Significant disease	Occasional assistance necessary	Normal or reduced	Full or Confusion
50%	Mainly Sit/Lie	Unable to do any work Extensive disease	Considerable assistance required	Normal or reduced	Full or Confusion
40%	Mainly in Bed	Unable to do most activity Extensive disease	Mainly assistance	Normal or reduced	Full or Drowsy +/– Confusion
30%	Totally Bed Bound	Unable to do any activity Extensive disease	Total Care	Normal or reduced	Full or Drowsy +/– Confusion
20%	Totally Bed Bound	Unable to do any activity Extensive disease	Total Care	Minimal to sips	Full or Drowsy +/– Confusion
10%	Totally Bed Bound	Unable to do any activity Extensive disease	Total Care	Mouth care only	Drowsy or Coma +/– Confusion
0%	Death	—	—	—	—

Reproduced with permission. Copyright Victoria Hospice Society, BC, Canada (2001) www.victoriahospice.org.

Figure 6. Palliative Performance Scale
(continued on next page)

Instructions for using the Palliative Performance Scale

(Instructions written by, and provided here, with the permission of Victoria Hospice Society, 2016.)

(See also definition of terms)

1. PPS scores are determined by reading horizontally at each level to find a 'best fit' for the patient which is then assigned as the PPS% score.

2. Begin at the left column and read downwards until the appropriate ambulation level is reached, then read across to the next column and downwards again until the activity/evidence of disease is located. These steps are repeated until all five columns are covered before assigning the actual PPS for that patient. In this way, 'leftward' columns (columns to the left of any specific column) are 'stronger' determinants and generally take precedence over others.

   Example 1: A patient who spends the majority of the day sitting or lying down due to fatigue from advanced disease and requires considerable assistance to walk even for short distances but who is otherwise fully conscious level with good intake would be scored at PPS 50%.

   Example 2: A patient who has become paralyzed and quadriplegic requiring total care would be PPS 30%. Although this patient may be placed in a wheelchair (and perhaps seem initially to be at 50%), the score is 30% because he or she would be otherwise totally bed bound due to the disease or complication if it were not for caregivers providing total care including lift/transfer. The patient may have normal intake and full conscious level.

   Example 3: However, if the patient in example 2 was paraplegic and bed bound but still able to do some self-care such as feed themselves, then the PPS would be higher at 40 or 50% since he or she is not 'total care.'

3. PPS scores are in 10% increments only. Sometimes, there are several columns easily placed at one level but one or two which seem better at a higher or lower level. One then needs to make a 'best fit' de-

cision. Choosing a 'half-fit' value of PPS 45%, for example, is not correct. The combination of clinical judgment and 'leftward precedence' is used to determine whether 40% or 50% is the more accurate score for that patient.

4. PPS may be used for several purposes. First, it is an excellent communication tool for quickly describing a patient's current functional level. Second, it may have value in criteria for workload assessment or other measurements and comparisons. Finally, it appears to have prognostic value.

Definition of Terms for PPS

As noted below, some of the terms have similar meanings with the differences being more readily apparent as one reads horizontally across each row to find an overall 'best fit' using all five columns.

1. Ambulation

The items '**mainly sit/lie**,' '**mainly in bed**,' and '**totally bed bound**' are clearly similar. The subtle differences are related to items in the self-care column. For example, 'totally bed 'bound' at PPS 30% is due to either profound weakness or paralysis such that the patient not only can't get out of bed but is also unable to do any self-care. The difference between 'sit/lie' and 'bed' is proportionate to the amount of time the patient is able to sit up vs need to lie down.

'Reduced ambulation' is located at the PPS 70% and PPS 60% level. By using the adjacent column, the reduction of ambulation is tied to inability to carry out their normal job, work occupation or some hobbies or housework activities. The person is still able to walk and transfer on their own but at PPS 60% needs occasional assistance.

2. Activity & Extent of disease

'**Some**,' '**significant**,' and '**extensive**' disease refer to physical and investigative evidence which shows degrees of progression. For example in breast cancer, a local recurrence would imply 'some' disease, one or two metastases in the lung or bone would imply 'significant'

Figure 6. Palliative Performance Scale

disease, whereas multiple metastases in lung, bone, liver, brain, hypercalcemia or other major complications would be 'extensive' disease. The extent may also refer to progression of disease despite active treatments. Using PPS in AIDS, 'some' may mean the shift from HIV to AIDS, 'significant' implies progression in physical decline, new or difficult symptoms and laboratory findings with low counts. 'Extensive' refers to one or more serious complications with or without continuation of active antiretrovirals, antibiotics, etc.

The above extent of disease is also judged in context with the ability to maintain one's work and hobbies or activities. Decline in activity may mean the person still plays golf but reduces from playing 18 holes to 9 holes, or just a par 3, or to backyard putting. People who enjoy walking will gradually reduce the distance covered, although they may continue trying, sometimes even close to death (e.g. trying to walk the halls).

3. Self-Care

'**Occasional assistance**' means that most of the time patients are able to transfer out of bed, walk, wash, toilet and eat by their own means, but that on occasion (perhaps once daily or a few times weekly) they require minor assistance.

'**Considerable assistance**' means that regularly every day the patient needs help, usually by one person, to do some of the activities noted above. For example, the person needs help to get to the bathroom but is then able to brush his or her teeth or wash at least hands and face. Food will often need to be cut into edible sizes but the patient is then able to eat of his or her own accord.

'**Mainly assistance**' is a further extension of 'considerable.' Using the above example, the patient now needs help getting up but also needs assistance washing his face and shaving, but can usually eat with minimal or no help. This may fluctuate according to fatigue during the day.

'**Total care**' means that the patient is completely unable to eat without help, toilet or do any self-care. Depending on the clinical situation, the patient may or may not be able to chew and swallow food once prepared and fed to him or her.

4. Intake

Changes in intake are quite obvious with '**normal intake**' referring to the person's usual eating habits while healthy. '**Reduced**' means any reduction from that and is highly variable according to the unique individual circumstances. '**Minimal**' refers to very small amounts, usually pureed or liquid, which are well below nutritional sustenance.

5. Conscious Level

'**Full consciousness**' implies full alertness and orientation with good cognitive abilities in various domains of thinking, memory, etc. '**Confusion**' is used to denote presence of either delirium or dementia and is a reduced level of consciousness. It may be mild, moderate or severe with multiple possible etiologies. '**Drowsiness**' implies either fatigue, drug side effects, delirium or closeness to death and is sometimes included in the term stupor. '**Coma**' in this context is the absence of response to verbal or physical stimuli; some reflexes may or may not remain. The depth of coma may fluctuate throughout a 24 hour period.

Symptom Assessment Tools

Many assessment tools focus on one symptom and collect detailed information that will help the health care team to treat or provide relief from the symptom.

Symptom Assessment Tool

The Symptom Assessment Tool (Table 1) is used to thoroughly assess a person's symptom, with the goals of determining its causes and the person's understanding and experience of the symptom, as well as to track changes in response to treatment or resulting from disease progression.

For this text, the Symptom Assessment Tool was adapted and extended from the Symptom Assessment Acronym (Fraser Health Authority, 2016b) for use as a standardized

way for assessing each symptom. The Symptom Assessment Tool uses the mnemonic "OPQRSTUV" to help ensure a thorough assessment.

Instructions: Assess a person for a symptom whenever it is reported in the ESAS or by the person or family. Rephrase and adapt as necessary the sample questions shown in the Symptom Assessment Tool for each symptom (see Chapter 5, "Enhancing Physical Comfort") and use the questions to assess the symptom in the person. Bulleted items in the tool are those that the HCP assesses through observation or measurement.

Record the assessment and report to the physician/nurse practitioner if requesting orders.

Table 1. Symptom Assessment Tool

	Symptom Assessment Tool	
O	**Onset**	When did you start experiencing this symptom? How long does the symptom last?
P	**Provoking/Palliating**	What triggers this symptom? How often do you feel this symptom each day? What decreases the symptom? Is there a pattern to the symptom's occurance? Does this symptom increase the severity of other symptoms? Do other symptoms make this symptom feel worse?
Q	**Quality**	Can you describe the symptom, what it feels like?
R	**Region/Radiating**	Where are you feeling the symptom? Any other areas? Does the symptom radiate to other regions? Does the symptom cause other symptoms?
S	**Severity**	Can you rate this symptom (discomfort) on a scale of 0 to 10, with 0 being no symptom and 10 being the worst symptom you can imagine? Would you prefer to rate your symptom with words such as "mild," "moderate," or "severe"?
T	**Treatment**	What medications have you used to control this symptom? What doses have you tried? What was effective? Did you experience any side effects when you took the medications? Have your medications for managing this symptom been changed recently?
U	**Understanding**	What do you think is causing the symptom? How is this symptom affecting your daily activities? Can you tell me how it is for you to experience this symptom?
V	**Values**	What are your goals managing this symptom? On a scale of 0 to 10, where would you like your symptom to be? What is most important to you today?

W	**What Else?**	• Physical assessment
		   ◦ Look for any changes
		 • Other relevant findings
		   ◦ Medications
		   ◦ Relevant lab and diagnostic results

Rating Scales

The numerical rating scale 0 to 10 (Figure 7), like that in the Symptom Assessment Tool (Table 1 on page 65), is a common way to have people rate the severity of their symptom (e.g., pain, nausea). Ensure that the person understands that 0 indicates that the symptom is not present and 10 indicates that the symptom is the worst the person can imagine it to be.

Can you give your pain a number between 0 and 10, with 0 being no pain and 10 being the worst pain you can imagine?

Sometimes people have difficulty rating their pain with a number and may find it easier to use words such as "mild," "moderate," or "severe," or "small," "medium," or "big." Using a rating scale like that in Figure 7, which includes colors as well as numbers and words, may be helpful. In Figure 7, green represents no pain and red represents severe pain.

When dying people are unable to rate or report pain, use the Facial Grimace and Behaviour Assessment Tool (see Figure 14 on page 75).

Figure 7. Sample number/word/color rating scale

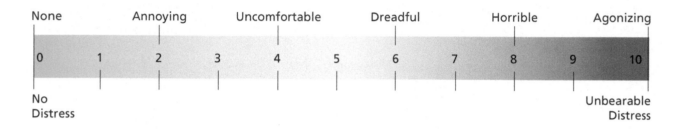

Body Map

The Body Map (Figure 8) can be used to help a dying person accurately communicate the location of pain in their body, whether the pain occurs at a single or multiple sites. People with mild or moderate cognitive impairment may be able to use a body map even if they are not able to respond well verbally (Weiner, Peterson, and Keefe, 1998).

Instructions: Provide the person with a body map, writing tools (e.g., pens, pencils, or markers), and some time to indicate on the map where they experience pain. If the

person's vision is limited, enlarge the body map. If a person is unable to draw on the map, they may be able to point to the areas where they feel pain and a family member or an HCP can draw the areas on the body map for the person. Using a body map to report the location of pain does not require any verbal skills but does require that the person have the cognitive skills to relate the body map to their own body. This tool should be used only to indicate the location of pain, not to rule out pain.

Figure 8. Body Map

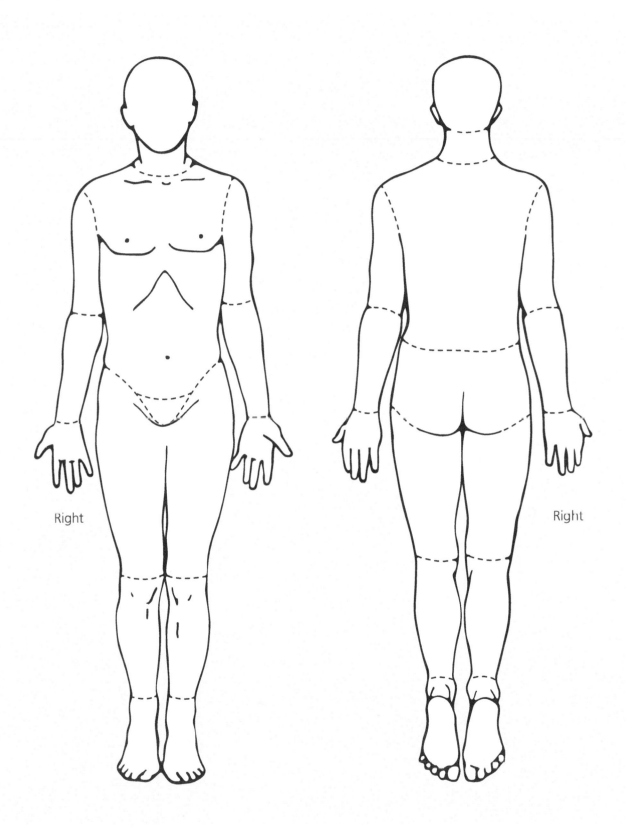

Right

Right

The Clinical COPD (Chronic Obstructive Pulmonary Disease) Questionnaire (Figure 9) (van der Molen, 1999) is used to gather information about the intensity, frequency, and duration of a person's dyspnea. This self-assessment questionnaire can help in determining the causes and triggers of dyspnea, and the effect of treatments and preventive measures on the severity and frequency of dyspneic episodes. The frequency of administering the questionnaire will decrease when the triggers and causes of the person's dyspnea have been determined and preventive measures and treatments are working effectively.

Instructions: Have the person who experiences dyspnea complete the questionnaire shown in Figure 9.

Figure 9. Clinical COPD Questionnaire

Patient number:_____
Date:_____

CLINICAL COPD QUESTIONNAIRE

Please **circle** the number of the response that best describes how you have been feeling during the **past week**.
(Only **one** response for each question).

On average, **during the past week**, how often did you feel:	never	hardly ever	a few times	several times	many times	a great many times	almost all the time
1. Short of breath **at rest**?	0	1	2	3	4	5	6
2. Short of breath **doing physical activities**?	0	1	2	3	4	5	6
3. **Concerned** about getting a cold or your breathing getting worse?	0	1	2	3	4	5	6
4. **Depressed (down)** because of your breathing problems?	0	1	2	3	4	5	6
In general, **during the past week**, how much of the time:							
5. Did you **cough**?	0	1	2	3	4	5	6
6. Did you **produce phlegm**?	0	1	2	3	4	5	6
On average, **during the past week**, how limited were you in these activities **because of your breathing problems**:	not limited at all	very slightly limited	slightly limited	moderately limited	very limited	extremely limited	totally limited /or unable to do
7. **Strenuous physical activities** (such as climbing stairs, hurrying, doing sports)?	0	1	2	3	4	5	6
8. **Moderate physical activities** (such as walking, housework, carrying things)?	0	1	2	3	4	5	6
9. **Daily activities at home** (such as dressing, washing yourself)?	0	1	2	3	4	5	6
10. **Social activities** (such as talking, being with children, visiting friends/ relatives)?	0	1	2	3	4	5	6

Assessing Delirium: Confusion Assessment Method (CAM)

The CAM (Figure 10) (VIHA, 2014) is used to identify the presence of delirium in a person and assess possible causes of the delirium.

Instructions: Answer the questions in Figure 10.

Figure 10. Confusion Assessment Method (CAM)

The diagnosis of delirium by CAM requires BOTH **A** and **B**	
A. **Acute onset** and **Fluctuating course**	Is there evidence of an acute change in mental status from patient baseline? Does the abnormal behavior: • come and go? • fluctuate during the day? • increase/decrease in severity?
B. **Inattention**	Does the patient: • have difficulty focusing attention? • become easily distracted? • have difficulty keeping track of what is said?
AND the presence of EITHER feature **C** or **D**	
C. **Disorganized thinking**	Is the patient's thinking • disorganized? • incoherent? For example does the patient have • rambling speech / irrelevant conversation? • unpredictable switching of subjects? • unclear or illogical flow of ideas?
D. **Altered level of consciousness**	Overall, what is the patient's level of consciousness: • alert (normal) • vigilant (hyper-alert) • lethargic (drowsy but easily roused) • stuporous (difficult to rouse) • comatose (unarousable)

Adapted with permission from: Inouye SK, vanDyck CH, Alessi CA, Balkin S, Siegal AP, Horwitz RI. *Clarifying confusion: The Confusion Assessment Method*. A new method for detection of delirium. Ann Intern Med. 1990; 113: 941–948. Confusion Assessment Method: Training Manual and Coding Guide, Copyright © 2003, Hospital Elder Life Program, LLC.

Assessing Changes in Bowel Function: Victoria Bowel Performance Scale (BPS)

The Victoria BPS (Figure 11) (Victoria Hospice Society, 2009) is used to assess a person's bowel function and changes in response to treatment for diarrhea or constipation, and provides treatment options.

Instructions: See Figure 11.

Figure 11. Victoria Bowel Performance Scale (BPS)

(continued on next page)

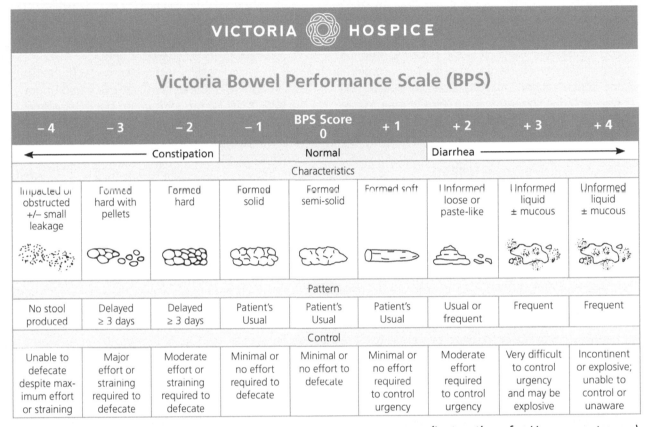

(Instructions for Use on next page)

Figure 11. Victoria Bowel Performance Scale (BPS)

Instructions for Use

1. BPS is a 9-point scale. It is a **single score**, based on the overall **'best vertical fit'** among the above three parameters [characteristics, pattern, control] and is recorded for example as: BPS +1, BPS –3 or BPS G.

2. Look vertically down each BPS level to become familiar with how the three parameters of **characteristics, pattern & control** change in gradation from constipation to diarrhea.

3. For the bowel pattern, it is the patient's **goal** that is the determining factor. The goal is recorded in the centre section, marked with the patient's desired goal for how often they would prefer to have a bowel movement. Based on their goal, then the **actual frequency** is either within that goal, delayed beyond the goal, or more frequent than the goal. If the goal is met, the score is **BPS G**.

4. Patients may use different words than above to describe their bowel activity. One must use clinical judgment in deciding which boxes are most appropriate.

5. For patients with ostomies or short bowel syndrome, all 3 parameters should be assessed according to closeness to the patient's desired goal.

6. In potential confounding cases, determination of the most appropriate BPS score is made using the following methods:
   - Two vertically similar parameters generally outweigh the third;
   - Single priority weighting among parameters is Characteristics > Pattern > Control

7. When recording BPS in hospital or facility patient charts where charting is required every shift or daily, a **BPS 'X'** is used to indicate no bowel assessment was done in that timeframe. Otherwise, the actual BPS number is recorded. **Do not write "0"** as it is misleading; the correct recording would be BPS X.

8. The BPS cannot be applied when there is no expected functioning bowel, as may occur with patients on TPN or if imminently dying with no oral intake. If this is the case, the correct recording is **BPS N/A**.

The Victoria Bowel Performance Scale (BPS), originally published in the Journal of Pain & Symptom Management 2007, has been slightly revised to incorporate the patients' goal for bowel pattern. Downing, Hawley, Barwich and Black, 2009. © Victoria Hospice Society, 2016.

For permissions, please send request via email to edu.hospice@viha.ca

Assessing Frailty: Canadian Study of Health and Aging (CSHA) Clinical Frailty Scale

Frailty refers to changes in a person's status that result from losses of energy, physical abilities, cognition, and health. Depending on their level of frailty, people are increasingly vulnerable and at risk of dying in the coming year or months. The CSHA Clinical Frailty Scale (Figure 12) (Rockwood et al., 2005) is a concise, efficient, and validated clinical tool for assessing frailty. Each of the seven values in the scale is highly correlated (r = 0.80) with the 70-item Frailty Index (Rockwood et al., 2005), and each increment in value signifies that the person is at an increased risk of dying and has increased needs that may require institutional care.

Instructions: Observe the person and their activities, and identify a frailty score between 1 and 7 (see Figure 12) that matches the person's energy, abilities, and health. People identified as frail or vulnerable (frailty values 4 to 7) would benefit from a palliative approach being integrated into their care.

Figure 12. CSHA Clinical Frailty Scale

1. *Very fit*—robust, active, energetic, well motivated and fit; these people commonly exercise regularly and are in the most fit group for their age.
2. *Well*—without active disease, but less fit than people in category 1.
3. *Well, with treated comorbid disease*—disease symptoms are well controlled compared with those in category 4.
4. *Apparently vulnerable*—although not frankly dependent these people commonly complain of being "slowed up" or have disease symptoms.
5. *Mildly frail*—with limited dependence on others for instrumental activities of daily living
6. *Moderately frail*—help is needed with both instrumental and non-instrumental activities of daily living
7. *Severely frail*—completely dependent on others for activities of daily living, or terminally ill.

Conversion between the CSHA Clinical Frailty Scale and the PPS

The PPS is used primarily in palliative care, whereas the seven-point CSHA Clinical Frailty Scale is used in geriatric medicine. Communication problems between HCPs in these two areas of specialty are common, because each understands only their own scale. Grossman and her team evaluated these two scales and developed a conversion tool (Figure 13) (Grossman et al., 2014) to help increase understanding of the scales. The proposed conversion tool facilitates communication between HCPs in geriatric medicine and HCPs in hospice and palliative care.

Figure 13. Proposed conversion between the CSHA Clinical Frailty Scale and the PPS

CSHA Clinical Frailty Scale	Palliative Performance Scale
3–4	70%–90%
5	60%
6	40%–50%
7	10%–30%

Facial Grimace and Behaviour Assessment Tool

The Facial Grimace and Behaviour Assessment Tool (Figure 14) (Brignell, 2009) is used to help identify, on the basis of a person's facial expressions or behaviors, when the person might be experiencing pain or distress. The tool provides reference drawings of facial expressions and a list of behaviors commonly associated with pain and distress. Developed for pediatric patients, the tool is also used for assessing adults who are not comfortable with or are unable to use other rating scales.

Instructions: When providing care, compare the facial expressions of the person to those in the tool. Record the value corresponding to the person's facial expression in the first part of the tool, in the column for the relevant time period. Then use the scoring system to assign values to any behaviors, listed in the second part of the tool, that may indicate that the person is in pain or distress. Assess the person before and after receiving medications or treatments, as well as daily to detect changes in their comfort.

Figure 14. Facial Grimace and Behaviour Assessment Tool

Facial Grimace and Behaviour Assessment Tool

Name: _____   Active ☐ Resting ☐ Time: _____

| 0 | 2 | 4 | 6 | 8 | 10 |
| no pain | mild | discomforting | distressing | horrible | excruciating |

Regular pain medication: _____   Rescue/PRN medication _____

Month:

Date or Time														
FACIAL SCORE														
10														
8														
6														
4														
2														
0														
PRN medication														

Facial Grimace Score: The facial grimace scale scores the level of pain (from 0-10 on the left) as assessed by the caregiver observing the facial expressions of the resident. Assessment is done once daily or more (14 days are indicated above). This assessment of the degree of discomfort should be done at the same time every day and during the same level of activity. **Note if rescue/PRN medication is given; yes (y), no (n) or dose.**

Behaviour Checklist

10 – always   8 – mostly   6 – often   4 – occasionally   2 – rarely   0 – never

Date or Time														
BEHAVIOUR														
Eats poorly														
Tense														
Quiet														
Indicates pain														
Calls out														
Paces														
Noisy breathing														
Sleeps poorly														
Picks														
PRN medication														

Behaviour Checklist: Behaviour changes can be used to assess pain or distress, and thereby evaluate the efficacy of interventions. At the top of the scoring graph, when the specific behaviour has been observed, it can be rated from 10 (always) to 0 (never). The behaviours being rated and scored over 24 hours are listed down the left column. This chart scores 9 different behaviours over 14 days. The caregiver can expand on the checklist, i.e., rocking, screams, etc. **Note if rescue/PRN medication given. Both tools may be adapted for individual use.**

Used with permission, Ann Brignell, 2016

Pain Assessment in Advanced Dementia (PAINAD) Tool

The Pain Assessment in Advanced Dementia (PAINAD) tool (Figure 15) (Warden, Hurley, and Volicer, 2003) is used to assess a person's pain on the basis of five parameters of observed behavior. This tool is used when people with dementia are no longer able to verbally communicate their pain.

Instructions: Observe the person for three to five minutes during an activity that includes movement (e.g., positioning or transferring the person), and assign a score between 0 and 2, as indicated in Figure 15, that reflects their current behavior.

Add the values to obtain a total score, ranging from 0 to 10. The score indicates whether the person might be experiencing pain; higher scores more accurately indicate pain than lower scores. The score does not indicate the severity of pain.

Compare the total score to a previous score obtained using the tool. An increased score suggests an increase in pain, while a lower score suggests that pain has decreased.

The PAINAD should be administered:
- At admission
- At each quarterly nursing review
- During every shift for people whose behaviors suggest their pain is not controlled
- Each time a change in a person's pain status is reported
- Following a pain intervention (within one hour) to evaluate treatment effectiveness

Figure 15. Pain Assessment in Advanced Dementia (PAINAD) Scale

	0	1	2	Score
Breathing Independent of vocalization	Normal	Occasional labored breathing. Short period of hyperventilation.	Noisy labored breathing. Long period of hyperventilation. Cheyne-Stokes respirations.	
Negative Vocalization	None	Occasional moan or groan. Low level speech with a negative or disapproving quality.	Repeated troubled calling out. Loud moaning or groaning. Crying.	
Facial Expression	Smiling, or inexpressive	Sad. Frightened. Frown.	Facial grimacing.	
Body Language	Relaxed	Tense. Distressed pacing. Fidgeting.	Rigid. Fists clenched, knees pulled up. Pulling or pushing away. Striking out.	
Consolability	No need to console	Distracted or reassured by voice or touch.	Unable to console, distract or reassure.	
			TOTAL	

Non-Communicative Patient's Pain Assessment Instrument (NOPPAIN)

The NOPPAIN tool (Figure 16) (Snow et al., 2004) is used while providing care to assess pain on the basis of observing a person's behaviors and facial expression. Using this tool daily to assess the person's pain can help to prevent pain from escalating and facilitates early detection of new pain.

Instructions: While providing regular care, observe the person's responses to repositioning, transferring, and so on, as well as verbal and facial cues and behaviors that might indicate the person is experiencing pain. Indicate on the body map included in the tool the location of suspected pain, or illustrate how the person's behavior suggests that the person is in pain. Use the thermometer in the tool to indicate the severity of the pain.

NOPPAIN

(Non-Communicative Patient's Pain Assessment Instrument

Activity Chart Check List

Name of Evaluator _____
Name of Resident: _____
Date: _____
Time: _____

DIRECTIONS: Nursing assistant should complete at least 5 minutes of daily care activities for the resident while observing for pain behaviors. Both pages of this form should be completed immediately following care activities

	Did you do this? (Check Yes or No)	Did you see pain when you did this? (Check Yes or No)		Did you do this? (Check Yes or No)	Did you see pain when you did this? (Check Yes or No)
(a) Put resident in bed OR saw resident lying down	☐ YES ☐ NO	☐ YES ☐ NO	(f) Fed resident	☐ YES ☐ NO	☐ YES ☐ NO
(b) Turned resident in bed	☐ YES ☐ NO	☐ YES ☐ NO	(g) Helped resident stand OR saw resident stand	☐ YES ☐ NO	☐ YES ☐ NO
(c) Transferred resident (bed to chair, chair to bed, standing or wheelchair to toilet	☐ YES ☐ NO	☐ YES ☐ NO	(h) Helped resident walk OR saw resident walk	☐ YES ☐ NO	☐ YES ☐ NO
(d) Sat resident up (bed or chair) OR saw resident sitting	☐ YES ☐ NO	☐ YES ☐ NO	(i) Bathed resident OR gave resident sponge bath	☐ YES ☐ NO	☐ YES ☐ NO
(e) Dressed resident	☐ YES ☐ NO	☐ YES ☐ NO			

ASK THE PATIENT: Are you in pain? ☐ yes ☐ no
ASK THE PATIENT: Do you hurt? ☐ yes ☐ no

Pain Response (What did you see and hear during care?)

Pain Words?
- "That hurts!" • "Ouch!"
- Cursing • "Stop that!"

☐ YES ☐ NO

How intense were the pain words?

0 1 2 3 4 5
Lowest Possible Intensity — Highest Possible Intensity

Pain Faces?
- grimaces • winces
- furrowed brow

☐ YES ☐ NO

How intense were the pain faces?

0 1 2 3 4 5
Lowest Possible Intensity — Highest Possible Intensity

Bracing?
- rigidity • holding • guarding (especially during movement)

☐ YES ☐ NO

How intense was the bracing?

0 1 2 3 4 5
Lowest Possible Intensity — Highest Possible Intensity

Pain Noises?
- moans • groans • grunts
- cries • gasps • sighs

☐ YES ☐ NO

How intense were the pain noises?

0 1 2 3 4 5
Lowest Possible Intensity — Highest Possible Intensity

Rubbing?
- massaging affected area

☐ YES ☐ NO

How intense was the rubbing?

0 1 2 3 4 5
Lowest Possible Intensity — Highest Possible Intensity

Restlessness?
- frequent shifting • rocking
- inability to stay still

☐ YES ☐ NO

How intense was the restlessness?

0 1 2 3 4 5
Lowest Possible Intensity — Highest Possible Intensity

Locate Problem Areas

Please "X" the site of any pain
Please "O" the site of any skin problems

FRONT   BACK

A U.S. Veterans Affairs METRIC™ Instrument. Snow, O'Malley, Kunik, Cody, Bruera, Beck, Ashton. Alteration of this instrument is prohibited. This instrument can be copied and distributed free of charge for clinical or scholarly use. Development was supported by VA HSR&D and NIMH. Contact Dr. Snow at asnow@bcm.tmc.edu.

Figure 16. Non-Communicative Patient's Pain Assessment Instrument (NOPPAIN) part 2

NOPPAIN
(Non-Communicative Patient's Pain Assessment Instrument)
Activity Chart Check List

Name of Evaluator _____
Name of Resident: _____
Date: _____
Time: _____

Rate the resident's pain at the highest level you saw it at during care. **(circle your answer)**

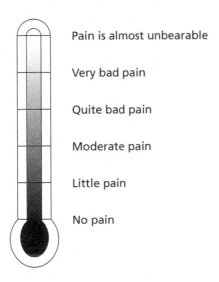

Pain is almost unbearable

Very bad pain

Quite bad pain

Moderate pain

Little pain

No pain

SBAR Communication Tool

Assessments need to be communicated between team members in a clear and concise way. The less involved with the dying person the team member receiving information is, and the less that team member knows about the person or their condition, the more important it is to provide a clear and through assessment.

Over the years I have heard the following comments:

I hear the health care worker say, "The practical nurse doesn't listen to me."

And sometimes I hear the practical nurse say, "The RN doesn't listen to me."

And sometimes I hear the nurses say, "The physician doesn't listen to me."

And sometimes I hear the person and family say, "No one listens to me!"

I suggest that sometimes people are not heard because the report is not clear and concise and it is difficult for the listener to understand what is needed and what should be done.

The SBAR (Situation, Background, Assessment, Recommendation) (Figure 17) is a communication tool that provides a framework to help you prepare and deliver a clear report. This tool is adapted from an aviation tool that pilots used for communicating urgent and important information in times of emergency.

Instructions: After completing an assessment, for example, by using the Symptom Assessment Tool (see Table 1 on page 65), use the SBAR tool to help you prepare and then present your report to the physician/nurse practitioner and other members of the health care team.

Figure 17. SBAR Communication Tool

Gather the following information for when you speak with the physician/nurse practitioner: chart, PPS, allergies, medications (current), new lab and radiology reports, recent weight, code status.

S **SITUATION**
My name is [insert your name] and I am working at [insert your place of work].
I am calling about: [insert the person's first and last name]
[Describe the problem and concerns].

B **BACKGROUND**
State briefly the pertinent **medical history/any recent changes/emergent issues.**
A brief synopsis of the **treatment to date and effectiveness.**

A **ASSESSMENT of ANY ISSUE/SYMPTOM**

Onset	
Provoking/Palliating	
Quality	
Region/Radiation	
Severity (0–10) (ESAS)	
Treatment	
Understanding/Impact on resident	
Values	

Any changes from prior assessments:

R **RECOMMENDATION**
Do you think we should: (State what you would like to see done)
- ☐ Order/increase analgesic/other medication?
- ☐ Request the physician/nurse practitioner to see the person at this time?
- ☐ Order diagnostic tests?
- ☐ Other:

If a change in treatment is ordered, then ask:
- ☐ If the patient does not improve, when do you want us to call again?
- ☐ Do you want to refer to the Palliative Care Physician/PCCT if there is no improvement?

Document the change in condition and the notification of the physician/nurse practitioner

Psychosocial Assessment Tools

Psychosocial Assessment Form

The Psychosocial Assessment Form on pages 83 to 88 was developed to help the health care team better understand the person and the family, prepare to address practical issues, and record and update goals-of-care conversations.

This form was adapted, with permission, from the Victoria Hospice Society's Psychosocial Assessment Tool (Victoria Hospice Society, 2016). Its current format was developed to support HCPs striving for best practice interactions. The open boxes used for gathering information can be used by the HCP, the person, and family to free-form write or draw their answers. Consider this as your template, and adapt and tailor it to best meet the needs of people in your care.

Instructions: Using the form, work with the person and family to gather information about the person, the family, their care needs, and their decision-making concerns and requests. The form is a living document and can be completed over time. It is helpful to attach additional pages to the form so that new changes and observations can be recorded.

Date of Assessment _____

Name _____ Address _____ Phone _____

Contact person _____ Address _____ Phone _____
(if different from above)

My family map (genogram) and support

SYMBOLS
☐ Male ◯ Female
——— Present bond
═══ Strong bond
∿∿∿ Stressing/negative bond
- - - - Superficial bond
—⫽— Separation
⇄ Good communication

Getting to Know You—The Person

My life review—interests and career

My strengths—coping strategies, decision-making style

My fears and concerns—physical, spiritual, emotional, financial, sexual, and other

My understanding of my illness

My cultural beliefs and practices

My community support

My goals of care

Date	Goals

My preferences concerning the time of death

My special requests for the time of death and following death

Getting to Know the Primary Caregiver

Name _____ Address _____ Phone _____

Caregiver's life—current demands, interests	Caregiver's strengths—coping strategies, decision-making style

Caregiver's fears and concerns—physical, spiritual, emotional, financial, sexual, and other	Caregiver's needs—physical, psychological, medical, spiritual

Caregiver's community support	Caregiver's cultural/spiritual beliefs

Getting to Know the Family

Caregiver's family map and community support

Communication, decision-making styles, family roles

Getting to Know Other Caregivers

Name	Contact information	Concerns

Forms, Facilitators, and Funeral

FORMS	Signed	Date	Document location	Notes
Advanced Directive form				
Do Not Resuscitate form				
Representation Agreement				
Will				

FACILITATORS			
Power of Attorney	Person(s) appointed	Relationship to dying person	Contact phone numbers
• Enduring			
• Bank/financial			
• Other			
Substitute Decision Maker			

FUNERAL			
Funeral planning	yes	no	Notes
Funeral home		Phone number	

Requests to be called or present		Call to be present for time of death		Call when death is imminent	
	Times available to be called	Anytime	Day or evening only	Anytime	Day or evening only
Name	Phone number				
Name	Phone number				

Request for religious or spiritual contact to be present when death is imminent, at the time of, or following death			
Person requesting	Phone number	Religious/spiritual contact requested	Phone number

Notes

Bereavement Risk Assessment Tool (BRAT)

Victoria Hospice Society created the BRAT (Figure 18) (Victoria Hospice Society, 2014) to help identify any person, who may be at risk of experiencing a difficult grief and bereavement process. The tool contains simple check boxes under headings that identify areas in which difficult grief might occur. When using the BRAT, it is important to remember that risks it identifies are not certainties that someone's grief process will be difficult or complicated, but rather are probabilities that it might be so. Identifying the risks helps to alert HCPs that a person may need monitoring over time to evaluate whether grief is becoming difficult for them. If it is, then greater bereavement support can be offered if it exists within the organization, or referrals to appropriate community agencies can be given.

Note: An Excel program and a user's manual available through Victoria Hospice Society can expand the use of the BRAT. Contact Victoria Hospice (victoriahospice.org) for further information.

Instructions: Using the information shown in Figure 18, assess a person for their risk of having a difficult bereavement, and then communicate any concerns to the health care team. This tool may also be used to help determine where best to allocate scarce bereavement services after a death.

Figure 18. Bereavement Risk Assessment Tool (BRAT)

Bereavement Risk Assessment Tool
© Victoria Hospice Society 2008

Assessment Date	Assessed by	ID#	Patient / Deceased Name	Bereaved Name

Risk Indicators and Protective Factors | Comments

I. Kinship
- ☐ a) spouse/partner of patient or deceased
- ☐ b) parent/parental figure of patient or deceased

II Caregiver
- ☐ a) family member or friend who has taken primary responsibility for care

III. Mental Health
- ☐ a) significant mental illness (eg major depression, schizophrenia, anxiety disorder)
- ☐ b) significant mental disability (eg developmental, dementia, stroke, head injury)

IV. Coping
- ☐ a) substance abuse / addiction (specify)
- ☐ b) considered suicide (no plan, no previous attempt)
- ☐ c) has suicide plan and a means to carry it out OR has made previous attempt
- ☐ d) self-expressed concerns regarding own coping, now or in future
- ☐ e) heightened emotional states (anger, guilt, anxiety) as typical response to stressors
- ☐ f) yearning/pining for the deceased OR persistent disturbing thoughts/images > 3 months*
- ☐ g) declines available resources or support
- ☐ h) inability to experience grief feelings or acknowledge reality of the death > 3 months*

V. Spirituality / Religion
- ☐ significant challenge to fundamental beliefs / loss of meaning or faith / spiritual distress

VI. Concurrent Stressors
- ☐ a) two or more competing demands (eg single parenting, work, other caregiving)
- ☐ b) insufficient financial, practical or physical resources (eg ⊠ income, no childcare, illness)
- ☐ c) recent non-death losses (eg divorce, unemployment, moving, retirement)
- ☐ d) significant other with life-threatening illness / injury (other than patient/deceased)

VII. Previous Bereavements
- ☐ a) unresolved previous bereavement(s)
- ☐ b) death of other significant person within 1 year (from time of patient's death)
- ☐ c) cumulative grief from > 2 OTHER deaths over past 3 years
- ☐ d) death or loss of parent/parental figure during own childhood (less than age 19)

VIII. Supports & Relationships
- ☐ a) lack of social support/social isolation (perceived or real - eg housebound)
- ☐ b) cultural or language barriers to support
- ☐ c) longstanding or current discordant relationship(s) within the family
- ☐ d) relationship with patient/deceased (eg abuse, dependency)

IX. Children & Youth
- ☐ a) death of parent, parental figure or sibling*
- ☐ b) demonstration of extreme, ongoing behaviours/symptoms (eg sep anxiety+, nightmares)
- ☐ c) parent expresses concern regarding his/her ability to support child's grief
- ☐ d) parent/parental figure significantly compromised by his/her own grief

X. Circumstances Involving the Patient, the Care or the Death
- ☐ a) patient/deceased less than age 35
- ☐ b) lack of preparedness for the death (as perceived or demonstrated by bereaved)*
- ☐ c) distress witnessing the death OR death perceived as preventable*
- ☐ d) violent, traumatic OR unexplained death (eg accident, suicide, unknown cause)*
- ☐ e) significant anger with OTHER health care providers (eg "my GP missed the diagnosis")
- ☐ f) significant anger with OUR hospice palliative care program (eg "you killed my wife")

XI. Protective Factors Supporting Positive Bereavement Outcome
- ☐ a) internalized belief in own ability to cope effectively
- ☐ b) perceives AND is willing to access strong social support network
- ☐ c) predisposed to high level of optimism/positive state of mind
- ☐ d) spiritual/religious beliefs that assist in coping with the death

Aug-08

FICA Spiritual Assessment Tool

The FICA Spiritual Assessment Tool (Figure 19) (Puchalski and Romer, 2000) is used to gather information about the person's spiritual beliefs, understanding, and needs. The information can be shared with members of the health care team and recorded to provide guidance on appropriate ways for all team members to integrate spirituality into the person's care.

Instructions: When a person enters a care facility or when home care begins, use the FICA tool to gather information on their spiritual care needs. The person's needs may change over time; therefore check in with the person regularly to confirm that the care team is meeting the person's spiritual care needs.

Choose a selection of the questions from the FICA tool, as appropriate for the person and family. Document their answers, and share this information with the health care team. All members of the team can use the information collected to integrate spiritual care into daily caregiving.

Figure 19. FICA Spiritual Assessment Tool

"FICA" can be a useful device to help HCPs and patients discuss the role of religion and spirituality as relevant to health and illness (Pulchalski, 2000). FICA is a device that can assist the HCP in taking a patient's spiritual history and facilitating discussions on the role of spirituality and religion in a patient's physical well being. By using FICA and addressing spiritual issues, an environment of intimacy and trust may be established, leading to patient comfort in revealing fundamental information about their worldviews and sources of personal meaning.

Faith or beliefs: *What is your faith or belief? Do you consider yourself spiritual or religious? What things do you believe give meaning to your life?*

Importance and Influence: *What influence does it have on how you take care of yourself? How have your beliefs influenced your behavior during this illness? What role do your beliefs play in regaining your health?*

Community: *Are you part of a spiritual or religious community? Is this of support to you and how? Is there a person or group of people you really love or who are really important to you?*

Address: *How would you like me, your healthcare provider, to address these issues in your healthcare?*

IDEA Ethical Decision-Making Framework

The fundamental purpose of ethics in health care is to guide the decision making to answer the question, "What should we do and why?"

The IDEA Ethical Decision-Making Framework (adapted) (Figure 20) can help HCPs make ethical decisions. The framework has four steps:
1. Identify the facts and the ethical question(s)
2. Determine ethical principles in conflict
3. Explore the available options
4. Act on the decision and evaluate

The IDEA Ethical Decision-Making Framework builds upon the Toronto Central Community Care Access Centre Community Ethics Toolkit (2008), which was based on the work of Jonsen, Seigler, and Winslade (2002); the work of the Core Curriculum Working Group at the University of Toronto Joint Centre for Bioethics; and incorporates aspects of the accountability for reasonableness framework developed by Daniels and Sabin (2002) and adapted by Gibson, Martin, and Singer (2005).

Figure 20. IDEA Ethical Decision-Making Framework

(continued on next page)

IDEA[1]

Ethical Decision-Making Framework

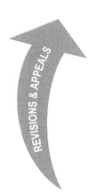

4. Act

- Recommend
- Implement
- Evaluate

<u>Ask</u>: *Are we (am I) comfortable with this decision?*

COMPLIANCE

1. Identify the Facts

- Medical Indications
- Patient Preferences
- Evidence
- Contextual Features

<u>Ask</u>: *What is the ethical issue?*

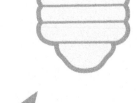

What is an ethical issue?

- *Am I trying to determine the right course of action?*
- *Am I asking a "should" question?*
- *Are values and beliefs involved?*
- *Am I feeling uncomfortable?*

If you answered yes to any of these questions, you may be encountering an ethical issue.

REVISIONS & APPEALS

EMPOWERMENT • PUBLICITY

3. Explore the Options

- Harms & Benefits
- Strengths & Limitations
- Laws & Policies
- Mission, Vision, Values

<u>Ask</u>: *What is the most ethically justifiable option?*

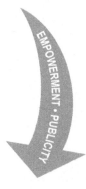

2. Determine the Relevant Ethical Principles

- Nature & Scope
- Relative Weights

<u>Ask</u>: *Have perspectives of relevant individuals been sought?*

RELEVANCE

---

[1] The IDEA: Ethical Decision-Making Framework builds upon the Toronto Central Community Care Access Centre *Community Ethics Toolkit* (2008), which was based on the work of Jonsen, Seigler, & Winslade (2002); the work of the Core Curriculum Working Group at the University of Toronto Joint Centre for Bioethics; and incorporates aspects of the accountability for reasonableness framework developed by Daniels and Sabin (2002) and adapted by Gibson, Martin, & Singer (2005).

Figure 20. IDEA Ethical Decision-Making Framework

(continued on next page)

Identify the facts and the ethical question

Determine the ethical principles in conflict

Explore your options

Act on your decision and evaluate

Submitted by (name):	
Manager's name:	
Team name:	
BRN:	
Other team members: (hospital partners/SPO, etc.)	

IDENTIFY THE FACTS

Medical Indications	**Person's Preferences**
State the person's medical problem, history, and diagnosis; is it acute, chronic, critical, emergent, and reversible? Goals of treatment? Probabilities of success? Plans in case of therapeutic failure? Potential benefits of care? How can harm be avoided? Medical risks if service is discontinued?	State the person's preferences. Do they have the capacity to decide? If yes, are the person's wishes informed, understood, voluntary? If not, who is the substitute decision maker? Does the person have prior, expressed wishes? Is person's right to choose being respected?
Quality of Life	**Contextual Features**
Describe quality of life in the person's terms, person's subjective acceptance of likely quality of life, and views and concerns of care providers. Examine the emotional factors influencing each individual, such as existing feelings, values, biases and prior experiences.	Any other family involved or significant relationships? Are any care plans in place? Relevant social, legal, economic, and institutional circumstances? Other relevant features, e.g. religious & cultural factors, limits on confidentiality, resource allocation issues, legal implications, research or teaching involved, provider conflict of interest? Organizational values to consider?

Adapted from Jonsen, Albert, Siegler, Mark and William J. Winslade. Clinical Ethics: A Practical Approach to Ethical Decisions in Clinical Medicine, Publisher: McGraw-Hill Medical; 5 edition (May 22, 2002).

Figure 20. IDEA Ethical Decision-Making Framework

(continued on next page)

IDENTIFY THE ETHICAL ISSUE

What is the distinct ethics question that concerns you? Be as concrete as possible about the specific ethics issue on which you are trying to deliberate. It is OK to revise this question as you move through the IDEA framework.

DETERMINE THE ETHICAL PRINCIPLES IN CONFLICT

What ethical principles are in conflict? Review each of the principles from the Code of Ethics for your workplace and practice, then explain any issues if they apply.

Principle	Explain the issue
Advocacy	
Person and Employee Safety	
Commitment to Quality Services	
Confidentiality	
Conflict of Interest	
Dignity	
Fair and Equitable Access	
Health and Well-being	
Informed Choice and Empowerment	
Relationships Among Community Agencies	

Figure 20. IDEA Ethical Decision-Making Framework

(continued on next page)

EXPLORE OPTIONS

Explore options and consider their strengths and weaknesses

Brainstorm and discuss options alone or with peers. Be creative and use your imagination. Consider a compromise. Predict the outcomes for each alternative. Does the alternative fit with the person/family values? Question whether the alternative meets the ethics, values, policies, directives and regulations of your workplace.

Option(s)	Strengths	Weaknesses
1)		
2)		
3)		
4)		
5)		

Figure 20. IDEA Ethical Decision-Making Framework (continued on next page)

ACT ON YOUR DECISION AND EVALUATE

Develop an action plan

Given all the information that you have, choose the best option available. Develop an action plan. Present your suggested alternative and action plan to the person and those involved. Re-examine the alternatives if other factors come to light, if the situation changes, or if an agreement cannot be reached. Determine when to evaluate the plan. Document and communicate the plan.

Self-evaluate your decision

How do you (individually and/or as a team) feel about the decision and the plan? What would you do differently next time? What would you do the same? What have you learned about yourself? What have you learned about this decision-making process?

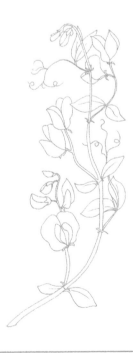

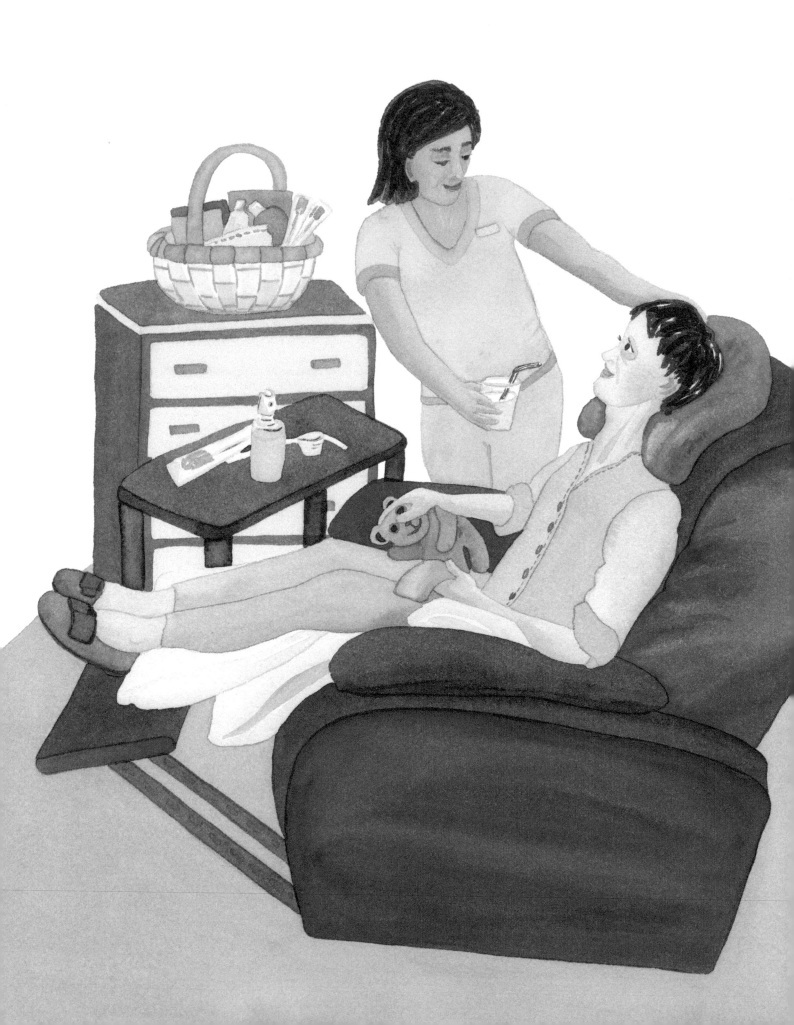

Enhancing Physical Comfort

Part 1: Principles and Practices

Death is inevitable. Pain, distress and other symptoms do not have to be.

A nurse

The principles for managing symptoms, using medications, and using opioids are key to increasing the physical comfort of the dying person. Physical comfort and symptom management are essential to improving the person's quality of life. When symptoms are not controlled, the dying person and their family may experience increased suffering and anxiety. The principles for symptom management can be integrated into care in any setting. Globally, the medications and guidelines for symptom management vary, but the principles remain the same.

Understanding the person's place in their illness trajectory will help guide investigations and treatments. Consider using the Gold Standards Framework Prognostic Indicator Guidance (GSF PIG) tool, the Supportive and Palliative Care Indicators Tool (SPICT), and tools for assessing frailty and one-year mortality (see Chapter 4, "Using Standardized Tools") to help inform goals-of-care conversations and determine whether investigations are appropriate.

Remember that physical symptoms are not managed in isolation. In order to manage symptoms in a way that meets the needs of the dying person and is appropriate for their decline, it is essential to address psychosocial issues. Using the Psychosocial Assessment Form (see Chapter 4, "Using Standardized Tools") will help the health care team to understand the dying person, in terms of who they are, what is important to them and their family, and their community support.

Principles of Symptom Management

Physical symptoms are managed by addressing the underlying disease causing the symptoms, by using medications and treatments to diminish or mask the symptoms, by using nonpharmacological measures to enhance physical comfort, and by addressing psychosocial needs. Apply these principles for symptom management:

- Focus on the person's goals of care.
- Educate the person and family.
- Prevent symptoms that can be prevented.
- Manage symptoms before they escalate.
- Use nonpharmacological comfort measures when possible.
- Support the family to participate in planning and providing care.
- Follow the care plan and administer medications as ordered.
- Evaluate, record, and report the person's responses to medications and comfort measures.

(Pallium Canada, 2013; WHO, 2012; ELNEC, 2015)

Ethics Touchstone
Principle 2
Licensed Practical Nurses provide safe and competent care for their clients.

Reflect on how nurses provide safe and competent care by integrating the principles of symptom management to help prevent and manage symptoms.

Code of Ethics for Licensed/Registered Practical Nurses (CCPNR, 2013)

Principles for Using Medications to Manage Symptoms

These principles guide the practice of health care providers (HCPs) who administer medications for managing symptoms in hospice and palliative care:

- Use the oral route when possible. Use an alternative route when necessary.

- Remember that a combination of medications may be more effective than a single one.
- Consider the needs of the person and their family, and the realities of the care setting when deciding which medication and route to use.
- Provide medications regularly and around the clock for ongoing symptoms. Ongoing symptoms will require ongoing medications.
- Titrate (increase or decrease) medications to the dose that meets the person's goals.
- Continue medications for as long as the symptom continues.
- Provide breakthrough doses to prevent pain, respond to breakthrough pain, and help with titration.
- Use nonpharmacological comfort measures to assist with symptom management.
- Evaluate and record the person's responses to medications and nonpharmacological comfort measures.
- Assess regularly and when the person's condition or behaviors change.

(CHPCA, 2013; Dahlin, 2013)

When using medications to manage symptoms, become familiar with the following characteristics of the medication so as to best evaluate its effectiveness and follow the care plan:
- Onset of effect
- Time to peak effect
- Duration of effect

 Ethics Touchstone
Reflect on Charlie's story below and, using critical thinking, consider how you might have proceeded differently, using the Symptom Assessment Tool to assist you to complete a thorough assessment, and the SBAR tool to consult with the physician/nurse practitioner to manage this symptom sooner and more effectively. What would you have reported?

Charlie

"Tell me about what is concerning you," I said.

We needed to understand as much about his suffering as we could in preparation for his transfer to hospice.

"The pain in my back," he said.

"Is it worse or better since the radiation?" I asked.

"It never helped. And it's worse now than ever. I can't move an inch." His radiation had happened over two weeks ago. He should have had some relief from the radiation by now.

It dawned on me in that second: he was still getting oral analgesics even though he had been nauseated and vomiting on and off over the past week. Maybe he had vomited or was not absorbing some of his pain

medications. The physician/nurse practitioner had left orders for a route change if required. We had not implemented a route change.

"I am confident that we can make you more comfortable right now, Charlie. If we put a tiny needle right here in your arm, just underneath the skin, we will be able to give your pain medications through the needle, and you won't have to swallow the pills. It is possible that your stomach is not absorbing the medication and that on occasion you have vomited your pain medications. That may be why you are having more pain. How does that sound? Is there anything else, Charlie?"

His long skeleton did not move behind the crinkled white bed sheet. With eye mask still intact, his lips moved in a whisper, "Thank you."

Using Opioids to Manage Symptoms

Opioids are compounds that bind to opiate receptors in the body. Using opioids to manage symptoms has revolutionized the capacity to improve quality of life and relieve suffering of people experiencing pain and dyspnea in hospice and palliative care. Use opioids when non-opioid medications are not effective and when it is not possible or no longer appropriate to treat the underlying disease causing the symptom (Pallium Canada, 2013; Fraser Health Authority, 2016a; Paice, 2015). This section discusses principles for using opioids, the side effects opioids cause, and fears the dying person, family, and health care team commonly express about opioids.

Mechanism of Opioid Action

Opioids work by decreasing a person's perception of pain. They bind to one or more opioid receptors in the body and decrease the transmission of pain messages to the brain. With dyspnea, it is thought that opioids might decrease the sensitivity of the carbon dioxide receptors in the respiratory centers, thereby diminishing the sensation of breathlessness. They may also relax the airways by binding to the opioid receptors in the airways, and increase oxygenation of the heart by causing cardiac vasodilation (UTHealth, 2016).

Common Opioids Used in Hospice and Palliative Care

The opioids commonly used for symptom management are either natural, semi-synthetic, or synthetic. Opioids that occur naturally, which are termed "opiates," are extracted from the resin of the opium poppy. Although there are more than 25 different opioid compounds present in opium, only morphine and codeine are used as opiate analgesics. Codeine is derived from morphine during manufacturing, and after codeine is administered the body converts it back into morphine (UTHealth, 2016).

Semi-synthetic opioids such as hydrocodone, hydromorphone, oxycodone, and oxymorphone are derived from the morphine molecule but are then restructured during manufacturing.

Fully synthetic opioids, such as methadone and fentanyl, are synthesized from chemicals that are not derived from the opium plant.

Morphine

Morphine is a natural opioid and the most commonly used and least expensive opioid available. Because morphine can be made into many different products, it is possible to tailor the dose and route to best meet the needs of the person. Morphine is usually used for people with moderate to severe pain. Morphine doses have no ceiling and can be increased as appropriate until pain is relieved (Kennedy, 2016).

Compared with semi-synthetic and synthetic opioids, natural opioids such as morphine are more likely to cause histamine-release reactions. These reactions may appear as allergy-like symptoms, including itching, sneezing, and worsening of asthma. Therefore, after administering morphine, observe for histamine reactions, which may occur immediately or up to a few days later. If a histamine reaction occurs, talk with the physician/nurse practitioner about changing the medication to a semi-synthetic or synthetic opioid that may be better tolerated (Fraser Health Authority, 2016a).

People with poor renal function may not be able to tolerate morphine. In particular, when morphine is given regularly, the accumulation of morphine and the metabolites increases the risk of toxicity.

Morphine is the opioid with which other opioids are compared in terms of potency. "Equianalgesia" is the degree of analgesia another opioid provides compared with the degree of analgesia that morphine provides.

Table 1 provides dosage equivalents for common opioids provided orally/rectally or subcutaneously, as compared with the strength or potency of morphine (Pharmacist's Letter, 2012). You can use these values to calculate an equivalent dose of the new opioid.

Table 1. Equianalgesia of Opioids and Different Routes of Administration

Opioid	Oral/Rectal Dose	Subcutaneous	Schedule
Hydromorphone	2 mg	1 mg	q4h
Oxycodone	5 to 7 mg	—	q4h
Morphine	10 mg	5 mg	q4h

True Opioid Allergy

People may say that they are allergic to opioids, but in fact what they often describe are side effects of the medication. Side effects occur in at least 60% of people.

People may experience a histamine release, primarily with morphine and less frequently with semi-synthetic opioids. In these cases, the person may experience a worsening of asthma, pruritus, or sneezing. This may occur in 2 to 10 in 100 patients (Gueant et al., 1998; Mertes and Laxenaire, 2000).

A true allergic response to opioids that includes Immunoglobulin E immune-mediated secretions accompanied by an anaphylactic reaction is rare and occurs in less than 0.001% of the population (1 in 91,000 people).

Codeine

Codeine is considered a weak opioid that, when combined with acetaminophen, provides relief of moderate pain. Because it has a lower potency than morphine, codeine may be perceived as a safer opioid for beginning opioid therapy. The codeine-acetaminophen-caffeine tablet formulation is a widely prescribed pain reliever partly due to its image as having low potency and being safe (Kennedy, 2016).

Unlike morphine, codeine has a ceiling dose at which pain relief does not increase but side effects continue to increase. The ceiling dose for codeine has been suggested to be between 240 mg and 600 mg per day (Sweetman, 2005). The ceiling might be lower for a codeine-acetaminophen combination, as the maximum daily dose of acetaminophen is 4 g or less.

Codeine's effectiveness can be unreliable. Codeine itself does not provide pain relief until the body metabolizes it in the liver into the primary active pain-relieving metabolite—morphine. The metabolic process depends on the presence of sufficient liver enzymes; an insufficiency of liver enzymes results in minimal production of morphine. Caucasians are more likely to be poor converters of codeine to morphine, yet this problem occurs in many other populations too. An elderly person may also be unable to tolerate opioid doses due to changes in metabolism and

clearance of opioids, comorbidities, and concurrent medication interactions (Ginsburg, Silver, and Berman, 2009). Therefore, it important to monitor the effectiveness of the pain relief in all people taking codeine (Kennedy, 2016).

The equianalgesic dose for codeine is:

morphine 10 mg PO = approx. codeine 100 mg PO

This conversion may be erroneous because the absorption and metabolism of codeine vary greatly from person to person. However, the equianalgesic dose does provide a general idea of what the equivalency might be. Just remember that using the equivalency chart for codeine to morphine may not be as reliable as using it to compare hydromorphone to morphine (Kennedy, 2016).

Hydromorphone

Hydromorphone is a semi-synthetic, potent opioid used for treating moderate to severe pain. Because of its potency, it is a high-risk medication and its use requires special attention.

Hydromorphone and its metabolites are cleared from the body through the kidneys more easily than morphine; therefore, hydromorphone is the opioid of choice for people with renal disease (Kennedy, 2016).

Because the words "hydromorphone" and "morphine" are somewhat similar, one may be mistaken for the other and consequently result in the wrong medication being given. If hydromorphone is mistakenly given instead of morphine, the person receives a five-fold higher dose. If repeated errors occur, serious toxicity and harm could result. Safety organizations recommend using TALLman lettering to bring attention to and to carefully distinguish medication names. TALLman lettering involves a mix of capital letters and lowercase letters within the same word (e.g., HYDROmorphone) (ISMP, 2011) that helps differentiate similarly named medications from each other.

The equianalgesic dose for hydromorphone is:

morphine 10 mg PO = hydromorphone 2 mg PO

Oxycodone

Oxycodone is a semi-synthetic opioid that is used for treating moderate pain when in combination with acetaminophen or acetylsalicylic acid, and for treating severe pain on its own. Some people may respond well to oxycodone compared with other opioids, including people who have allergic reactions to other opioids, such as morphine and codeine.

Oxycodone is available in immediate-release and sustained-release tablets at varying strengths (Fraser Health Authority, 2016a). New formulations of sustained-release oxycodone have been produced to decrease abuse of the more rapidly acting preparation. However, both of these new formulations, Oxycontin and Oxyneo, are not safe or indicated for people who have difficulty swallowing.

The equianalgesic dose for oxycodone is:

morphine 10 mg PO = oxycodone 5 to 10 mg PO

Fentanyl

Fentanyl is 80 to 100 times more potent than morphine. It is a true synthetic opioid—a medication manufactured to interact with opioid receptors. Similar to methadone, fentanyl presents a lower risk of histamine reaction. Even fentanyl patches containing the smallest dose provide too much opioid and are unsafe for a person who is opioid naive (Kennedy, 2016). According to a recent study, fentanyl patches are safe to prescribe only for people with adequate prior exposure to opioids (Friesen, Woelk, and Bugden, 2016).

Fentanyl in a transdermal (TD) patch form releases the medication through the epidermal skin layer into the subcutaneous fat layer, where the medication is absorbed slowly into the circulatory system. Consistent absorption requires continual adherence of the patch to the skin at normal skin temperature. If the skin temperature increases, medication absorption will increase (Pallium Canada, 2013). When changing or discontinuing fentanyl, medication continues to be released from the deposit area below the skin for up to three days; about 50% of the medication is gone within about 17 hours (range of 13 to 22 hours) (Kennedy, 2016).

In some people, fentanyl TD may cause less drowsiness and constipation than equivalent doses of sustained-release morphine. Fentanyl TD is considered when pain is persistent and severe, and when regular oral administration is not possible. Fentanyl is also considered for people with renal failure, as there are no known active metabolites.

Fentanyl TD should not be used for a person who is less than 18 years of age or is opioid naive. An opioid naive person is someone who has received less than 60 mg PO

total daily dose (TDD) morphine equivalent for seven days. Use of fentanyl TD should also be avoided if the person is:

- Receiving either codeine or tramadol (for which determining the morphine equivalent is difficult)
- Experiencing mild, unstable, or poorly controlled pain
- Diaphoretic, cachexic, or morbidly obese
- Experiencing significant respiratory depression or has acute or severe bronchial asthma

(Kennedy, 2016)

The equianalgesic dose of fentanyl is not clearly established. Instead, a range of fentanyl doses is usually stated.

Procedures for applying a fentanyl patch

Fentanyl is a potent medication. When applying or removing a fentanyl patch, HCPs and other people should observe these careful handling procedures to avoid direct contact with the patch (Fraser Health Authority, 2016a; Kennedy, 2016):

- Wear gloves to apply and remove the patch.
- Place the patch on the person's chest, back, flank, or upper arm, in an area that is dry, hairless, and not inflamed or radiated, and in which no cuts or sores are present. (Body hair can be clipped, but do not shave the area because doing so could irritate the skin.)
- Apply the patch to the skin and hold the palm of the hand over the patch for 30 seconds to ensure good connection with the skin. Apply a transparent adhesive film dressing over the patch if necessary. Record the date and time of application on the label provided, but do not write on the patch itself.
- Remove old patches before applying a new patch.
- Change patches every 72 hours as ordered. (Some people may require a new patch every 48 hours.)
- Avoid placing the patch in areas of the body where the clothing or the person might rub the patch off.
- Avoid placing the patch on tattoos, which may alter absorption.
- If your skin comes into contact with the fentanyl patch, rinse the skin with water and do not use soap.
- Apply patches to different sites on the body to avoid causing irritation (try to avoid using an already used site for seven days before reusing it).
- Monitor carefully if the person is diaphoretic, which can cause the patch to fall off and possibly result in a change in the amount of medication absorbed.
- Assess the positioning of the patch at least every 24 hours.
- Educate the person and family about the following:
  - Avoid involving children in the application of the patch. (Incidents of a fentanyl patch falling off and being handled by children have occurred, resulting

in death.) Do *not* call the patches "stickies," "Band-Aids," or "tattoos."

  ○ Avoid applying heat (e.g., a heating pad or hot water bottle) to the area, as doing so may result in too much opioid being absorbed at one time.

* Remove patches from a person who has died before transferring the body to the morgue or funeral home.

Facilitating transitions to/from a fentanyl patch and to/from other opioids

When administering fentanyl patches, ask the physician/nurse practitioner to provide an immediate-release opioid, such as morphine or hydromorphone, for breakthrough doses.

* When switching *to* the fentanyl patch *from* an immediate-release opioid, follow the physician/nurse practitioner's order and, until the fentanyl takes effect, provide a determined number of immediate-release opioid doses before discontinuing the immediate-release opioid.
* Similarly, when switching *from* the fentanyl patch *to* an immediate-release opioid, follow the schedule the physician/nurse practitioner and organization provide for delaying the initial use of the an immediate-release opioid until enough time has passed for the person's system to become clear of fentanyl.

Safe procedures for disposing of a fentanyl patch after use

Teach all people who might come into contact with the fentanyl patches—HCPs, the person, and their family—how to safely dispose of patches after their removal. Everyone needs to be aware that discarded patches contain sufficient medication to seriously harm or kill someone, even after the dying person has worn the patch for 72 hours. Adhere strictly to these safety measures to avoid serious injury or death:

* Use gloves when applying, removing, and disposing of fentanyl patches.
* Fold the patch in half, with the sticky sides together.
* Place the patch in a secure, locked location, away from children.
* Return unused patches to the pharmacist.
* Do not flush patches down the toilet—this practice contaminates the environment.

Sufentanil

Sufentanil is a true synthetic opioid that is 1,000 times more potent than morphine. Sufentanil can be given sublingually and is quickly absorbed through the mucous membranes. The medication takes effect in approximately 5 to 10 minutes and reaches its peak effect in 15 to 30 minutes; the effect lasts for 30 to 40 minutes. The short duration of its effect is ideal for using prior to painful procedures (e.g., dressing change, burn debridement, repositioning a person).

After administering the medication with a syringe under the person's tongue, instruct the person to hold the solution in their mouth for two minutes. Holding the medication under the tongue for this duration enables absorption of the medication through the mucous membrane into the bloodstream. People with cognitive impairment may have difficulty holding the medication in their mouth.

Follow the physician/nurse practitioner's orders, as well as the organization's guidelines and policies, to determine the dose that will best meet the needs of the person. Too high a dose can depress respiration. Do not administer sufentanil to people who are opioid naive.

Sufentanil is very potent, and its name may be confused with fentanyl. Therefore, again consider using TALLman lettering (e.g., SUFentanil and fentanyl) to avoid the possibility of one name being mistaken for the other.

Methadone

Methadone is a true synthetic opioid that can be used as an alternative if a person has had an allergic reaction to other opioids, both natural or semi-synthetic. When used correctly, methadone can provide pain relief for both nociceptive and neuropathic pain (Pallium Canada, 2013).

Methadone is a complex opioid to use because it is slow to build up to its peak effect, so there is a greater risk of over- or underestimating the correct dose needed to provide pain relief. Not only do physician/nurse practitioners require a special license to prescribe methadone because of the complexity of this medication, but the person using this medication must be closely monitored to avoid unwanted side effects and toxicity. Methadone accumulation may appear within the first 3 to 14 days. People changing from another opioid to methadone often require hospital admission for close supervision.

Opioid Toxicity

Opioid toxicity can occur when the person accumulates an opioid because their body is unable to eliminate it and its metabolites fast enough. This can happen when opioids are administered regularly either for a long period of time or in too large a dose. When opioids accumulate, the person may display these symptoms:

- Increased agitation
- Increased dreaming
- Hallucinations
- Drowsiness that does not diminish over the first few days on the medication
- Jerking or twitching movements
- Seizures
- Hypersensitization/hyperalgesia, which is when being touched, even gently, is painful to the person (the risk of developing this symptom increases with higher doses of opioids, e.g., TDD > 200 mg morphine equivalent)

The health care team can prevent opioid toxicity by first ensuring that the person's organ function, primarily renal function, is sufficient to eliminate opioids and metabolites. Nurses can also ensure that administered doses are increased in appropriate steps to avoid toxicity.

When opioid toxicity is suspected, consult with the physician/nurse practitioner. Opioid-induced toxicity can be treated by using different opioids in rotation and flushing out the metabolite accumulation with hydration (often by hypodermoclysis, which involves administering fluid subcutaneously), if this is in alignment with the person's goals of care. When a person is receiving opioids and is able to swallow and tolerate fluids, encouraging fluid intake is helpful for preventing opioid toxicity.

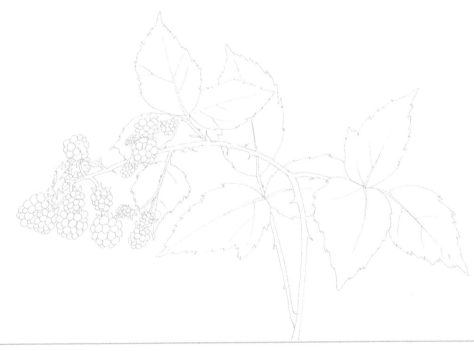

Addressing the Side Effects of Opioids

Before discussing how to use opioids to manage symptoms, this section addresses the side effects of opioids, and concerns and fears that people have about using them.

 Ethics Touchstone
Provision 4
The nurse has authority, accountability, and responsibility for nursing practice; makes decisions; and takes action consistent with the obligation to promote health and to provide optimal care.
Code of Ethics for Nurses (ANA, 2015a)

Consider how fears and concerns about administering opioids might interfere with a nurse's ability to provide optimal care.

Common Side Effects of Opioids

People who take opioids may experience several common side effects, which can be anticipated and managed (ELNEC, 2015; Fraser Health Authority, 2016a).

Constipation

Constipation is the most common side effect of and fear about taking opioids because of their action in decreasing the motility of the intestines, thus causing constipation. Dr. Jim Wilde, a dear colleague, has said, "The hand that writes the opioid order writes the laxative order!" Information on managing constipation is presented in the "Changes in Bowel Function" section in Part 2 of this chapter.

Nausea and Vomiting

Nausea and vomiting are my number one fear about using opioids! They cause nausea and vomiting either through the central nervous system (CNS) or through the gastrointestinal (GI) tract.

When people are nauseated and vomit within minutes, hours, or a few days of starting to take opioids, it is usually because the CNS has identified opioids as a foreign compound that needs to be eliminated from the body. The body may become tolerant of the opioid, and nausea and vomiting may settle after a period of time. Until then, anti-emetics will be required to control the nausea and vomiting.

Other people become nauseated after the opioid slows the peristaltic movements of the GI system. Digestion slows and undigested food remains in the stomach. When this happens, the person may vomit undigested food. A medication such as metoclopramide will stimulate the GI system to "get back to work" and move food through the digestive tract.

Information on managing nausea is available in the "Nausea and Vomiting" section in Part 2 of this chapter.

Confusion

Some people who take opioids experience an increase in dreams and misperceptions, and sometimes experience delirium. Such symptoms may necessitate a switch to an alternative opioid; for example, a person may experience less confusion if the medication is switched from morphine to hydromorphone or a fentanyl patch. Other people become confused if the opioid dose is increased too rapidly.

Drowsiness

When a person starts taking an opioid and when the dose of the opioid is increased, it is normal for the person to be drowsier for a few days. Anticipate this and prepare the person and the family for this side effect. You may say:

When a person starts receiving an opioid, such as morphine, they can expect to feel more drowsy and may want to sleep more for the next few days. This is normal and will pass in about three days.

If death is imminent, it may be helpful to say to the person or the family:

If a person is dying in the coming days and weeks, then they will sleep more because of the dying process. If that is the case, they may not recover from the increased drowsiness associated with starting or increasing the opioid medication.

Opioid-Induced Respiratory Depression

Opioids can slow respiration. Many people fear that opioids will cause respiratory depression and death.

People at increased risk for developing significant opioid-induced respiratory depression are the elderly, those who are opioid naive, those with compromised respiratory systems (e.g., people with COPD), and those receiving concomitant sedating medications. Respiratory depression may also occur if the opioid dose is increased very rapidly to manage severe distress, and if the medication accumulates in the bloodstream past the point needed for symptom management.

Respiratory depression seldom happens in people who receive regular doses of opioids titrated to meet their specific need for symptom management. Pain is usually relieved, and a decreased level of consciousness usually occurs before respiratory depression does.

The Pasero Opioid-Induced Sedation Scale (Pasero scale) (Pasero, 2009) (Figure 1) will help you identify sedation that may precede respiratory depression and help you know when to withhold medication. Using the Pasero scale, monitor the person's respiratory rate, and respond and report if the person's level of consciousness is declining. Administer oxygen *if* oxygen saturation decreases to less than 90%. The treatment to reverse opioid-induced respiratory depression is to administer naloxone (Fraser Health Authority, 2016a). Become familiar with the practice guidelines in your care setting and consult with your team about any concerns you have.

The Pasero scale was not developed to be used with people who are actively dying of their disease. For example, in such people, it is expected that the level of consciousness will decline and respirations may become irregular and sporadic. It is very appropriate to consult with the team and discuss whether the level of consciousness is decreased because of medication or because of disease progression.

Figure 1. Pasero Opioid-Induced Sedation Scale with Interventions

Level	State	Dosing Guidance
S = Sleep	Easy to arouse	Acceptable—*No action necessary; may increase opioid dose if needed*
1	Awake and alert	Acceptable—*No action necessary; may increase opioid dose if needed*
2	Slightly drowsy, easily aroused	Acceptable—*No action necessary; may increase opioid dose if needed*
3	Frequently drowsy, arousable, drifts off to sleep during conversation	Unacceptable *Monitor respiratory status and sedation level closely until sedation level is stable at less than 3 and respiratory status is satisfactory* *Decrease opioid dose 25% to 50%[1] or notify prescriber or anesthesiologist for orders* *Consider administering a non-sedating, opioid-sparing non-opioid, such as acetaminophen or an NSAID, if not contraindicated*
4	Somnolent, minimal or no response to verbal or physical stimulation	Unacceptable *Stop opioid* *Consider administering naloxone[2,3]* *Notify prescriber or anesthesiologist* *Monitor respiratory status and sedation level closely until sedation level is stable at less than 3 and respiratory status is satisfactory*

Appropriate action is given in italics at each level of sedation.

[1] Opioid analgesic orders or a hospital protocol should include the expectation that a nurse will decrease the opioid dose if a patient is excessively sedated.

[2] Mix 0.4 mg of naloxone and 10 mL of normal saline in syringe and administer this dilute solution very slowly (0.5 mL over two minutes) while observing the patient's response (titrate to effect) (Source: Pasero, Portenoy, McCaffery M. Opioid analgesics. In: *Pain: Clinical Manual*. 2nd ed. St. Louis, MO: Mosby; 1999:161–

299; American Pain Society (APS). *Principles of Analgesic Use in the Treatment of Acute Pain and Chronic Cancer Pain*. 5th ed. Glenview, IL: APS; 2003.)

[3] Hospital protocols should include the expectation that a nurse will administer naloxone to any patient suspected of having life-threatening opioid-induced sedation and respiratory depression.

Copyright © 1994, Chris Pasero. Used with permission. Source: Pasero C. *Acute Pain Service: Policy and Procedure Manual*. Los Angeles, CA: Academy Medical Systems; 1994.

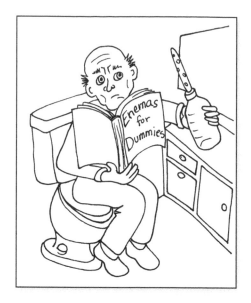 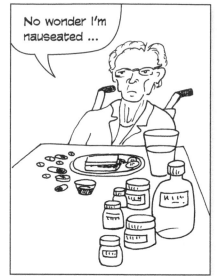 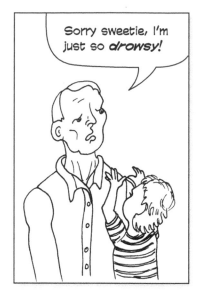

Other Side Effects of Opioids

Dry mouth, urinary retention, pruritus (itching), dizziness, and diaphoresis (sweating) are other side effects that may occur with opioids. However, these side effects may occur independently of taking opioids and may be unrelated to the medication. Remember these key points about the side effects of opioids:

- Dry mouth is common, especially in people who take morphine. Good mouth care and frequent sips of liquids are usually effective in treating dry mouth.

- Urinary retention may occur as a result of increased bladder sphincter tone, which reduces the ability of the bladder to empty. This side effect may lessen with ongoing use of the opioid.
- Pruritus may occur as a result of the histamine released in response to medications, especially morphine. An antihistamine or opioid rotation may be required.
- Dizziness may be caused by the histamine release, resulting in a pooling of the venous blood supply. Repositioning and standing up slowly may be helpful.

Addressing Concerns and Fears about Opioids

In addition to being concerned about the side effects opioids cause, a dying person and their family may fear the symbolism of using opioids, worry that their use should be postponed until the pain is severe, and worry about developing tolerance of, dependence on, and addiction to opioids. Sharing information may help the person and family make informed decisions about taking opioids.

Symbolism

A common fear stems from associating the use of opioids with imminent death. You may hear:

If he starts on morphine, he will die!

She will die sooner if this medication is given.

Remember these key points when addressing this fear:

- Opioids are no longer reserved for use in a person's last days and hours, as they were previously.
- Opioids are now used much earlier in the disease process to provide comfort for the person.
- Among people who receive opioids to manage pain, many report improved quality of life and some live longer than people who did not receive opioids.

Postponing Use of Opioids Until Later

Some people fear that starting opioids early in the disease process may leave the person without sufficient options to manage increased pain in the future. You may hear:

If I take morphine now, what will I take when the pain gets really bad?

I need to save taking the morphine for when I really need it.

Remember these key points when addressing this fear:
* The dose of the morphine can be increased if and when the pain increases.
* There is no ceiling on the amount of pain relief that opioids can supply.

Tolerance

Just as people think they should postpone using opioids until pain or dyspnea becomes "really bad," they may fear that the opioids will stop working if they are used too long or too often. You may hear:

What if my mom becomes used to the morphine and it is not effective anymore?

Remember these key points when addressing this fear:
* When a person becomes used to the opioid, they have developed a tolerance to that specific opioid. When the pain has not increased but the body requires more of the same medication to reach the same pain relief threshold, tolerance has occurred.
* Tolerance develops in people at different rates. If tolerance occurs, the opioid dose can be increased or a different opioid can be used to provide sufficient pain relief.

Dependence

The person and family may fear becoming dependent on the opioid. You may hear:

Will my mom become dependent on the morphine if she takes it every day?

Remember these key points when addressing this fear:
* Dependence occurs when the body becomes accustomed to receiving the opioid. Dependence is reversible.
* If a new treatment relieved the person's pain, and the opioid was no longer needed after a lengthy period of treatment, then the opioid dose would need to be reduced slowly to prevent withdrawal symptoms. This does *not* indicate an addiction.

Addiction

Historically it was thought that addiction was rarely an issue for people who received opioids in the treatment of cancer-related pain. However, the provision of opioids in hospice and palliative care for people with chronic illnesses obligates HCPs to learn about the use of opioids in this population.

People considering taking opioids may express a fear of becoming addicted. You may hear:

Will I become a drug addict if I take morphine regularly?

I don't want to turn into an addict.

Remember these key points when addressing this fear:
* Addiction is a psychological issue.
* A person who is addicted has an overwhelming preoccupation with taking more medication than necessary.
* Addiction results in compulsive drug-seeking behavior.

Help the person and family understand their fears, and connect them with the physician/nurse practitioner or the palliative care consultant with whom they can discuss their fears.

Pain does not protect people from developing addiction to opioids. Talk with the health care team and consider the person's prognosis:
* Is the person going to need pain management for years?
* Is the risk of addiction a concern for this person?
* What medications and modalities can help to decrease the dose of opioids required to manage the pain?

If the person has a history of addiction, it will be expected that they will need a higher dose of opioid to manage pain or dyspnea. When supporting pain management, keep the following principles in mind:
* When a person has a history of addiction, behaviors may appear that are not related only to addiction (e.g., seeking more than one physician/nurse practitioner to obtain multiple prescriptions) but also to the pain associated with the disease state.
* Pain management for a person with a past or current addiction may require consultation with a palliative specialist to ensure that pain is adequately controlled.
* The titration of opioids and administration of prescriptions should be closely monitored and controlled (Pallium Canada, 2013).

Sharing Information with Families to Address Fears and Concerns about Opioids
- Listen!
- Allow both the person and their family to tell their story and express their concerns.
- If needed, ask questions to help identify fears.

Diversion

It is important to administer opioids with caution and prevent their diversion or misuse (Smith and Passik, 2008).

"Diversion" occurs when prescriptions for opioids, written for a person in pain, make their way to the illegal market. This can occur if the person gives or sells medications, or medications are stolen. Dr. Sharon Koivu, a palliative care physician, is passionate about providing education to decrease both addiction and diversion. She suggests that "diversion is the last elephant in the room."

Use due diligence to prevent diversion. The following protocols will help prevent medications from being diverted:
- Avoid dispensing large quantities of opioids at one time.
- Advise all HCPs, the person, and the family to store opioids in a secure and locked location.
- Educate the person and family about returning unused opioids to a pharmacy.
- Ensure that the person is taking and receiving the opioids prescribed.

Opioids will always be an important tool in palliative care. However, *administering opioids with caution is the new normal.*

HCPs' Fears about Opioids

It is not uncommon for members of the health care team to have concerns and fears about administering opioids, as illustrated in the following story, in which the nurse exacerbates Mr. Brown's suffering by withholding the opioids.

The Story of Mr. Brown

Mr. Brown is in bed, in a semi-Fowler's position. He is short of breath at rest. Accessory muscles engage with the work of breathing. He speaks a few words, pauses for a breath, and then speaks again, but only a few words. His respiratory rate is 36/minute. I ask him to rate the difficulty of breathing. He says, "5 out of 10."

What can I do to help him?

He was started on morphine a week ago. He was a bit drowsy for the first few days, but is certainly not drowsy now. He receives morphine 10 mg PO q4h. His last dose was one hour ago. There is an order for morphine 5 mg PO q1h PRN, but, I am not comfortable giving it.

If I give him another dose, it may cause respiratory depression, it may lower the oxygen levels in his blood, it may be his last dose ... What if he takes it and dies?

I turn the fan on and position it toward him. I squeeze his hand and tell him that I will check in on him in a half hour.

Ethics Touchstone

Use the IDEA Ethical Decision-Making Framework to examine the ethical questions raised in the story about Mr. Brown. What are the options? What are the strengths and weaknesses of the different options?

Best Practices for Relieving Symptoms with Opioids

The following concepts and practices guide the development of a care plan when using opioids for symptom management. Similar practices can be used in titrating other medications to relieve other symptoms, such as nausea and vomiting or constipation (Fraser Health Authority, 2016a; Pallium Canada, 2013; ELNEC, 2015).

Provide Enough Opioid to Surpass the Symptom Relief Threshold

Pain occurs because a stimulus, such as a tumor pressing on a bone, provides neural input that causes the neurons to fire, sending a signal (in this instance a signal of pain) to the brain. Remember that nerves work on an "all-or-nothing" basis, sending a signal only when the input surpasses the threshold for neurons to fire. In the case of pain, the stimulus must cause sufficient neural input to surpass the threshold, causing neurons to fire and the person to feel pain. When a medication relieves the pain, it can be said that the medication surpassed the pain relief threshold.

When working with medications, and specifically opioids, the goal is to administer sufficient medication to surpass the pain relief threshold and thereby enhance physical comfort.

Figure 2 illustrates the pain relief threshold in relation to increasing doses of opioids. The arched lines represent serum opioid levels after the administration of three different oral opioid doses. The first dose of medication is not sufficient to reach the pain relief threshold. The second dose surpasses the threshold and relieves the symptom. The third dose relieves the pain but is also high enough to cause excessive side effects. In this scenario, the middle dose is the ideal dose for this person.

The space between the pain relief threshold and the increasing side effects is called "the therapeutic window." The ideal dose of any medication raises serum levels of the medication to the therapeutic window—sufficient to relieve the symptom without causing excessive side effects.

For some medications and for some people, the therapeutic window can be quite shallow. When the therapeutic window is shallow, frequent doses may be necessary to maintain serum levels within the therapeutic window, thereby avoiding fluctuations of serum levels that cause side effects or breakthrough pain.

Sustained-release medications are useful for keeping serum levels of medications consistently within the therapeutic window, over a long period of time. These can be used after the person's ideal dose of medication has been titrated. Pumps that provide continuous subcutaneous infusion of medications—that is, small amounts of the medication at frequent intervals—can be useful for keeping people in the therapeutic range.

Figure 2. Effects of different doses of oral opioids on serum levels of opioids

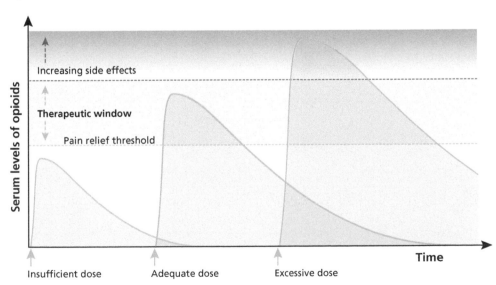

When a dying person regularly receives immediate-release opioids, such as morphine by the oral route, the medication reaches the peak level in the blood in about one hour. Within two to three hours, the level of opioid in the blood decreases as the opioid is excreted through the kidneys.

Historically, people were given medication for pain on a PRN (which means *pro re nata*, or "as needed") basis. When medications are given as needed, the person experiences a cycle of recurring and possibly increasing pain. For example, a hospitalized person receives a dose of opioid, and an hour later the pain is relieved. A few hours later, the pain returns, but the person is reluctant to request medication. When the person finally asks for medication, the nurse may be busy, so the person waits longer for pain relief. The nurse gives the medication, and the person waits for it to take effect. The cycle begins again.

In addition to the problem of the person needing to ask for the medication, the nurse may not think that the medication is needed or may feel uncomfortable providing it. Depending on who is providing the care, the dying person may encounter delays in receiving medication.

Best practice is to provide medication for ongoing pain regularly, around the clock. Therefore PRN orders are *not* an effective way to provide opioids.

Figure 3 illustrates that when the opioid is provided regularly around the clock, serum levels of opioids remain above the pain relief threshold, ensuring ongoing pain relief.

The goal is to find the right dose that has the desired effect on pain or dyspnea, and then to give that dose regularly to prevent the symptom from recurring. Immediate-release opioids, such as morphine or hydromorphone, are administered regularly every 4 hours to prevent the symptom from recurring. Medications such as sustained-release morphine are administered every 8 to 12 hours.

Continuous pain or dyspnea requires that medication be given regularly around the clock.

Figure 3. Continuous symptom relief provided by opioids administered regularly and around the clock

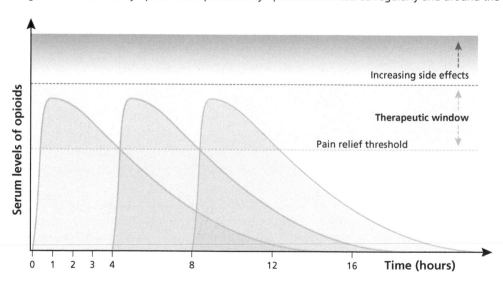

Provide Breakthrough Doses PRN

When a person's pain is controlled, breakthrough pain is pain that "breaks through" regular pain management. Breakthrough pain can occur spontaneously or predictably with a specific incident (e.g., a dressing change). Breakthrough pain can also occur when the pain is not well controlled and can more accurately be called "end of dose failure."

Figure 4 shows the value of giving the breakthrough dose (BTD) prior to a painful procedure. In this case, the person is given the BTD an hour before a painful procedure. The extra medication causes a temporary increase in the serum level of opioids to provide pain relief before the painful procedure. BTDs are also given while titrating medications to find the correct dose.

BTDs are often called "incident doses," "booster doses," and "bolus doses" or "interim doses." An order for regular opioids should always include an order for a BTD. The same opioid should be used for the BTD as for the regular dose whenever possible. For example, if the person is taking morphine every 4 hours or sustained-release morphine every 12 hours, the breakthrough medication will be an immediate-release morphine. However, if the person has a fentanyl transdermal patch, then the medication used for BTDs will be either hydromorphone or morphine.

When breakthrough pain occurs spontaneously, respond promptly to provide the BTD.

When incident pain or dyspnea can be anticipated, provide a BTD in advance. For example, if personal care and a dressing change are known to be painful or cause an increase in respiratory distress, schedule and provide a BTD an hour or two before care is provided.

Newer rapid-onset transmucosal opioid preparations are available that can be very useful in treating people whose pain comes on very quickly, too fast for morphine or hydromorphone to take effect in time. These medications include fentanyl sublingual tablets and sublingual sufentanil liquid, both of which must be held in the mouth until absorbed, and not swallowed. Though expensive, these medicines can be very helpful and cost-effective in certain situations. As well, these rapid-onset medications can be provided immediately before anticipated procedures that cause pain.

Various formulas are recommended for determining the BTD. The BTD is often calculated as either 50% of the q4h dose or 10% of the total daily dose (TDD). When a new regular opioid dose is ordered, a new BTD will also need to be calculated and ordered.

Figure 4. Effects of an immediate-release opioid BTD on serum levels of opioids

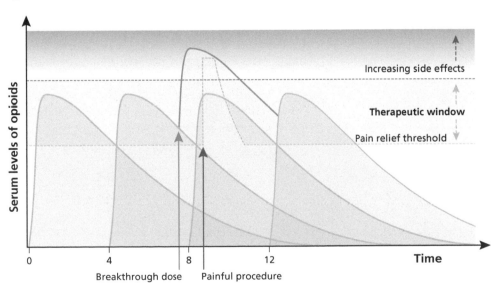

Sample Calculations: BTD

Ming is receiving hydromorphone 2 mg PO q4h. She requires a BTD.

50% of q4h Dose Method
Calculate her new BTD by dividing the q4h dose by 2.
* The new order will be hydromorphone 1 mg PO PRN for BTD.

10% of TDD Method
Calculate the BTD by dividing her 24-hour TDD by 10.
* The TDD is 2 mg x 6 doses = 12 mg.
* 10% of 12 mg = 1.2 mg PO.

Hydromorphone comes in 1 mg and 2 mg tablets, so the BTD will also be hydromorphone 1 mg PO PRN.

BTDs can be used to inform the titration process.

Titrate to the Most Effective Dose

The goal is to determine the dose of opioid required to reach the symptom relief threshold (or to reach the person's individualized goal for symptom management), while not causing excessive side effects. The process of increasing, and sometimes decreasing, the dose of medication to meet the desired effect is called "titration."

Follow these guidelines for titrating opioids:
* Use an immediate-release form of opioid to find the right dose.
* Start low and go slow—especially when caring for frail, elderly, or opioid naive people.
* Switch to a sustained-release medication once the symptom has settled if the condition is stable.
* Increase the oral dose of medication every 24 to 72 hours until the person is comfortable and their goals for symptom management are reached.
* Anticipate side effects and respond when they occur.
* Record and report a follow-up assessment.

While nurses are not expected to calculate or order medications, the information provided in this text will help you understand the physician/nurse practitioner's rationale, identify a mistake if one is made, feel more comfortable in administering opioids, and share information with the person and the family.

When the symptom is not managed adequately, or when the symptom recurs before the next regularly scheduled medication is due, then the ongoing dose is titrated, in this case increased.

In the following case study, Sam has required several BTDs in the past 24 hours. The regular dose is insufficient and needs to be increased.

Sample Calculation: New Opioid Dose

Sam is taking morphine 30 mg PO q4h (i.e., the regular dose). He receives morphine 15 mg PO as needed for breakthrough pain. For the past two days, Sam took 5 or 6 BTDs in each 24-hour period. His pain is dull and continuous. He rates his pain at 7 out of 10. His pain is relieved to 1 out of 10 only following the BTD.

There are several methods for calculating the new q4h dose. One common method is to increase the regular dose by the amount of the BTD. In Sam's case, the calculation would look like this:

Sample titration calculation

q4h dose	+	BTD	=	new q4h dose
30 mg	+	15 mg	=	45 mg q4h

Follow up and reassess Sam one hour and three hours after he receives his new q4h dose. If appropriate, ask Sam or his family to rate and record his pain levels regularly for the next several doses. Offer BTDs if necessary. Remind Sam to call if he requires another BTD.

Switch to Sustained-Release Opioids When Symptom Is Relieved and Stable

When symptom relief appears to be stable, the person may benefit from sustained-release opioids. Long-acting preparations of morphine, hydromorphone, and Oxycontin are administered every 8 to 12 hours. When a sustained-release opioid is used for the regular medication, then the immediate-release opioid is used for the BTD, and the formula for calculating the BTD is the same. For example, Sariah receives sustained-release morphine 15 mg q12h, and morphine 2.5 mg PRN for breakthrough pain.

Switch Routes of Administration When Necessary

When the person is not able to tolerate oral medications (e.g., due to vomiting) or is unable to swallow (e.g., due to physical decline), the person will need to receive medication by an alternative route. A route change will require a physician/nurse practitioner's order (if not already received) and access to the new form of medication.

It is helpful to anticipate the need for a route change. People who live in isolated communities may not have easy access to a pharmacy, people who live in the city may not have a pharmacy available, and not all facilities stock medication in different forms. If you are working in a facility, you can arrange for common medications to be kept in stock in a variety of different forms for administration by different routes. It is helpful to have a selection of medications that can be delivered by oral, buccal, suppository, topical, transdermal, and subcutaneous routes. In a home setting, you may want to have available sufficient alternative route medications as the person's condition declines.

The medication delivery routes discussed below can be used for a wide range of medications.

Oral

The oral route is the preferred route because of the ease of administration and gradual increase and decrease in the concentration of the medication in the blood. When a person takes opioids orally, the immediate-release opioids usually take effect within the hour and peak within two hours.

If the person is not able to swallow tablets, the immediate-release opioids can be crushed. Sustained-release opioids cannot be crushed or chewed. Ask the pharmacist or physician/nurse practitioner if the capsules can be opened.

Subcutaneous

Subcutaneous injections are given when the oral route is not available (e.g., the person is dying imminently and is no longer able to swallow, or is vomiting and unable to hold medications in their stomach). Keep the volume of the injection to less than 1 mL. There is limited formal research information on this, but considerable practice suggests than volumes between 0.5 and 1 mL are less painful to patients than larger volumes.

Topical

The topical application of morphine may be helpful for treating painful skin ulcers. The morphine is mixed with an aqueous gel at 0.125% (ELMMB, 2013).

Transdermal

The transdermal route is effective for people experiencing:
* Poor absorption of oral medications
* Swallowing difficulties
* Nausea and vomiting
* Difficulty in taking medications regularly by mouth

This route should not be used for people who are cachectic, as absorption is poor.

Parenteral

Consider administering medications parenterally when the person:
* Is unable to swallow
* Is vomiting
* Has a GI obstruction or impaired absorption
* Has severe pain that requires quick relief

Buccal

The route for medications placed between the inside of the cheek and the gum is called the "buccal route." It is often used when the person is no longer able to swallow. The medication is best absorbed when it is given in volumes of 1 mL or less, to prevent incidental swallowing or choking.

Medications that are highly lipophilic, such as sufentanil, are absorbed through the mucosal membrane directly into the bloodstream. The medication starts to take effect approximately 10 minutes after being administered. As absorption is not predictable, the effectiveness of this route is variable. In addition, non-lipophilic medications such as morphine are poorly absorbed, thereby limiting the potential use of this route.

Sublingual

When using the sublingual route, medication is placed under the tongue to be absorbed through the mucosa. This method is useful when administering sufentanil or lorazepam.

Rectal

Like the oral route, the rectal route provides a steady absorption of medication. The rectal route may be useful when the person has difficulty with absorption of the medications by mouth; however, families might not like to use this route because of the difficulty in positioning the person for insertion of the suppository containing the medication.

Intravenous

The intravenous route is the least preferred route, because it is often limited to certain settings due to the competencies required to use it. This route can be used when other routes do not give adequate pain relief. One example of benefits of this method of medication delivery is the continuous infusion of opioids when intermittent dosing does not provide adequate pain relief.

Epidural or intrathecal

Epidural or intrathecal delivery is the delivery of medications directly into spaces surrounding the spinal cord through a very small catheter inserted between specific vertebrae. Medication is delivered into the catheter using a small computerized pump. The medication mixes with the epidural or cerebral spinal fluid, is absorbed, and relieves pain with greater effectiveness than when administered by the oral, subcutaneous, or intravenous routes. These routes are being researched for use with people whose pain is not controlled when other medication delivery routes are used.

Intramuscular

The intramuscular route is not recommended, because frequent injections can be painful and because the person may lack the muscle mass injections require.

Recalculate the Dose When Changing Routes

If the person is not able to tolerate oral medications, either due to nausea, vomiting, or decreasing ability to swallow, changing routes may be necessary.

Route Change: New Dose Calculation—Oral to Subcutaneous

A medication is twice as effective when administered through the subcutaneous (SC) route versus orally. Therefore the SC dose is only 50% of the oral dose.

Sample Calculation: Route Change Oral to SC

Eva is vomiting and not able to take morphine 10 mg PO q4h, or morphine 5 mg PO PRN for BTD for breakthrough pain. The policy is to divide the oral dose by 2 to determine the new dose for SC administration.

Sample titration calculation:
Oral dose ÷ 2 = SC dose
10 mg ÷ 2 = 5 mg SC dose

The SC dose is morphine 5 mg SC q4h, with morphine 2.5 mg SC PRN for breakthrough pain.

Route Change: New Dose Calculation— Subcutaneous to Oral

When switching opioid delivery from the SC route to the oral route, the SC dose is multiplied by 2, or doubled, to determine the oral dose.

Sample Calculation: Route Change SC to Oral

Two days later Eva is no longer experiencing nausea or vomiting. She is swallowing well and taking fluids without experiencing any nausea. The physician/nurse practitioner provides the order to switch her medication back to oral morphine. She is currently on morphine 5.0 mg SC q4h, with morphine 2.5 mg SC PRN for BTD.

Sample titration calculation:
SC dose × 2 = oral dose
5 mg   × 2 = 10 mg oral dose

The oral dose is morphine 10 mg PO q4h, with morphine 5 mg PO for PRN for BTD.

Route Change: New Dose Calculation—Oral to Rectal and Vice Versa

When the delivery route is changed from the oral to the rectal route or from the rectal to the oral route, the absorption is considered the same and the dose is not changed.

Use Equianalgesia Conversions When Switching Opioids

People may need to switch to a different opioid if, for example, they experience side effects or develop a tolerance to a particular opioid. When switching to a new opioid, it is important to give the person an equivalent dose of the new opioid. As mentioned earlier, this is obviously not something that you as a nurse will order, but it is something that you will want to know about to ensure that an appropriate dose is ordered. You can also help explain it to the person and family. Use Table 1 (see page 101) to calculate an equivalent dose of a new opioid.

Case Study

Eli, a 51-year-old man, has a history of liver failure from advanced cirrhosis, and a recent GI bleed from esophageal varices. He has pain from ascites and from a bedsore acquired before admission to the unit. He has stated that he does not want any further blood transfusions and has asked to be allowed to die peacefully and naturally. He is taking morphine 20 mg PO q4h, with morphine 10 mg PO PRN for BTD.

Eli is now experiencing delirium, is unable to provide clear answers, and moans and grimaces when repositioned. The care team wonders if he is confused because of the morphine.

Orders

The physician/nurse practitioner provides the following orders:
1. Discontinue the morphine.
2. Start hydromorphone 2 mg PO q4h and hydromorphone 1 mg PO PRN for BTD.

The nurse reviews the equianalgesic chart and confirms that morphine 10 mg PO is equivalent to hydromorphone 2 mg PO. Therefore, morphine 20 mg PO q4h is equivalent to hydromorphone 4 mg PO q4h. The nurse realizes, on the basis of the equianalgesic chart, that the dose the physician/nurse practitioner ordered is half the dose that should be ordered.

Information Sharing

The nurse phones the physician/nurse practitioner, reviews the equianalgesic chart with her, and provides a brief assessment of Eli, including that he appears to be having discomfort with turns and repositioning. The physician/nurse practitioner provides the following order:
1. Give hydromorphone 4 mg PO q4h, and hydromorphone 2 mg PO PRN for relief of breakthrough pain.

Nonpharmacological Comfort Measures—Comfort Basket

The "comfort basket" is an image I use for the collection of nonpharmacological items HCPs and family members can use to help decrease a dying person's discomfort and provide support. Comfort measures help people relax, distract them from discomfort that symptoms cause, and can help medications be more effective. Comfort measures can help relieve discomfort while the person waits for medication to take effect. And comfort measures can communicate compassion, with or without the use of medication.

Most nonpharmacological comfort measures can be provided by any person, without a prescription or specialist. You may need to check the policies of your agency, facility, or unit to clarify what strategies can be used and who on the team can use them.

Consider these guidelines when providing nonpharmacological comfort measures:
- Respect the dying person and individualize the care.
- Be flexible when offering comfort measures, because those that work now may not work at another time, and vice versa.
- Invite the family to participate in providing comfort measures.
- Provide the family with information about the comfort measures you use and how the family can integrate them into caring for the person.
- Encourage the family to think of things the person used to do that brought them comfort. Consider whether those things could be adapted to be comfort measures now.
- Keep in mind that family members might want to lie next to or snuggle with the person or want time for intimacy. They may want permission to lie on the bed. Side rails can prevent people from falling out of bed. Closing the door can provide some privacy.
- If appropriate, invite family and friends to share their comfort measures.
- Be open to adding new tools to your comfort basket.
- Invite the dying person to teach you new comfort measures.

It is important to choose comfort measures that will best meet the needs and preferences of this person at this time. You might ask questions like those below:

I understand that you studied therapeutic touch together. Have you thought of offering a treatment to Bob?

I hear that you and Sam used to sing together. Would you consider singing for him now?

Comfort Basket—Creativity in Caregiving

Consider creating your own "basket" of comfort measures from your life, talents, and experiences. People may sing, distract, massage, energize, or tell funny stories to bring comfort.

You can also get ideas about what is important to the person you are caring for in the home setting by looking at what is on their shelves, walls, and countertops. In the residential care setting, you may find hand cream on the bathroom counter, pillows in the closet, and a music player on the shelf. If you integrate these items into your care of the person, you are more likely to provide comfort than if you use something from another person's shelves. I remember a woman whose love was music, and she taught the caregivers to arrange different songs to set different moods, depending on her need.

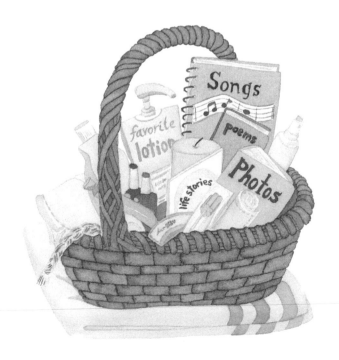

Part 2: Common Symptoms

Part 2 of this chapter describes the most common symptoms a dying person might experience and strategies for enhancing the person's physical comfort. Symptom-specific assessment tools are identified. Consider also using the GSF PIG, the SPICT, a one-year mortality prognostic tool, and/or the CSHA Clinical Frailty Scale to help inform goals-of-care conversations and determine needs for investigations.

Psychosocial factors are integral to enhancing a person's physical comfort and may change as symptoms progress. Use the Psychosocial Assessment Form to help address changes in the person's psychosocial needs.

Anorexia and Cachexia

Jack, 84 years old, was admitted a month ago. His condition is declining, and he has repeated chest infections, frequent falls, progressive dementia, and lung cancer. Since admission Jack is sleeping more, is withdrawn and refusing food, and is having some difficulty swallowing.

Megan, Jack's wife, visits daily, brings homemade custard, and encourages Jack to eat. Megan is concerned that if Jack does not eat, he will die.

Jack's daughter Mary arrived today from out of town. Alarmed by his weight loss, Mary promptly declared, "He is starving!" She believes that decreased nutritional intake is responsible for his declining condition.

Food is a basic need and a fundamental preoccupation of human beings. Many social gatherings and cultural rituals involve food and eating as a way of "being together." Preparing and serving food is one way to communicate love.

The nutritional needs and therefore the dietary intake of a person change from birth to adulthood to the senior years and through the dying process as a normal function of living and dying. The type of food a 2-year-old eats would cause a newborn to choke, and the quantity of food required to nourish and satisfy a 25-year-old male would cause an older adult to feel bloated or nauseated.

Regardless of changing nutritional needs, and regardless of whether decreasing intake is normal when a person is living with a life-limiting illness, their declining interest in food and decreasing dietary intake may become the primary concern for the family. Different understandings of what is happening and how to respond may cause conflict within families and within the health care team, as well as between the family and the health care team, in the last months, weeks, or days of a person's life.

What Are Anorexia, Cachexia, and Anorexia-Cachexia Syndrome?

Anorexia in the context of this text for a person living with a life-limiting illness is defined as decreased appetite or lack of interest in food and eating. Cachexia is defined as substantial weight loss comprising muscle (skeletal) and fat tissue losses that do not respond to increased intake or supplementation; bone mineral losses; and overall weakness and inflammatory processes (Wholihan, 2015). In this context, anorexia or cachexia can occur in the absence of the other. Primary anorexia-cachexia syndrome (ACS), in which both anorexia and cachexia are present, is caused by multiple endogenous abnormalities, possibly related to the perceived threat of increasing chronic progressive illness. The presence of primary ACS indicates a poorer prognosis than if either anorexia or cachexia is absent. Secondary anorexia or cachexia result from factors that reduce intake or absorption of nutrients (e.g., nausea, diarrhea, pain).

Prevalence

Primary ACS has been reported in up to 86% of people with cancer-related illnesses. Among people with COPD, 30%–70% experience ACS, as do 30%–60% of people with end-stage renal disease. HIV and CHF are also associated with anorexia and cachexia, affecting 10%–35% of people with those conditions (Wholihan, 2015).

Causes of Secondary Anorexia and Cachexia

Factors causing secondary anorexia and cachexia include:
* Oral discomfort (e.g., dry mouth, sore mouth, stomatitis, difficulty or pain with swallowing)
* Aversion to food odors and tastes
* Uncontrolled pain, dyspnea, and nausea and vomiting
* Fatigue
* Psychosocial issues (e.g., depression, anxiety or stress)
* Cognitive impairment
* Side effects of medications
* Side effects of treatments (e.g., chemotherapy, radiation therapy)

While it might be assumed that anorexia (decreased appetite) causes cachexia (involuntary weight loss), in many cases the biochemical changes of cachexia contribute to anorexia (Morley, Thomas, and Wilson, 2006; Wholihan, 2015).

A thorough assessment can help to determine which factors are contributing to anorexia and cachexia.

Causes of Primary ACS

Primary ACS is a complex multifactorial syndrome that affects many people with life-limiting illnesses, including cancer (Wholihan, 2015). People with ACS present symptoms that vary depending on the initial illness but are similar in terms of decreased intake, lack of appetite, skeletal muscle loss, fat loss, fatigue, weakness, altered immunity, and chronic inflammatory processes. The GI symptoms associated with ACS include nausea, vomiting, constipation, belching, abdominal pain, bloating, indigestion, and hiccups. Related symptoms include food aversions, changes in the ability to smell and taste, and early satiety (Arensmeyer, 2012).

Cachexia occurs due to increased protein catabolism (breakdown), lipid (fat) catabolism, and changes in carbohydrate metabolism. The release of cytokines, even at low levels, and the immune system's response to disease are thought to initiate the metabolic changes. Cytokines involved are tumor necrosis factor, interleukin-1, interleukin-6, and protein cachexia factor (Morley, Thomas, and Wilson, 2006).

The initiation of ACS is not yet clearly understood; however, a simplified understanding of the processes involved can help when talking with the person and family. Current research suggests that severe progressive illness decreases food intake and causes fatigue. As illness progresses, peripheral inputs alert the body to the increasing threat of the progressive illness (e.g., tumor, renal failure), creating a catabolic effect that includes inflammation and the release of cytokines (immune system messengers). The person's basal energy expenditure, which has already increased to deal with progressive illness, increases further because of the inflammatory reactions. The ensuing inflammation, cytokines release, and metabolic abnormalities lead to disrupted neuro-hormonal signaling. These changes, along with the release of disease-specific molecules such as tumor necrosis factor and the ACS-specific protein (proteolysis-inducing factor), and fat (lipid-mobilizing factor) degrading factors (Dodson et al., 2011), produce a catabolic state in which the person suffers significant muscle and fat tissue losses. The person is using significantly more energy now than normal; their muscle and fat stores are being broken down, but the person is unable to take up or use ingested or supplemented nutrients because of the development of glucose intolerance, insulin resistance, and GI issues (Wholihan, 2015).

It may help the family to understand the difference between cachexia and starvation and to understand that their loved one with cachexia is not starving. Table 2 shows differences in the body's response to starvation and cachexia. Notice how energy output is decreased in starvation but increased in cachexia, and how differently the body's resources are conserved or used in these two conditions.

Table 2. Differences in the Body's Response to Starvation and ACS

Starvation	Anorexia-Cachexia Syndrome
Intake • Limited or no intake	Intake • Decreased intake due to difficulty or inability to digest and metabolize nutrients
Energy Use • Body uses less energy by reducing non-essential functions	Energy Use • Body uses more nutrients and energy because of inflammation and immune response
Change in Primary Energy Source • Body uses fat stores to produce energy, preserving internal organs and muscle tissues	Change in Primary Energy Source • Body uses protein and fat stores equally to produce energy, and *does not* preserve muscles or organs

Assessment

Anorexia and cachexia are remarkably common among people with progressive serious illnesses. It is imperative that nurses screen regularly for signs of anorexia and cachexia. Early detection provides the greatest opportunity for improving quality of life for the dying person.

Assess for anorexia and cachexia when the person or family expresses concerns about decreased appetite, decreased dietary intake, or weight loss. A thorough assessment for ACS includes assessing the person's appetite, their dietary intake, and, if warranted, their nutritional status. Weight loss, regardless of etiology, has a decidedly negative effect on survival (Wholihan, 2015).

Screen for Anorexia with the Edmonton Symptom Assessment System

Use the Edmonton Symptom Assessment System (ESAS) as a regular screening tool for anorexia. Follow up with an assessment when the ESAS question about dietary intake returns a value greater than 0 (Cancer Care Ontario, 2010; Wholihan, 2015), indicating decreased appetite. When the person cannot self-report, frontline HCPs and family members who help with meals can assist with assessment. A general guideline suggests that ESAS scores from 1 to 3 indicate mild anorexia/pre-cachexia, scores from 4 to 6 may suggest moderate anorexia/cachexia, and scores from 7 to 10 indicate severe anorexia and cachexia (Cancer Care Ontario, 2010).

Assess with the Symptom Assessment Tool Adapted for Anorexia and Cachexia

When anorexia, cachexia, or ACS are suspected, assess the person for primary and secondary causes using the Symptom Assessment Tool adapted for anorexia and cachexia (see Table 3). If the person is unable to self-report, front-line HCPs and family members can help provide answers. When secondary causes of anorexia or cachexia are discovered, treatments can be discussed.

The assessment of muscle and fat-tissue losses and edema is crucial to understanding the severity of ACS (Patient Global Platform, 2014). A person with less than 5% weight loss in the past six months may have early signs of ACS. At the other end of the spectrum, when a person shows weight loss greater than 5% in the past six months and significant losses of muscle and fat tissue, and edema is present, the person may have severe ACS.

Assess Frailty and Inform Goals-of-Care Conversations

Assess the person's frailty using the CSHA Clinical Frailty Scale or the Palliative Performance Scale (PPS). Consider using the GSF PIG, the SPICT, or tools for prognosticating one-year mortality (see Chapter 4, "Using Standardized Tools") to inform goals-of-care conversations and determine whether investigations are appropriate.

Investigate to Identify or Confirm Causes

The physician/nurse practitioner may order blood work, specifically serum albumin levels, to determine the person's nutritional status. If severe ACS has been identified, testing serum albumin levels may not provide additional information.

Table 3. Symptom Assessment Tool Adapted for Anorexia and Cachexia

	Symptom Assessment Tool Adapted for Anorexia and Cachexia	
O	**Onset**	Anorexia: When did you first notice your appetite decreasing? Cachexia: When did you first notice that you were experiencing weight loss?
P	**Provoking/Palliating**	Anorexia: Do you know what has caused you to lose interest in eating and food? Is there anything that stimulates your appetite or makes you hungry? Does your loss of appetite cause any other symptoms? Are there other symptoms [secondary causes] that may be causing your lack of appetite, such as nausea, vomiting, constipation, diarrhea, sore or dry mouth, taste changes, unpleasant food odors, problems swallowing, early feelings of fullness, pain, shortness of breath, depression, anxiety, and fatigue? Cachexia: What do you think might be causing you to lose weight?
Q	**Quality**	Can you describe the symptoms you have been experiencing? On a scale of 0 to 10, can you rate your current appetite, with 0 being no change in appetite and 10 being great changes in appetite?
R	**Region/Radiating**	Can you describe how your loss of appetite is affecting your body? Can you describe your experience with weight loss? Are you losing weight from specific areas of your body?
S	**Severity**	How severe are your symptoms related to anorexia? Can you rate their severity on a scale of 0 to 10? How much are you able to ingest in terms of fluids and solids? How much weight have you lost, and over how much time has this weight loss occurred?
T	**Treatment**	Have you tried any supplements or medications in the past to help you with your loss of appetite? Weight loss? What doses have you tried? What was effective? Did you experience any side effects when you took the medications? Have any of your medications changed recently?
U	**Understanding**	What do you think is causing the loss in appetite? Weight loss? How is this affecting your daily activities? Can you tell me how you feel about your loss of appetite and weight?
V	**Values**	What are your goals for managing your weight loss and loss of appetite? On a scale of 0 to 10, where would you like your appetite to be?
W	**What Else?**	• Physical assessment

The dramatic changes in the appearance of a person with anorexia, cachexia, or ACS can be difficult for family members to witness and for HCPs to understand and explain.

Ethics Touchstone
Principle 2.1
Respect the right and responsibility of clients to be informed and make decisions about their health care.
Code of Ethics for Licensed/Registered Practical Nurses (CCPNR, 2013)

Use the IDEA Ethical Decision-Making Framework to identify ethical issues to address for a person with anorexia and/or cachexia, given the right of the person to be informed and make decisions about their health care. What ethical issues might arise if the family does not want the person to be told that they are dying?

With the Family

For a person who is losing weight, looking in a mirror and not recognizing yourself is disturbing. It may be helpful for the person and family to understand that the physical changes are not from starvation and instead result from metabolic changes causing muscle wasting, fat loss, and increased energy expenditure. Just as the disease process cannot be changed, the altered metabolism will not change. Cachexia cannot be reversed.

Help the family to understand that cachexia and anorexia are part of the normal dying process resulting from severe progressive illness. Anorexia and cachexia are related to decreased survival in people with progressive illnesses, including cancers (Wholihan, 2015). In some cases, the nurse may need to advocate for the dying person to help the family understand why the person is not eating (Brady, 2016).

The family may be concerned that the person is starving or is at risk of dying sooner and may not understand that increased dietary intake will not slow weight loss. Early in the disease process, a dying person is encouraged to eat foods that give them the most nutrition. As disease progresses, however, eating may cause the person discomfort if food is forced into a GI system that cannot digest and metabolize adequately.

When intake decreases further, the family may want to discuss the possibility of tube feeding or parenteral nutrition. Help the family understand that current research does not support parenteral nutrition, tube feeding, or nutritional supplements, as they do not increase survival, reduce pressure ulcers, limit the risk of aspiration, or enhance functional capacity. In some cases, these measures may cause more discomfort for the person with ACS (Dy, 2006).

Hand feeding has been identified as the best method for feeding a person with dementia and ACS (Wholihan, 2015). This supports a holistic approach to care, opening new avenues for family members to interact with their loved one. Help family members shift their focus from ensuring sufficient nutrition to providing what the person prefers and allowing them to eat what their body can tolerate. It is important to cater to the person's preferences so as to prevent food from becoming a source of stress or conflict.

Support the person and family in learning new ways to spend time together that do not involve food and eating. Reviewing the goals of care with the person and family may help facilitate the family's understanding of the person's goals of care and what is important to the person at the time. It is also important to create a comfortable and stimulating environment for dying people when they do eat and, even if they are not hungry, to encourage them to be with the family during meals to enjoy the time together.

It may help for the person and family to meet with a dietician to help determine tolerable food options and suggestions for altering food intake.

Common Questions about Anorexia-Cachexia Syndrome

Nurses can adopt the following answers to common questions and concerns that family members might express about ACS.

What are anorexia, cachexia, and ACS?

Anorexia is decreased appetite, and cachexia is involuntary weight loss. A person who has both has ACS.

What causes cachexia and anorexia?

When a person is very ill, their body's immune system triggers an inflammatory response. When illness is progressive and long-term, systemic inflammation develops. Current research indicates that the systemic inflammation may trigger processes that cause weight loss and decrease the appetite. It is important to note that weight loss may occur regardless of how much a person eats.

What causes weight loss?

The weight loss is partly the result of a poor appetite and decreased intake. It also results from the systemic inflammation and increased energy expenditure of cachexia, which causes the body to consume energy faster than normal. The body uses its own muscles to meet its nutritional needs, which results in weight loss.

Is cachexia the same as starvation?

Cachexia is different from starvation (see Table 2 on page 121). When a person is starving, their body processes slow down to conserve nutrients, using fat stores for energy. With cachexia, the body processes speed up in response to the inflammation, consuming more energy than normal. In contrast to what happens in starvation, in the case of cachexia the body burns muscle and fat tissues for energy. The significant loss of these tissues greatly changes the appearance of the person, giving rise to the wasted look of cachexia.

Is she dying because she is not eating?

No. She is not eating because she is dying.

Is the dying person not eating due to discomfort?

A dying person does not experience hunger in the same way that a healthy person does. Therefore, decreased intake in a dying person does not give rise to feelings of hunger. A dry mouth or other types of problems in the mouth can cause discomfort, so regular mouth care will be helpful for a person with anorexia and cachexia.

How can you support and care for the person?

You can provide nurturing care in the form of skin care, massage, and mouth care. You can explore how to simply "be with" the person, providing companionship—for example, by reading to or telling the person stories. Ask the family how they would like to help.

Are there any treatments or medications that would help?

Medications can stimulate the appetite. Because there are many causes of anorexia and cachexia, the person may need a combination of medications. Medications such as steroids do not increase weight over the long term, nor do they build muscle mass or prolong life.

Nonpharmacological Comfort Measures

Consider these strategies for managing comfort with anorexia and cachexia (Arensmeyer, 2012; Morley, Thomas, and Wilson, 2006; Wholihan, 2015).

Offer Dietary Counseling

Proactively offering nutritional counseling may slow or delay the person's weight loss, helping to maintain their functional status and quality of life (Arensmeyer, 2012).

Offer Nourishment as Tolerated

Provide the person with small amounts of food frequently throughout the day, always bearing in mind the person's interest in food. Remember to include foods that the person can tolerate and enjoys. Add extra calories or additional protein to foods, if tolerated.

Offer Fluids as Tolerated

With anorexia and cachexia, fluid intake may become more important than solid intake. Early in the disease process, it is helpful to encourage the person to take in fluids, especially if the person is receiving high doses of opioids. This helps to facilitate metabolite excretion. See the section on dehydration in Chapter 7, "Caring in the Last Days and Hours."

Support the Family and the HCP to Nurture in New Ways

There are many ways that the HCP and the family can nurture the person that do not involve food. Shifting the focus away from food and toward enjoyable activities, such as massages, music, reading, and recording memories, is helpful.

Prevent Pressure Ulcers and Other Secondary Issues Related to Cachexia

As the person loses their muscle and fat tissues, they will lose their natural cushion. Their skin also becomes more susceptible to breakdown. This can make staying in one position for any length of time uncomfortable for the person. Help to maintain the person's comfort by repositioning them as often as needed. Assess skin regularly for sores and provide comfort measures, such as gentle massage, to help prevent skin breakdown.

Pharmacological Measures

Medications can help increase appetite and energy in the short term but will not result in the rebuilding of muscle tissue or strength. Because anorexia and cachexia are caused by a combination of many factors, no single medication or treatment will be effective (Arensmeyer, 2012; Morley, Thomas, and Wilson, 2006; Wholihan, 2015).

Megestrol Acetate

Megestrol acetate, a female hormone taken orally, is reported to improve appetite and produces a small weight gain. It is also reported to improve the person's sense of well-being and decrease fatigue, and may improve quality of life. Megestrol acetate does not increase survival time.

Gastric Motility Agents

When nausea, vomiting, or gastric stasis cause issues leading to anorexia, medications such as metoclopramide or domperidone may be helpful.

Corticosteroids

Dexamethasone has been used in people suffering with cancer, with varying levels of success. Improvements are subjective and last less than three or four weeks. This medication does not increase survival.

Growth Hormone Receptor Agonists

Growth hormone receptor agonists (e.g., anamorelin) are being trialed in people with cancer-related ACS and show promise for increasing muscle tissue (Temel et al., 2016).

Cannabinoids

There is insufficient research, specifically quality controlled studies, to evaluate the potential of cannabinoids for increasing appetite and decreasing weight loss in people with ACS (Reuter and Martin, 2016).

Evaluating and Confirming

Nurses will need to check with the dying person regularly to assess the progress of anorexia, cachexia, or ACS. As pharmacological treatment options for these symptoms are severely limited, follow-up focuses primarily on providing nonpharmacological comfort measures for the person and psychosocial support for the person and family, helping the family to adapt and find new ways of nurturing their loved one as the symptoms progress.

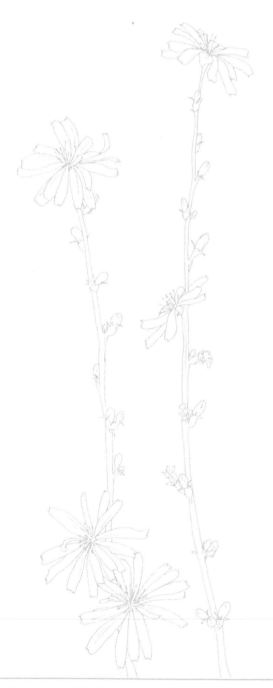

Truths of Nutrition at the End Of Life

What a patient can eat now will become less.

What a patient can drink now will become less.

Both eating and drinking will stop.

Cessation of eating and drinking is natural to the dying process, as is the fighting against it.

What is nutritionally of value at one stage is not at another.

When dying, eating food that you like becomes more important than eating food for nutritional value.

What "works" in terms of food is not necessarily either what one likes or good nutrition.

The atmosphere around eating is more important that what is ingested.

What is nutritionally right at one stage may be very wrong at another.

Aggressive nutritional therapy in advanced disease often contributes to difficulty in symptom control.

In advanced disease, food can cause more discomfort than pleasure.

(Adapted from Downing and Wainwright, 2006)

Changes in Bowel Function

Mr. Johnson was recently admitted to acute care and has end-stage heart failure and severe osteoarthritic pain in the hips and knees. Today, he advised me about his abdomen being tender and at times painful. I palpated his abdomen. It was firm and tender. He told me that his last bowel movement was four days ago and he had to strain to have only a small, hard BM that further aggravated his hemorrhoids.

Changes in bowel function, such as constipation and diarrhea, occur commonly in the last months of life. A person who experiences any of the following symptoms may be constipated: decreased frequency of bowel movements (BMs), increased hardness of the stool, or increased effort needed to pass the stool. Given that the normal length of time between BMs varies greatly from person to person, constipation may be identified after different lengths of time without passing stool.

Prevalence

People over the age of 65 with decreased mobility or decreased dietary and fluid intake or who are dehydrated are at higher risk for changes in bowel function. It is estimated that 30–100% of people receiving palliative care may be experiencing constipation (Economou, 2015). People receiving opioids are at high risk for constipation, as are people with tumors in the adominal/pelvic region who may have masses pressing on the bowels, causing changes in function.

Causes

Constipation can be caused by factors affecting the content of the bowel (e.g., changes in diet or fluid intake), the function of the bowel wall muscle (e.g., medications, obstruction, physical immobility), and the function of the bowel (e.g., tumor compression, ascites) (Fraser Health Authority, 2016c; Pallium Canada, 2013). Complications resulting from constipation include abdominal pain or discomfort, gastrointestinal symptoms such as nausea and vomiting, bowel obstruction, rectal pain, and hemorrhoids.

When a person experiences diarrhea, their large intestine is not reabsorbing water, resulting in the stools being liquid rather than solid and formed. A person may have multiple loose BMs in a day that may be accompanied by cramping and abdominal discomfort. Fluid losses with diarrhea can be severe and result in dehydration, leading to physical weakness, electrolyte imbalance, or delirium. Causes of diarrhea include medications, radiation and/or chemotherapy treatments, malabsorption of food, surgeries, infections (e.g., VRE, MRSA, C. diff.) and some cancers.

It is important to know that sometimes when a person becomes very constipated, liquid stool from behind a partial blockage can bypass a lump of hard stool (fecal impaction) lodged in the rectum, giving the appearance of diarrhea.

Pathophysiology

The colon's function is to provide a conduit for stool from the small intestine to the anus and to remove excess fluids from stool. The average transit time for the stool to move through the colon is two to three days. When stool remains in the colon longer and fluids continue to be extracted, the stool becomes drier, harder, and difficult to move. When stool passes too quickly through the colon, it is watery and unformed; the person has diarrhea (Economou, 2015; Pallium Canada, 2013).

Constipation occurs when peristalsis slows and the stool remains in the colon longer than usually, becoming increasingly dehydrated. Factors that affect peristalsis are input from the enteric nervous system, the person's intake of fluids and fiber, the person's activity level, and changes in the person's bowel routine (e.g., lack of time and privacy for defecation):

- Medications (e.g., opioids) interfere with the enteric neural input to the colon, decreasing the rate of peristalsis.
- Disease progression may decrease a person's overall activity level, which means their muscular activity decreases. Ambulation, overall movement, and contractions of abdominal muscles all contribute to initiating and promoting peristalsis. Low levels of activity mean that peristalsis is stimulated less.
- Decreased intake may affect both dietary fiber and fluid intake. The balance between dietary fiber and fluid intake helps initiate peristalsis by distending the colon walls. It also helps move stool along by maintaining appropriate consistency. An imbalance in fiber or water intake will affect peristalsis in the colon, contributing either to constipation or diarrhea.

- Decreased privacy may result when a person moves from one place of residence to another, for example, to a long-term care facility. The resulting change to a bowel routine, including insufficient time or opportunity at the appropriate time, can inhibit peristalsis. Anxiety and distress can also affect bowel function.

When the peristalsis rate increases and/or when the colon's capacity to remove water from the stool decreases, the person experiences diarrhea. Side effects of radiation and chemotherapy can damage epithelial cells of the GI tract, preventing water absorption in the colon. Digestive abnormalities as well as excessive blood in the intestinal lumen can cause diarrhea (Economou, 2015).

Assessment

Changes in bowel function can be assessed using the Victoria Bowel Performance Scale (BPS) (Victoria Hospice Society, 2009) in conjuction with the Symptom Assessment Tool adapted for changes in bowel function. Investigations will be required to confirm or identify causes of constipation or diarrhea.

Assess with the Victoria BPS

This tool provides criteria and visual images for assessing the severity of constipation or diarrhea, in comparison to the person's usual bowel movements. Figure 5 shows the assessment portion of the tool. The complete tool (see page 71 in Chapter 4, "Using Standardized Tools") includes guidelines for bowel management, as well as recommendations for intake, medications, investigations, and physical care that correspond to each score on the scale.

Figure 5. Victoria Bowel Performance Scale

VICTORIA HOSPICE

Victoria Bowel Performance Scale (BPS)

–4	–3	–2	–1	BPS Score 0	+1	+2	+3	+4
← Constipation				Normal		Diarrhea →		
Characteristics								
Impacted or obstructed +/– small leakage	Formed hard with pellets	Formed hard	Formed solid	Formed semi-solid	Formed soft	Unformed loose or paste-like	Unformed liquid ± mucous	Unformed liquid ± mucous
Pattern								
No stool produced	Delayed ≥ 3 days	Delayed ≥ 3 days	Patient's Usual	Patient's Usual	Patient's Usual	Usual or frequent	Frequent	Frequent
Control								
Unable to defecate despite maximum effort or straining	Major effort or straining required to defecate	Moderate effort or straining required to defecate	Minimal or no effort required to defecate	Minimal or no effort to defecate	Minimal or no effort required to control urgency	Moderate effort required to control urgency	Very difficult to control urgency and may be explosive	Incontinent or explosive; unable to control or unaware

Assess with the Symptom Assessment Tool Adapted for Changes in Bowel Function

Use the questions provided in this Symptom Assessment Tool adapted for changes in bowel function (Table 4) as a guide when gathering information about a person's bowel changes.

Assess Frailty and Inform Goals-of-Care Conversations

Assess the person's frailty using the CSHA Clinical Frailty Scale or the PPS. Consider using the GSF PIG, the SPICT, or tools for prognosticating one-year mortality (see Chapter 4, "Using Standardized Tools") to inform goals-of-care conversations and determine whether investigations are appropriate.

Table 4. Symptom Assessment Tool Adapted for Changes in Bowel Function

Symptom Assessment Tool Adapted for Changes in Bowel Function		
O	*Onset*	How are your bowels working? Are there problem with constipation? Diarrhea? When did you have your last BM? What is/was your normal bowel pattern?
P	*Provoking/Palliating*	What makes the constipation/diarrhea worse? Better? Is there nausea or vomiting?
Q	*Quality*	• Use the Victoria Hospice BPS to collect information on stool consistency and effort required.
R	*Region/Radiating*	Have you noticed changes in the amount of gas you are passing? • Auscultate bowel sounds and pitch in four quadrants. • Palpate abdomen for distention, bloating, asymmetry, masses, pain, discomfort. Is there pain or discomfort when having a BM? • If yes, consider a perirectal assessment for hemorrhoids or fissures.
S	*Severity*	Can you rate your constipation/diarrhea on a scale of 0 to 10? • Observe the person for signs of dehydration. What fluids have you taken in today?
T	*Treatment*	Have you used medications in the past or are you currently using medications that affect your bowels? Have you taken laxatives recently? Are you taking laxatives currently?
U	*Understanding*	What do you think is causing the problems with your bowels? How is this for you?
V	*Values*	• Ask "What are your goals and hopes for bowel management?" • Review goals of care with the person.
W	*What Else?*	• Physical assessment ○ When was last head-to-toe assessment? ○ If the person has not had a BM in three days or is leaking stool, has a rectal check been completed? Contraindications to a rectal check are severely impaired immunity, such as a very low white cell count (may occur with chemotherapy, the presence of a tumor, or impaired blood coagulation). • Relevant lab and diagnostic results • Medications

These tips may be helpful to understanding the cause of constipation and diarrhea:

- If a person expels liquid stool after a period of constipation, they may have fecal impaction in the rectum. A rectal examination may be required to assess for impaction.
- Stools passed with blood or mucus may suggest the presence of a tumor, hemorrhoids, fissures, or pre-existing colitis.
- Investigations are required to confirm or identify the causes of constipation or diarrhea.

Information Sharing

It is important for HCPs to share information with the person and their family about how constipation or diarrhea develop in the body. You can adapt the following information about how the GI tract works or provide printed information, depending on the preferences of the person and family.

How the GI Tract Works

The body processes food in the following manner:
- Food goes into the mouth, down to the stomach, and through to the small intestine, where nutrition is extracted from the digested food mass. The remaining liquidy mass moves next into the large intestine—the colon—which is the last section of the intestine. The colon works like a drying tube, removing moisture from the mass as it moves along the length of the colon. As moisture is removed, stool is formed and moved along to the rectum for evacuation. Liquid is removed from the stool as long as it remains in the colon.
- If the mass moves very slowly through the colon, the stool dries out and becomes hard, resulting in constipation. Opioids, other medications, disease, or the person's immobility can reduce motility in the colon.
- If the mass moves too quickly through the colon, too little liquid is removed, resulting in diarrhea.

The goal is to keep the mass moving through the intestines so that the stool is formed (not hard or dried out) and is easily evacuated without excessive strain.

Precautions When Using Laxatives and Stool Softeners

When laxatives are required, they must be taken regularly to keep everything moving and prevent constipation. Taking large doses of laxatives infrequently is counterproductive, as they may initiate a very unpleasant cycle of diarrhea followed by constipation.

Stool softeners are rarely effective for constipation in palliative care settings, and osmotic laxatives may make BMs very difficult to control. Stimulant laxatives, such as sennosides, are the preferred treatment.

Decisions about managing bowel function must reflect the person's goals of care. Nurses can proceed by asking questions such as these:

What are your goals for this symptom?

How often would you like to have a BM?

What is normal for you?

Is that what you would like to work toward? Is that possible?

The family can answer if the person is unable to speak or communicate effectively.

Nonpharmacological Comfort Measures

Preventing

Limited mobility and decreased dietary intake can significantly affect bowel function. If possible, include measures to address these causes (Larkin et al., 2008).

Limited mobility
Maintaining abdominal muscle strength and activity in a person with limited mobility can help prevent bowel problems. To encourage intestinal mobility, involve the person in chair or bed exercises that use abdominal muscles and require moving the legs. These may include range of motion exercises, with or without assistance, to the person's ability and tolerance.

Decreased dietary intake
When overall dietary intake decreases, insoluble fiber can be incorporated into the person's diet, but only if the person also ingests sufficient fluids. Many people approaching the end of life cannot drink enough fluids to enable fiber to work as a laxative. In such cases, fiber should be avoided, as it can make constipation worse.

When the person's energy or mobility is limited, dietary modifications and ensuring adequate fluid intake are important. When controlling urgency is an issue, providing quick and convenient access to a commode is a priority.

In the Moment

Use these strategies to provide comfort in the moment:
- Answer call bells as soon as possible.

- Provide privacy for the person, such as curtains and background noise, when the person is using the commode.
- Provide easy access to toileting facilities.
- Remove and clean the commode immediately after use.
- Assist the person with moving to and from the commode, and help to clean the person when necessary.
- Protect the person's skin from irritation.
- Use incontinence products if appropriate.
- If odour is bothersome to the person, provide air flow by opening a window or activating a fan.

With the Family

Share information with the family about:
- Ways to provide comfort (as above)
- Strategies for providing privacy when a person is using a commode in the room
- The importance of record keeping (documenting)—recording the date and quality of the person's BMs, including a description of stool

With the Care Team

Take these actions in conjunction with the care team:
- Follow bowel protocols as ordered, including recording and reporting response to treatment.
- Discuss options with the care team if the bowel protocol is not effective.
- Share assessments with the physician/nurse practitioner to discuss possible changes to medication orders.
- Follow up with the physician/nurse practitioner if constipation or diarrhea do not resolve.

Pharmacological Measures

Principles for Using Medications to Manage Bowel Function

Follow these principles for managing changes in bowel function:
- Be proactive. Remember that "the hand that writes the opioid order writes the laxative order."
- Administer medication regularly. The person may require laxatives or a bowel routine on an ongoing basis. Ensure that the agency-specific bowel protocol is being followed as ordered.

- Avoid overly complicated medication schedules by maximizing the dosage of the first-choice laxative before adding a second agent to help with constipation.
- Use the Victoria Hospice BPS (or a tool currently used in your facility) regularly to identify effectiveness of treatments.

Pharmacological Treatments for Constipation

Use pharmacological treatments to reduce constipation and increase comfort (Economou, 2015; Larkin, et al., 2008; Victoria Hospice Society, 2009).

Dietary fiber
Increase the person's intake of dietary fiber to help treat constipation by increasing the bulk in the bowel. This treatment is successful only if fluid intake is also increased and therefore is not an appropriate treatment for people unable to drink sufficient fluids.

Bowel stimulants
Administer bowel stimulant laxatives (e.g., bisacodyl) to increase peristaltic activity in the bowel. Exercise caution if you suspect the person's stool may be hard or impacted.

Laxatives
Administer laxatives to soften the stool and help with evacuation. Consider which type of laxative will work best for the person:
- **Osmotic laxatives** (e.g., lactulose): Hyperosmotic laxatives are unabsorbable compounds that remain in the colon, attracting water and softening the stool. The person may experience side effects such as cramping or abdominal discomfort.
- **Saline laxatives** (e.g., magnesium citrate): These laxatives also pull water into the colon to help soften the stool.
- **Lubricant laxatives** (e.g., oil-retention enema): This type of laxative coats the stool and may also help soften it by helping the colon retain water.

Enemas
Administer enemas to irritate and/or distend the colon to activate peristalsis in the colon.

Subcutaneous injectables
Use medications of this type (e.g., methylnaltrexone), which are highly effective for treating opioid-induced constipation. This treatment is contraindicated when a bowel obstruction is present.

Pharmacological Treatments for Diarrhea

Anti-diarrheal agents
Use medications of this type (e.g., loperamide) to slow peristalsis in a person experiencing diarrhea. Check the contraindications thoroughly and use only if indicated.

Bismuth subsalicylates
Use medications of this type to reset the fluid balance by affecting water loss and permeability throughout the intestines.

Evaluating and Confirming

Ask the person questions such as these to evaluate the treatment and confirm that it is having the desired effect:
- How is your bowel function affecting your well-being now?
- Are your goals for managing your bowel function being met?
- Does the care plan need to be adapted or updated?
- Do you need any more information about changes in bowel function and the plan for controlling it in the coming days?

Case Study

Information Sharing with the Physician/Nurse Practitioner

I am calling about Mr. Johnson. He is 54 years old, has end-stage heart failure, and has severe, bilateral osteoarthritic pain in the hips and knees. He is constipated. Here is my assessment:
- Onset: Last BM 4 days ago.
- Quality: Small, hard pellets, maximum effort to pass.
- Normal bowel pattern: Formed, minimal or no effort, regular BMs every 1 to 2 days.
- Constipation aggravates hemorrhoids, increased pain but no bleeding.
- Pain: Abdomen is tender and sometimes painful, and pain is associated with hemorrhoids and with passing firm stool.
- Decrease in gas passed in the last 4 days.
- Auscultation: Bowels active in all 4 quadrants.
- Palpation: Abdomen firm and tender to touch, no distinct masses.
- Intake has not changed. Managing food and fluids with no difficulty. Drinking 7 glasses of water per day.
- PPS currently 40%, was 50% on admission last week.
- Activity: Mainly in bed or chair but up a few times a day to go to the bathroom.
- Current medications: Sennosides 12 mg PO BID, morphine SR 15 mg PO q12h.
- Rectal check done, hard stool present in rectum.
- No recent X-ray available.

Mr. Johnson is getting very concerned and anxious about his bowels, particularly about pain with defecating and preventing constipation in the future.

Orders

The physician/nurse practitioner orders the following:
- Administer a sodium phosphate enema.
- Increase the sennosides to 24 mg BID.
- Provide ongoing assessments.

Delirium

What Is Delirium?

Shannon has always been predictable, but this person I have known and who knows me ... is unpredictable. She is agitated, she does not know me, and then she knows me. It is confusing. She looks just the same.

One minute she is clear, the next minute confused, and a few hours later clear again.

One minute she wants to stand up, and then she wants to sit down. She asks for something but is not sure what she wants. She opens her mouth to speak—she who was gifted with words—but her words are muddled.

She feeds herself, but suddenly she drops her cup. She is restless—she is awake all night ... just fussing and moving things around, and sorting papers at her desk. Then drowsy and sleeping for most of the day ... and it is difficult to wake her.

When she is awake, she is easily distracted and asking what is happening in the next room. The worst thing is that she has become paranoid. Suddenly she was scared, and she thought that I was poisoning her. She became aggressive and tried to hit me.

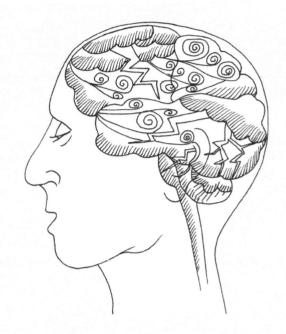

She is terrified. She sees spiders on the wall and strange creatures in the closet. She is fearful. She is terrified. What am I supposed to do? I told her I would care for her ... but I think I need to call 911. She does not feel safe here.

Delirium is an acute state of confusion that presents as a sudden, severe change in a person's cognition, affecting their awareness, attention, thinking, perception, and, subsequently, their behavior (Pallium Canada, 2013). The brain of a person who is delirious cannot send and receive information correctly (Lawlor and Bush, 2014).

The fifth edition of the *Diagnostic and Statistical Manual of Mental Disorders* describes delirium and presents the criteria used to diagnose it (American Psychiatric Association, 2000). They include the following:

- A disturbance of consciousness—reduced clarity of awareness of the environment and reduced ability to focus, sustain, or shift attention
- A change in cognition—memory deficit, disorientation, and language disturbances or the development of a perceptual disturbance that is not better accounted for by a pre-existing, established, or evolving dementia

- A disturbance that develops over a short period of time (usually hours to days) and tends to fluctuate during the course of the day
- A disturbance for which the history, physical examination, or laboratory findings provide evidence that it is caused by the direct physiological consequences of a general medical condition

Delirium is a frequent complication in the palliative setting, but recognition and documentation of delirium is low (Lawlor and Bush, 2014). It is estimated that approximately one-half of delirium episodes in people with advanced cancer are reversible. Nurses can help decrease the frequency and duration of delirium episodes by learning the risk factors for developing delirium, screening regularly to detect delirium early, and treating causes when possible (Pallium Canada, 2013).

Delirium from the Perspective of the Brain

In order for me (the brain) to work, the rest of my body parts and organs have to be working properly! When they don't do their job, that can stop me from being able to do my job. When the brain isn't working well, I appear to be confused. "Confused" means a lot of different things. It might mean I can't find the correct words, pay attention, or make good, clear decisions. It might mean I have difficulty remembering and sorting out what is in the past, the present, or the future. It might be that I am really sleepy when I am supposed to be awake, while at other times I am awake when everyone else is trying to sleep. Sometimes it makes me feel agitated and upset, and other times I am just sleepy and wonder what the fuss is all around me. I hallucinate and misunderstand what I am seeing, hearing, or experiencing. Sometimes I try to make sense of what I see, like the time I mistook the nurse for my daughter, or the time I thought the bells were the fire alarm. But other times what I see or think is happening is scary, and I feel scared. Today I saw spiders on the wall and thought that people were trying to hurt me and capture me. No one understands me. And I am afraid. I am not in control anymore.

I understand that what I experience is called "delirium." When I am in the midst of this delirium, I am completely confused, and then an hour later I am clear again. Sometimes I can remember the confusion, and other times I can't tell you anything about it.

When I ask the nurse why delirium occurs, I am told a whole list of things. But one thing that no one mentions is dying. Did you know that most causes of delirium are part of the dying process? Did you know that medications are one of the common causes of delirium? Now my body and I, we often need these medications to manage the common symptoms of dying, even though these medications can cause delirium. So as I see it, dying causes delirium.

Let me tell you why …

My body and I, we are connected. My body is sick right now. As the disease progresses through my body, my desire for food and my ability to swallow and digest food decreases. My organs, including my kidneys and liver, are not functioning well, so the toxins are building up. My heart is not doing well either, so I am low on oxygen and sometimes have too much carbon dioxide. I'm not swallowing well, so I'm low on water and energy. My metabolism is changing, and my electrolytes are out of balance. Even my immune system is weak. I get more infections—urinary tract infections and pneumonia are my constant companions. In order to do their job well, the antibiotics need a healthy immune system, so in my body they can't do their job well. I expect that at some point the antibiotics will stop working altogether!

Oh, and my bladder and bowels aren't working well, and with the side effects of medications, the bowels get constipated. Let me tell you, when the bowels are constipated, I can't see straight! The long and short of it is, you can look at the list of all the different things that cause delirium, but dying … well, dying is the "perfect storm" for delirium.

Three Types of Delirium

The three types of delirium are characterized as follows:
- **Hyperactive delirium:** The person shows outward signs of confusion, restlessness, agitation, and hallucinations. Restlessness and agitation can be verbal or motor in nature.
- **Hypoactive delirium:** The person is confused, but because the person is inactive and is sleeping more, the confusion may not be noticed. The person may appear depressed.
- **Mixed delirium:** The person may alternate between hypo- and hyperactive states, between being responsive and less responsive, awake and sleepy. For example, the person is difficult to rouse one minute and is climbing out of their bed the next (Heidrich and English, 2015).

Prevalence

The prevalence of delirium increases as people age. Approximately 1% to 2% of people over 65 years of age experience delirium. The prevalence increases to 10% among people aged 85 or older and is highest among people with dementia—22%. In addition, people who have a cognitive impairment, especially one that affects memory, who are taking multiple medications (five or more), especially psychotropic medications and sedatives, and who experience a sudden withdrawal of medications, and people who regularly use alcohol are at risk of developing delirium. The prevalence of delirium among people in residential care ranges from 1.4% to 70%, depending on comorbidities. For example, organ failure, multiple medical problems, undertreated pain, undergoing investigations, being immobilized, malnutrition and frailty, advanced cancer, sleep deprivation or disturbances, and the death of a loved one can increase a person's risk of developing delirium. Risk factors for developing delirium include being over 65 and having sensory deficits (e.g., poor eyesight or hearing), being in the intensive care unit, being hospitalized, and being in a residential or post-acute care setting (ANA, 2015b; Heidrich and English, 2015).

HCPs, including nurses, are not always able to recognize or monitor for delirium; consequently, approximately 60% of people with delirium are not identified as having delirium.

Causes

For most people, at least three factors contribute to the development of a delirium (Pallium Canada, 2013). The most common cause of delirium at the end of life is medications, (e.g., opioids, anticholinergics, benzodiazepines). Often these medications are essential for comfort and cannot be withdrawn. Metabolic insufficiency resulting from organ failure is the next most common cause of delirium. Other causes of delirium are shown in Figure 6.

The following acronym from Cancer Care Ontario (Cancer Care Ontario, 2010) may help nurses to remember common causes of delirium in the palliative setting:

D – Drugs, drugs, and more drugs! Dehydration and depression

E – Electrolyte imbalance, endocrine disorders, EtOH (alcohol) or drug abuse or withdrawal

L – Liver failure

I – Infection—urinary infection, pneumonia, sepsis

R – Respiratory problems (hypoxia), retention (urinary retention or constipation)

I – Increased intracranial pressure

U – Uremia—urinary issues (renal failure), undertreated pain

M – Metabolic disease, metastasis to the brain, medications, malnutrition

Figure 6. Causes of delirium

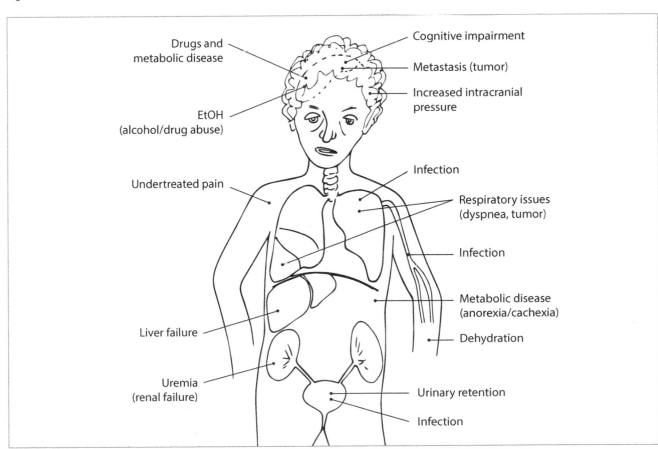

Pathophysiology

Delirium is *not* a psychological issue. Delirium is caused by pathophysiological changes in the body or brain that affect brain functioning.

Delirium is not a psychological issue, and it is not a mental health issue. It is caused by pathophysiological changes in the body that affect the brain. Imbalanced levels of neurotransmitters are implicated in delirium, causing reduced cholinergic function and increased dopaminergic and gabaergic function. Other neurotransmitter systems (e.g., serotoninergic, noradrenergic, glutaminergic, histaminergic) may also be involved. Areas of the brain affected are the thalamus and the basal ganglia, especially in the non-dominant hemisphere. Levels of neurotransmitters may become imbalanced in response to medication toxicity, metabolic toxicity, and systemic inflammation, and as a consequence of an acute stress response. Many of these processes are irreversible in the dying person.

Delirium is more likely to be reversed if it is detected early and acted on quickly, and if the causes are identified and can be treated.

Dementia and Delirium—How Are They Different?

In delirium, the brain tissue is usually intact; the changes occur elsewhere in the body and cause neurochemical changes in the brain. In dementia, the brain tissue itself is deteriorating. Table 5 shows the differences between the two conditions (Huang, 2016).

Table 5. Differences between Dementia and Delirium

Dementia	Delirium
Gradual onset	Sudden onset
Primary CNS etiology	Secondary CNS etiology
Chronic, progressive	Temporary, fluctuating
Slow decline of communication skills	Rapid decline of communication skills
Attention/alertness stable	Attention/alertness poor
Activity level preserved	Hyper-/hypoactivity
Rarely reversible	Often reversible

Reflections of a Nurse

I have learned about delirium, and I know that it is a bad thing! I have attended in-service sessions about delirium. I learned that delirium can cause debilitating complications such as dehydration, immobility due to fractures and falls, skin breakdown, infection, and potential loss of independence. I know that I am supposed to watch for delirium, screen for delirium, and treat it as an emergency. I know that early identification is often crucial to effective management. But, here is the challenge:

When the person is experiencing delirium, they may not know they have a problem, and if I do not know them, I may not know there is a problem. In addition to that, the family may be perplexed and confused themselves, not understanding what is happening. And in a busy medical unit, it is so easy for things to be missed, until the night shift. Then, during the night shift, the person does not settle and starts to walk the halls. In the morning, the person is sound asleep, and the day staff wonder what we on the night shift did to them and accuse us of overmedicating the person. I wish they would come and work the night shift on occasion!

How do I tell the difference between dementia and delirium?

I know that in palliative care, except in cases of people who are dying imminently, 60% of first occurrences of delirium may be successfully reversed. I know that subsequent deliriums are not reversed as frequently. But how do we decide whether or not to investigate when we do not have the "decision maker," when the person is no longer able to make decisions? And how can we manage the symptoms that are distressing to the person and the family? How do we help the family to have closure with the person when that person is so confused? That is the most difficult thing for me, that we no longer have the person as the primary decision maker. It is so difficult for the substitute decision makers to grasp all the complexities and possibilities and to suddenly have to step up to the plate and take on that role. It is especially difficult if they have not talked about these possibilities in advance!

Assessment

Screen with the Confusion Assessment Method (CAM)

The Confusion Assessment Method (CAM) is a screening tool developed specifically to identify delirium (VIHA, 2014). The CAM tool identifies four features of delirium:

A. Acute onset and fluctuating course
B. Inattention
C. Disorganized thinking
D. Altered level of consciousness

If the person has both A and B, plus either C or D, they should be assessed for delirium. The complete tool is in Chapter 4, "Using Standardized Tools" (see page 70).

In the case study about Shannon (see page 139), it is clear that she meets all four criteria for delirium identified in the CAM tool, which strongly suggests she is experiencing delirium. The onset of her fluctuating delirium was acute, she is unable to pay attention at times, her thinking is disorganized, and her level of consciousness is altered (her sleep-wake cycles are disturbed).

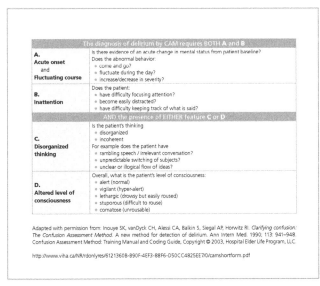

Confusion Assessment Method

Assess Frailty and Inform Goals-of-Care Conversations

Assess the person's frailty using the CSHA Clinical Frailty Scale or the PPS. Consider using the GSF PIG, the SPICT, or tools for prognosticating one-year mortality (see Chapter 4, "Using Standardized Tools") to inform goals-of-care conversations and determine whether investigations are appropriate.

Assess with the Symptom Assessment Tool Adapted for Delirium

Use the Symptom Assessment Tool adapted for delirium (Table 6) to assess it. As the person is unlikely to be able to help complete the assessment, ask the family and members of the health care team to gather information. Ask only questions that are appropriate for the person.

Investigate to Identify or Confirm Causes

Investigate underlying causes of delirium if it is appropriate to do so and consistent with the person's goals of care. Common laboratory and radiological tests may include the following: CBC, electrolytes, calcium, albumin, renal/liver function, blood cultures if sepsis is suspected, uric acid, oxygen saturation, and chest X-ray. Sometimes tests showing the brain via CT or MRI are helpful. The initial blood work and X-ray will identify infections, hypercalcemia, dehydration, and organ failure, often providing enough information to identify next steps.

Information Sharing

A family conference might be a good way to share information about delirium, the possible causes, investigations that can be done, and options for reversing the delirium and for treating its underlying cause. The case study about Shannon (see pages 139–140) highlights information sharing.

Table 6. Symptom Assessment Tool Adapted for Delirium

	Symptom Assessment Tool Adapted for Delirium	
O	**Onset**	• When was the person's confusion or delirium first noticed? • Has the person ever experienced confusion or delirium before?
P	**Provoking/Palliating**	• What seems to increase, decrease, or otherwise affect the confusion or delirium? • Recently, has the person moved in or been relocated, or experienced a significant loss?
Q **R**	**Quality/Radiating**	• Did the person's mental state change suddenly? If yes, explain. • Does the person have a normal sleep-wake cycle? If not, explain. • Is the person inattentive and easily distracted? Does the person have difficulty paying attention and following a conversation? • Is the person alert? Hyperalert? Drowsy? Stuporous? Non-responsive? • Does their level of consciousness fluctuate? Explain. • Is the person showing signs of perceptual disturbances and misperceptions, illusions, or hallucinations (tactile, visual, or auditory)? • Is the person demonstrating behaviors (e.g., picking at the air) that suggest perceptual disturbances? • Is the person expressing delusional ideas or inferring that they have such ideas?
S	**Severity**	• Is the person agitated? Hyperactive? Combative? A threat to self or others?
T	**Treatment**	• Is the person taking any medication that seems to affect confusion or level of consciousness? • Has medication been used in the past to help resolve confusion or delirium?
U	**Understanding**	• Does the family have any thoughts about what is causing this delirium? • What has the family been told about the person's condition?
V	**Values**	• Does the person or family have any beliefs or concerns specifically about delirium? • Does the person have any anxiety or spiritual distress?

W	**Physical Assessment**	• Physical assessment
		  ○ Vital signs
		  ○ Signs of fever, diaphoresis
		  ○ Chest sounds—presence of sputum
		  ○ Urinary retention/distended bladder
		  ○ Voiding—frequency, urgency, odor, urinary catheter
		  ○ Constipation
		  ○ Myoclonic twitching

Ethics Touchstone

Reflect on the family conference described in the case study about Shannon and, using critical thinking, suggest how the discussion might be different if the family were adamant about treating the infection and trying to restore their mom to her "old self." What ethical questions would this raise? What would the options be?

Case Study

Including the physician, the nurse practitioner, or both in family meetings about a person experiencing delirium can be especially helpful. Shannon's husband, Matthew, and daughter, Alicia, meet with the physician, Dr. Rajnic, and the nurse, Carmen, to discuss Shannon's delirium.

The physician welcomes everyone and identifies the reason for the meeting—to provide information so that family members understand what is happening and what steps can be taken to help Shannon.

Dr. Rajnic: Let's review Shannon's condition and talk about how she has been doing and how she is doing now.

Shannon is 85 years of age and has metastatic breast cancer, a history of mild cardiac problems for which a stent was inserted, and a long history of insulin-dependent diabetes. She is experiencing what physicians call "delirium." I understand that you are concerned about how she is functioning. We have some information to share with you about Shannon.

First of all, can you tell me what you see?

[Input from family]

Dr. Rajnic: What are you most concerned about?

[Input from family]

Dr. Rajnic: There are some decisions to make.

We need to decide how to proceed with some therapeutic options and decide on treatments. I would like to give you some information so that you can make a decision for Shannon, based on what you think she might have chosen for herself under these circumstances if she were able to speak for herself. Did you ever have conversations with her about how she might want to proceed under these circumstances?

Matthew: I know that my wife did not want to be kept alive artificially.

Alicia: My mom did want to live longer if she is going to be back to her "old self." If you can do something that will bring her back to her old normal, then we would want you to do that.

Dr. Rajnic: It's good to know that information. Let me review how Shannon is, and then let's consider those thoughts again ... First of all, she has cancer, and it has spread to her bones and lungs. She also has heart problems and a history of diabetes. These conditions complicate the treatment options. Also, she has a number of risk factors, including her age.

Some of the causes of delirium are medications, dehydration, infection, organs not functioning well, and urinary retention or constipation. According to her urine sample and her blood work, it appears that she has a urinary tract infection.

Considering Shannon's age and health, she is much more susceptible to conditions that cause delirium. We know that if we can successfully treat the urinary tract infection, then we should be able to clear the delirium. And she will return to what she was like before this particular infection.

We also know, given her history of recurring urinary tract infections in the past few months, that with all the conditions in her body she may not be able to fight the infection anymore. If that is the case, then the chances of reversing this delirium decrease.

What are your thoughts?

Matthew: Well, she is getting recurring infections, they are occurring more frequently, and I understand that the infections are harder to treat.

Dr. Rajnic: It sounds like the infection is part of her end-stage process.

Carmen: If she is not going to get better, if she is dying, what do you think we should do to keep her as comfortable as possible? What are your main priorities right now?

Alicia: Well, we want her to be ... we don't want her to have pain. How will we know if she is comfortable? We don't want her to be short of breath. We don't want her to lose her dignity. How much time do you think she has?

Carmen: So being pain free is important to her. And you have some good questions. Let's talk about those next.

Case Study

Dr. Rajnic: I understand that Shannon's strength has decreased in the past weeks, that she is getting up less and is in bed most of the time now … As her disease is advancing, she is having increased pain. In order to treat the pain, we have increased the medication. The increase in her pain medication has caused the delirium.

We can't decrease the medication if we want to keep her comfortable. We can switch her to a different pain medication. We can give her some fluids. But we cannot completely stop giving her something for the pain. So the challenge then is how to manage the delirium so that she is not agitated and is comfortable.

What are your thoughts?

Matthew: Well, she was clear that she did not want to die in pain. If you can't stop the pain medication, what can you do about her confusion … delirium?

Dr. Rajnic: We can switch her to a different medication. We can also give her fluids to help clear her system of the medication. And we can give her medication to decrease her agitation. If the delirium clears, then we can decrease the medication for the agitation and the hallucinations. If it does not clear, then the medication will make her comfortable and help her sleep.

Alicia: If she sleeps more, will she be able to talk with us? Is there anything that we can do to keep her comfortable and stop the delirium? How long do you think she has to live?

Dr. Rajnic: It sounds like the first priority is for her to be pain free. The next priority is for her to regain some clarity if at all possible, so you have a bit more time with her before she dies. Is that correct?

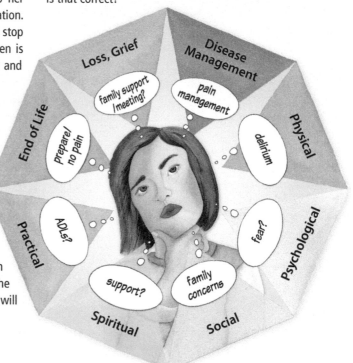

Nonpharmacological Comfort Measures

Preventing or Detecting Early

Many of the physical changes of dying (e.g., infections, dehydration, medication side effects, constipation, electrolyte imbalances) can cause delirium (ANA, 2015b; Pallium Canada, 2013). These measures may help prevent delirium:

- Provide continuity of caregivers and HCPs when possible.
- Support the person to accurately sense their surroundings by providing adequate lighting and helping them use their glasses and hearing aids.
- If the person is receiving opioids and is still swallowing fluids well, encourage the person to drink liquids to help the body excrete byproducts of the medication. Consider giving fluids by hypodermoclysis.
- Communicate using language appropriate for the person's abilities and cognition.
- Provide familiar sounds, smells, and textures that convey warmth and caring for that person. For example, lavender oil eases anxiety for many people. Reduce levels of stimuli.
- Provide music if it is helpful for the person.
- Try using guided imagery or relaxation techniques with the person, but only in the early phases of restlessness.
- Give the person something soft and comforting to hold (e.g., toy stuffed animal).

Use these strategies to detect delirium early:

- Be alert for signs of delirium. Report the delirium as soon as it is suspected or detected—do not wait for the delirium to escalate.
- Screen regularly for delirium. Monitor for acute changes in mentation.
- Record and report the person's history of delirium, as well as their history of traumatic themes that emerge in dreams.
- Differentiate delirium from "transitional talk" (see the discussion of "final gifts" and "nearing death awareness" in Chapter 7, "Caring in the Last Days and Hours").

In the Moment

During delirium, the person is not able to direct their own care, cannot manage their own safety, and may be in an altered state of consciousness. Consider the following strategies to help provide comfort and decrease the severity of delirium in a person (ANA, 2015b; Heidrich and English, 2015).

Ensure safety
Keep the person safe with these measures:

- Remove objects that the person could use to harm themselves or others (e.g., scissors, knives, sharp tools, medications).
- Keep the side rails of the bed down and lower the bed if the person keeps trying to get out of bed on their own. If necessary, use hip pads or place a mattress on the floor beside the bed to reduce consequences of a fall.
- Report immediately if a delirious person shows signs of harming themselves or others.
- Avoid physical restraints, as these may increase a person's physical aggression and compromise safety. Consider alternative strategies such as these:
  - Using a motion-sensor alarm or in-room camera to monitor the person
  - Removing or camouflaging tubes and catheters when possible if these upset the person.

Attend regularly to general care needs
The person is less likely to communicate their general care needs verbally when experiencing delirium. Nurses can provide support by regularly attending to these needs, such as providing support for toileting, providing mouth care, and ensuring hydration with sips of fluid if the person can swallow.

Manage agitation immediately
Agitation is a common symptom accompanying delirium (hyperactive delirium), although withdrawn behaviors (hypoactive delirium) can also occur. Remember that an agitated person is suffering. Ensure that you minimize discomfort; for example, help if the person needs to void, provide a breakthrough dose of medication if the person is in pain, and so on. Report if agitation does not decrease.

Provide constant observation
Use companions—trained or untrained volunteers or family members who "sit with" the person experiencing delirium (Carr, 2013). Sitters can reassure the person in the moment, as well as monitor the person and report changes in behavior and the delirium.

Ensure appropriate communication
Delirium affects the person's ability to speak and to understand language. Supporting a person with delirium requires that you speak in simple, clear, short sentences. Be patient when speaking, ask one question at a time, and wait for an answer before proceeding.

Orient the person to reality
Explore the dying person's reality to determine what they are experiencing. If possible and appropriate, orient them to reality. If the person is in a "happy place," it may not be necessary to orient them to the current reality.

Reassure the person
Delirium will make it difficult for the person to remember and understand what is happening. You can help them through the difficulties of delirium by reminding them frequently that they are not alone. Say, for example,

I am here with you. I will make sure you are safe.

Support the person during hallucinations
Hallucinations can terrify a person. You will need to work to understand what the person is experiencing and then reassure them that you are there to help. Acknowledge the person's feelings:

I don't see the spiders, but I know that you see them and I am here to help make them go away.

You can also help in these ways:

- Use calming phrases such as "I know this is frightening for you. I am going to help you through."
- Ask "What are you seeing, hearing? What are your worries about this?"

- Try to gently orient the person to reality if possible (remember that the delirium experience is the person's reality).

Encourage relaxation

Helping a person with delirium to relax can be comforting and provides a break for the family. Offering these comfort measures may help the person relax:
- Warmed blankets
- Soft items (e.g., toy stuffed animal, soft fleece blanket)
- Reiki, massage, or Healing Touch
- Favorite music
- Aromatherapy

For the Family

A loved one's delirium can be frightening for family members to witness, and the family may need as much support as the dying person to understand the experience of delirium. Anticipate that families will be experiencing grief (feeling the loss of who the person was), especially if symptoms are not resolving and the person's condition declines despite attempts to treat it. You can help the family by:
- Listening to their concerns and recording these to inform the health care team
- Providing a space for family members to nap and regain their strength during the delirium or after the person settles
- Providing warm blankets or other comfort items

The family may also want to talk with the nurse about themes that come forward in the delirium, or may have questions for the nurse or health care team about the differences between delirium and predeath awareness. Prepare yourself to answer these questions, and know how to refer the family to sources of more information.

Delirium and Final Gifts

It is not uncommon for people who are near death to "see" loved ones who have previously died. In their book *Final Gifts: Understanding the Special Awareness, Needs, and Communications of the Dying*, Callanan and Kelley refer to this as "predeath awareness" (Callanan and Kelley, 1993). It is different from hallucinations and is not considered delirium. More information on predeath awareness is available in Chapter 7, "Caring in the Last Days and Hours."

Following Delirium

When the delirium has settled, it may be possible to talk with the person and hear about what they remember from the time they had the delirium. It may be helpful to explore the themes that surfaced during the delirium. You may want to consider the concept of suffering associated with delirium and the concept of total pain.

Continue to assess and prevent delirium in these ways:
- Monitoring frequently. A sitter may be required to ensure that the person will stay settled in order to avoid injury or harm.
- Limiting noise, visitors, bright lights, and mirrors (which can distort images for the person).
- Avoiding changes and keeping familiar items within sight and reach.
- Monitoring hydration, nutrition, and swallowing.
- Maintaining skin integrity if the person has limited mobility, by regularly repositioning.
- Mobilizing the person to move as much as they are able.

Pharmacological Measures

Pharmacological measures may treat the causes of delirium and help to control the symptoms (ANA, 2015b; Heidrich and English, 2015; Pallium Canada, 2013).

Treat the Cause

If investigations have successfully identified a cause or causes of delirium, consider using the treatments shown in Table 7 to manage it. Ensure that treatments meet the person's goals of care.

Table 7. Causes and Treatments for Delirium

Cause	Treatments to Consider
Opioid toxicity	Change opioids
Sepsis	Start antibiotics
Drugs	Stop the offending medications
Dehydration	Provide fluids
Urinary tract infections	Administer antibiotics and remove the urinary catheter if appropriate
Hypercalcemia	Provide artificial hydration, then bisphosphonates
Hypoxia	Provide oxygen

Manage the Symptom

Medications can help manage symptoms of delirium, such as paranoia, agitation, hallucinations, and insomnia. Depending on the cause of the delirium and its severity, the medications required to manage the symptom may cause the person to be less alert and may even decrease responsiveness.

The person's goals of care will direct the physician/nurse practitioner, health care team, and family when they make decisions about medications. Consider the care plans in these two scenarios:

My dad just wants to be comfortable. He does not want any further tests or treatments.

Dad was clear this morning and he wants to live for the anniversary party this weekend. I think it is important to him for this delirium to be investigated and treated if possible.

Neuroleptic (antipsychotic) medications such as haloperidol are used to reduce moderate to severe agitation or psychotic symptoms associated with delirium. These medications may reduce the suffering of the person, enable investigations and treatments to proceed, and prevent the person from hurting themselves or others (Canadian Coalition for Seniors' Mental Health, 2006). These medications are used in lower doses than in the psychiatric setting; therefore, they cause fewer extrapyramidal side effects. Assess the person using the CSHA Clinical Frailty Scale (see Chapter 4, "Using Standardized Tools") when considering which medications to use.

The medications used to manage a particular symptom differ depending on the physician/nurse practitioner, community, and country. It matters less whether the physician/nurse practitioner chooses this medication or that medication, this dose or that dose. What matters most is that the person becomes comfortable. You may want to consult with a palliative care consultant for additional pharmacological strategies (Pallium Canada, 2013; Cancer Care Ontario, 2010).

Primary neuroleptic medications used to manage delirium include:

- Haloperidol—the first medication of choice because it is the least sedating
- Methotrimeprazine and chlorpromazine—more sedating than haloperidol, which can be advantageous if the person needs sedation to settle
- Loxapine—prescribed for very elderly and frail people and much less sedating than haloperidol or methotrimeprazine but also less effective

Newer neuroleptic medications are used when the prognosis is longer than a few days, because they have fewer extrapyramidal side effects. These medications include olanzapine, quetiapine, and risperidone.

Benzodiazepines (lorazepam, midazolam) often contribute to delirium and consequently are rarely used when a person has delirium; however, if used in conjunction with routinely administered neuroleptics, benzodiazepines may help control delirium (Pallium Canada, 2013).

Additional pharmacological options include using corticosteroids to reduce swelling if brain metastases are present, rotating opioids to help reduce or reverse opioid neurotoxicity, and hydrating the person to help flush out the buildup of metabolites.

Treating Unresolved Delirium

When the health care team is not able to control delirium, contact the palliative care consultant for additional support.

If the delirium cannot be reversed, that could indicate the person is entering the final stages of life. If the person is dying, the HCPs should meet with the family and inform them that the person is dying (Bush et al., 2014).

Palliative sedation may be considered if the person is dying imminently and the delirium cannot be treated. The goal is to provide sedation to the point where the person is comfortable. If the person is receiving pain medications, they are continued in conjunction with the sedative. Refer to your organizational policy on palliative sedation to better understand its use in your facility.

Dyspnea

The following story of difficult breathing is typical of people who have chronic obstructive pulmonary disease (COPD) or congestive heart failure (CHF).

Karl is a 77-year-old man who was diagnosed with COPD 10 years ago. In the past four months he has been in hospital three times for exacerbation of the COPD. He is declining in strength and has lost nearly 20 pounds. Karl is very short of breath when he exerts himself, is no longer able to care for himself, and requires help with bathing. He is on oxygen full-time, 3L/minute, and refuses to leave the house because doing so is too difficult with the oxygen. At night he sleeps in the recliner chair because it is difficult to sleep lying flat in bed. Tonight he became very short of breath again and called the ambulance to take him to emergency. When admitted, he expressed fears about the difficulty he is experiencing with breathing and stated that he is not sure what is happening and why he is not getting better.

What Is Dyspnea?

Dyspnea is the sensation of struggling to breathe. Dyspnea is what the person says it is; it is a subjective experience and cannot be measured solely on the basis of objective signs (Pallium Canada, 2013). People who have a life-limiting respiratory illness cite dyspnea as one of the symptoms they fear the most. Dyspnea can be distressing for the person experiencing it and for the family to witness. However, this symptom can be effectively managed.

Prevalence

Occurring primarily in people with pulmonary diseases, dyspnea is experienced by 95% of people with COPD and by 61% of people with CHF, the two leading causes of death in adults. Among people with lung cancer, 70% report dyspnea, as do 50% of people with amyotrophic lateral sclerosis (ALS). Dyspnea also affects 70% of people with dementia and 37% of people who have suffered a stroke. As weakness and fatigue increase with advancing illness, the risk and severity of dyspnea increase too (Dudgeon, 2015; Pallium Canada, 2013).

Causes

Dyspnea is triggered when the structure or function of the lungs or the exchange of gases is compromised. In a person with advanced disease, dyspnea, like many other symptoms, can have more than one cause. Figure 7 shows the causes of dyspnea, and Table 8 lists observable characteristics of dyspnea (Cancer Care Ontario, 2010; Downing and Wainwright, 2006; ELNEC, 2015).

Pulmonary Causes

A person may experience dyspnea when their lungs are compressed or restricted when expanding, or when gas exchange is inhibited. Causes include tumors, cardiomegaly, and superior vena cava syndrome that compress the lungs; edema, COPD, fatigue, muscle weakness, bronchitis, embolism, emphysema, and fibrosis that decrease lung capacity by restricting expansion of the lungs; and pneumonia or fibrosis that decrease gas exchange.

Cardiovascular Causes

Issues that diminish the heart's capacity to pump blood, such as CHF, coronary artery disease, and increased pulmonary artery pressure, can cause dyspnea. When the blood flow to the lungs decreases, gas exchange decreases and less oxygen is transported into the blood and to the tissues.

Neuromuscular Causes

Dyspnea may occur as a consequence of living with chronic life-limiting diseases, such as ALS, which weaken muscles and limit air movement. Disease treatments may cause temporary dyspnea, such as in chemotherapy-induced anemia, or chronic dyspnea, such as reduced lung capacity after lobectomy. Heart treatments, such as digoxin toxicity, or radiation pericarditis may also result in dyspnea. In some instances, pain can exacerbate dyspnea.

Life-limiting illnesses such as dementia cause fatigue, which results in muscle weakness that contributes to dyspnea. As the body works harder to function, the overall work of breathing becomes more difficult and dyspnea begins.

Figure 7. Causes of dyspnea

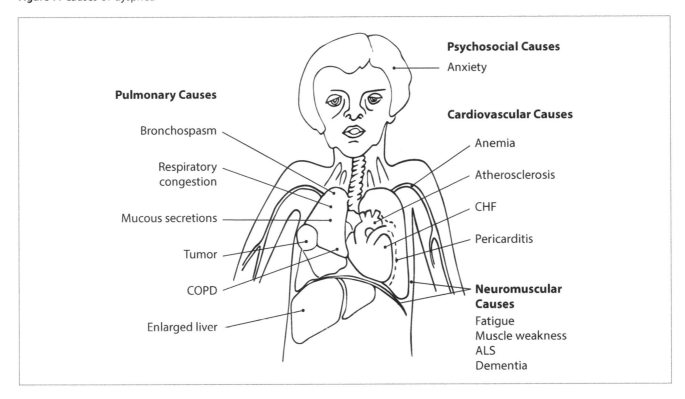

Psychosocial Causes

Psychosocial factors such as anxiety and panic episodes can cause rapid shallow breathing and the sensation of dyspnea. Shortness of breath is a frightening experience and can precipitate anxiety, which in itself will affect breathing.

(Downing and Wainwright, 2006; ELNEC, 2015)

Experiencing Dyspnea—an Activity

Dyspnea is a subjective experience defined as "What the person says it is." Experience it with this exercise!

Materials
One plain drinking straw

Procedure
1. While seated, put the end of the straw in your mouth, seal your lips around it, pinch your nostrils closed, and breathe using only the air from the straw for one minute.
2. Continue to pinch your nostrils closed and breathe only through the straw, but now increase your activity by walking around the room, slowly at first, and then at a faster pace. Discontinue pinching your nose and remove the straw from your mouth after one minute.

3. Breathe deeply and allow your breathing to return to normal.

Reflection
1. How do you feel now that you are not breathing through the straw?
2. Describe the experience of breathing through the straw. Did you feel that you were getting enough air? What words would you use to describe how you felt?
3. Most people feel relieved at being able to breathe so easily when the exercise ends. What might it feel like to have airways that always limited your air intake, affecting your activities of daily living?
4. What might it feel like to experience limited air intake suddenly, without warning and without knowing the cause?

Pathophysiology

Dyspnea is the sensation of breathlessness produced as an integrated response from the respiratory centers, located in the medulla and pons of the brain stem (Buchanan and Richerson, 2009; Burki and Lee, 2010; Dudgeon, 2015). These centers are activated by signals from the following:

- Mechanoreceptors in the upper or lower airways, lung parenchyma, or chest wall that signal increased work of breathing. Input to these receptors comes from stretched breathing muscles (diaphragm and intercostal), increased resistance to lung inflation, higher airflow, and increased interstitial and capillary pressure.
- Chemoreceptors located in blood vessels and the medulla of the brain stem, which signal changes in carbon dioxide, oxygen, and pH levels in the blood. This information is sent from the central and peripheral nervous systems to the respiratory centers. The sensation of breathlessness is triggered primarily when central chemoreceptors detect rising levels of carbon dioxide and notify the respiratory center that ventilation is inadequate. That dyspnea is triggered when carbon dioxide levels are elevated explains, in part, why supplemental oxygen might not diminish the sensation of dyspnea.

Both the chemoreceptors and mechanoreceptors send signals to the respiratory centers via respiratory muscle through vagal afferents. The centers respond by changing the depth and rate of respiration in order to meet the body's needs.

It is noteworthy that three descriptive qualities are now firmly linked with dyspnea: "air hunger," "work," and "tightness" (Dudgeon, 2015). These three terms may represent three distinct origins of dyspnea, with air hunger indicating insufficient ventilation, work reporting increased rate of, depth of, or impediment to breathing, and tightness signaling bronchoconstriction.

Assessment

"The only reliable measure of dyspnea is the patient's self-report" (Pallium Canada, 2013). It is essential to accept the person's assessment of dyspnea, regardless of whether objective physical measures corroborate this symptom (Dudgeon, 2015). People who may not appear dyspneic might report dyspnea as one of the symptoms of greatest concern for them.

People often use different terms, such as "breathless," "suffocating," "choking," "gasping," or "out of breath," to describe how they are feeling. They may not recognize their problem as being a breathing problem; they may just consider they are "weak" or "tired." When asked about their breathing, they may reply, "Oh I am just so out of breath when I do anything." A person may answer negatively to the question "Are you short of breath?" because they have limited their activities sufficiently that they are not short of breath. Ask instead "Are you short of breath when walking? Doing activities? Eating?" as a way to determine whether dyspnea is a problem.

Characteristics of Mild, Moderate, and Severe Dyspnea

Table 8 describes the observable characteristics of mild, moderate, and severe dyspnea. Note the progression of breathing difficulty, changes in talking with and without pauses, and the appearance of cyanosis as the severity of dyspnea changes. The descriptors in this table may help you to identify a person who may be having trouble breathing and to describe their experience when documenting and reporting.

Table 8. Observable Characteristics of Dyspnea

Severity of Dyspnea			
Mild	**Moderate**	**Severe**	
Person's Symptoms • Breathing not labored • Talks without pausing • No cyanosis • Can sit or lie with no short-ness of breath (SOB) • Worsens upon exertion Dyspnea is: • New or chronic • Intermittent or persistent	Person's Symptoms • Breathing is mildly difficult but not labored • Pauses while talking, q30 secs • No cyanosis • Worsens with walking or exertion; decreases partially with rest Dyspnea is: • New or chronic • Usually persistent	**Progressive Severe Dyspnea** Person's Symptoms • Breathing is labored when awake and asleep • Pauses while talking, q15–30 secs • +/– Cyanosis • Anxiety is present • Often wakes suddenly with dyspnea • Cough is often present • +/– New confusion • Worsens over a few days to weeks Dyspnea is: • Acute or chronic	**Sudden Severe Dyspnea** Person's Symptoms • Breathing is labored • Pauses while talking • Cyanosis is present • Has high levels of anxiety and fear • Is agitated • +/– Congestion • +/– Chest pain • +/– Diaphoresis • +/– Confusion Dyspnea is: • Sudden onset

(Cancer Care Ontario, 2010; Downing and Wainwright, 2006)

Screen for Dyspnea with the Edmonton Symptom Assessment System

Use the Edmonton Symptom Assessment System (ESAS) (see Chapter 4, "Using Standardized Tools") to screen for dyspnea when you suspect a person is experiencing breathing problems or the person reports feeling breathless. If the person is not able to complete the ESAS alone, the family may be able to share their observations of the person's shortness of breath and difficulty breathing.

Assess with the Symptom Assessment Tool Adapted for Dyspnea

When a person is identified as experiencing difficulty with breathing, use the Symptom Assessment Tool adapted for dyspnea (Table 9) to complete a thorough assessment. This tool provides specific questions for assessing dyspnea and identifying possible causes. As with other symptoms, choose a selection of questions from each section, and do not use questions that are redundant or do not apply.

Be aware that a person's dyspnea may interfere with their ability to answer questions. If they are experiencing an episode of dyspnea, you may need to complete a thorough assessment after you have implemented a few comfort measures.

When you want to understand about the work and the effort of breathing, you may want to use the word "exertion" instead of "breathlessness." Similarly, when you want to understand more about the fatigue related to breathlessness, you may want to substitute the word "fatigue" for "breathlessness."

Table 9. Symptom Assessment Tool Adapted for Dyspnea

		Symptom Assessment Tool Adapted for Dyspnea
O	*Onset*	When did the breathlessness begin? Is this a new experience or has this happened before? Did it begin suddenly or slowly?
P	*Provoking/Palliating*	What makes the breathlessness worse (e.g., lying down)? Is any specific time of day worse or better (e.g., morning, end of the day)? How does breathlessness affect your daily activities and functioning (e.g., dressing, moving about, conversing)? Can you identify any triggers of breathlessness (e.g., standing, exerting yourself, specific feelings, spiritual or emotional stresses, new scents or smells)? What helps relieve your breathlessness? Resting? For how long? Does using pillows, taking a certain position (e.g., sitting up), using oxygen, or having fresh air help with the breathlessness? How does your breathlessness affect your ability to sleep?
Q	*Quality*	How do you feel (e.g., gasping, choking, drowning) when you experience breathlessness?
R	*Region/Radiating*	Where does the breathlessness seem to originate? Does your breathlessness cause any other symptoms? Do you have any chest pain? Is the breathlessness related to a cough, fever, chest tightness, palpitations, nausea, light-headedness, COPD, heart failure, arrhythmias, or anemia? How does your breathlessness affect your ability to care for yourself and to participate in activities?
S	*Severity*	Can you rate the severity of your breathlessness when you are at rest on a scale of 0 to 10, with 0 being no symptom and 10 being the worst experience of breathlessness you can imagine? Can you rate the severity of your breathlessness when you are moving? Have you ever had a similar experience of breathlessness?
T	*Treatment*	Are there any recent treatments (e.g., radiation) that could be causing your breathlessness? Do you take any medications (e.g., steroids, antibiotics, opioids) to help decrease breathlessness?
U	*Understanding*	What do you think is happening when you experience breathlessness?
V	*Values*	In terms of your breathlessness, what level of comfort are you hoping for? What is your goal?

W	*What Else?*	• Physical assessment
		  ○ Check vital signs (e.g., blood pressure, pulse and respiratory rate [one full minute]).
		  ○ Auscultate lungs and upper airways. Are there breath sounds or grunting at the end of expiration?
		  ○ Observe for use of accessory muscles (e.g., use of clavicle muscles on inspiration, abdomen moving in on inspiration).
		  ○ Observe for cough, sputum, pedal edema.
		  ○ Measure oxygen saturation with an oximeter.
		  ○ Observe for gasping, pausing in conversation, nasal flaring.
		  ○ Observe the effect of dyspnea on the person's ability to speak, walk, or perform an activity.
		  ○ Observe for restlessness.

Assess Changes in Dyspnea Using the Clinical COPD Questionnaire

The Clinical COPD Questionnaire (CCQ) (see page 69 in Chapter 4, "Using Standardized Tools") is a well-established assessment tool that provides the HCP with information about the person's comfort level, their ability to tolerate activities, their experience of dyspnea itself, and their response to treatment (van der Molen, 1999).

Clinical COPD Questionnaire

Assess Frailty and Inform Goals-of-Care Conversations

Assess the person's frailty using the CSHA Clinical Frailty Scale or the PPS. Consider using the GSF PIG, the SPICT, or tools for prognosticating one-year mortality (see Chapter 4, "Using Standardized Tools") to inform goals-of-care conversations and determine whether investigations are appropriate.

Investigate to Identify or Confirm Causes

The person's goals of care will help the physician/nurse practitioner and the health care team determine which tests are most appropriate to help identify or confirm the cause of dyspnea. The physician/nurse practitioner may order the following investigations:

- Chest X-ray to rule out pneumonia, collapsed lung, or masses in lungs
- Blood work, including CBC, to measure hemoglobin to check for anemia, WBC count to check for infection, and electrolyte levels to evaluate renal function
- Spirometry test to evaluate how much and how effectively the person can hold air in their lungs and empty air out of their lungs
- Electrocardiogram to check the heart muscle and determine if there has been a cardiac event
- Less common investigations, such as a CT of the chest, bronchoscopy, and blood gases

As with all symptoms, it is essential to record your assessment and report when further assessment or intervention is required. With dyspnea, it is imperative to respond immediately when the person is struggling to breathe. Severe dyspnea is a crisis and requires an urgent response.

Nonpharmacological Comfort Measures

Remember that dyspnea is what the person says it is and cannot be measured by objective tools alone. The person is the expert. When managing dyspnea, clarify the person's hopes and goals for this symptom, and then personalize a plan of care (Dudgeon, 2015; Pallium Canada, 2013).

Preventing

Use these strategies to prevent dyspnea:
- Move slowly when providing care. Do not rush!
- Teach the family about the benefits of pacing activities, ways to manage breathlessness, controlling breathing, and breathing exercises, as well as relaxation and distraction techniques as appropriate.
- Pace activities by:
  - Ensuring that there is sufficient time for activities, including travel to and from locations
  - Providing breathing stations where the person can pause and sit when they are short of breath
  - Ensuring that the person has sufficient time to recuperate between activities.
- Work with the person to plan the day's activities: determine the person's priorities and focus on these.
- Encourage the family to provide as calm an environment as possible.
- Prevent constipation, as the person may become more breathless if they have to strain.
- Identify and record early signs of dyspnea that require medical, pharmacological, or nonpharmacological

interventions as a means to prevent or minimize episodes of respiratory distress.

- Review the information on the comfort basket (see page 118) in this chapter to explore or identify ways to increase comfort.

Manage the environment

Use these strategies to manage the environment:
- Identify triggers that cause dyspnea for this person, such as movement, scents, emotions, and exertion.
- Ensure that the person's living space is kept free of perfume and other scented products.
- Suggest that the person wear or provide the person with non-restrictive clothing that is loose around the neck and chest.
- Provide sufficient airflow to reduce the sensation of dyspnea.

In the Moment

Know that a person who is experiencing difficulty breathing may feel frightened or anxious. Offer a calming presence and validate the person's experience. Reassure the person that you will stay with them until they feel better. Responding quickly with nonpharmacological comfort measures can decrease the discomfort of dyspnea and limit the severity of the dyspneic episode. After the acute dyspnea has been managed, identify and record comfort measures that were helpful.

Try these strategies to decrease dyspnea in the moment:
- Direct the person to stop any activity.
- Guide or move the person to a position (e.g., sitting upright with arms raised in front of the body and resting on pillows or a table) that maximizes lung space and respiratory function while reducing physical effort.
- Coach the person to help slow their breathing (see "Coaching a Person Experiencing Difficulty with Breathing" on this page).
- Encourage people with COPD to use pursed-lip breathing, which slows the respiratory rate and helps keep small alveoli from collapsing.
- Open a window or provide a fan to increase airflow on the person's face.
- Provide moist air for a distressing cough. Saline may help loosen thick secretions that may be blocking the airway.
- Provide a cool moist cloth to freshen the person's face and allow them to better feel the airflow.
- Be a calm and gentle presence.

Coaching a Person Experiencing Difficulty with Breathing

You can offer a gentle, supportive presence, a calm voice, and an invitation to focus on your eyes as you model how to breathe more slowly and deeply. Following these instructions when coaching a person with dyspnea can be an effective way to decrease their dyspnea and may also help you manage your own stress:
- Provide a gentle and supportive presence.
- Reposition the person so they can maximize their lung capacity.
- Open a window or turn on a fan if possible.
- Kneel or bend close to the person. Gently touch under the arm or elbow if appropriate.
- Look into the person's eyes and, using a calm and gentle tone, coach the person to breathe with you:
  Look into my eyes ... focus on my eyes, my breathing ...
  Breathe with me ...
  That's right, breathe in, and out ...
  Your breathing is getting deeper, slower ...
  The oxygen is reaching to the tips of your fingers and the ends of your toes ...
  I am with you, and will stay with you until you are comfortable ...
  Your breathing is getting slower ...

When Dyspnea Has Settled

Talking with the person and the family once the dyspnea has settled can help them understand the experience and learn how to prevent dyspnea and respond should another episode of dyspnea occur. Consider these strategies:
- Teach the person and the family relaxation exercises.
- Consult with health care team members such as a physiotherapist, respiratory therapist, palliative care consultant, or specialist regarding disease or symptom management.
- Provide the family with information about pacing activities, managing breathlessness, controlling breathing, breathing exercises, relaxation techniques, and distraction, as appropriate.
- Connect the person with their spiritual leader or community to help address questions and anxiety, and/or to provide measures to manage dyspnea, such as prayer or meditation.

The Huffing/Coughing Technique

The huffing/coughing technique helps the person remove sputum from their lungs with less effort than normal coughing. It saves the person's energy and helps prevent infections caused by an increase of sputum in the lungs. Invite the person to use the technique, as described below:

1. Seat yourself in a comfortable position.
2. Lean your head slightly forward.
3. Place both feet firmly on the ground.
4. Inhale deeply through your nose.
5. Exhale in short, non-forceful bursts while keeping your mouth open, as if you were trying to make a mist on a window.
6. Repeat once or twice.

(Living Well with COPD, 2008)

Pharmacological Measures

While implementing nonpharmacological comfort measures to reduce dyspnea, collaborate with the health care team about pharmacological measures to treat the underlying disease (if appropriate) and manage the sensation of dyspnea. Use the SBAR tool to communicate assessment findings and goals of care when consulting with the physician/nurse practitioner.

Acute treatments might include antibiotics, chest physiotherapy, radiation or chemotherapy, pleural tap, abdominal paracentesis, and blood transfusions. Keep the person's goals of care in mind when considering such interventions.

Nurses and other HCPs can help maintain the person's airways by:
- Scheduling medications to reach optimal blood levels when they are needed, for example, having the person use their inhaler at least 15 minutes before an activity, and providing opioids sufficiently early to be effective during activity
- Checking the person's inhaler technique to ensure medication is being delivered appropriately

The physician/nurse practitioner and other members of the health care team will consider disease progression when changing medications and exploring whether to treat underlying causes of dyspnea. Medications that might be helpful include bronchodilators to decrease bronchospasm, diuretics to decrease fluid volume related to CHF,

steroids to decrease weakness and inflammation, and oxygen to relieve hypoxia. If dyspnea is still not relieved after these medications are added or doses are adjusted, then opioids, phenothiazines, and anxiolytics may be required. In the last days and hours, when the person's goals of care may be focused on symptom management alone, the opioids, phenothiazines, and anxiolytics may be the primary medications used to manage the symptom.

Opioids

Opioids can effectively treat dyspnea caused by cancers, COPD, heart failure, ALS, and renal failure. Twycross and Wilcock suggest that "early use of opioids, rather than hastening death in dyspneic patients, might actually prolong survival by reducing physical and psychological distress and exhaustion" (Twycross and Wilcock, 2001).

Opioids are believed to relieve dyspnea by:
- Reducing the sensitivity of the carbon dioxide receptors in the respiratory centers, thereby diminishing the sensation of breathlessness
- Binding to airway opioid receptors to relax the airways, thereby decreasing air pressure and the work required for breathing, and diminishing the mechanoreceptor messages sent to the respiratory centers about dyspnea
- Increasing oxygenation of the heart by causing cardiac vasodilation, thereby decreasing the chemoreceptor signals sent from the aorta about dyspnea

Finding the optimal dose and schedule for opioids

The frequency and dose of the opioids administered will depend on the frequency and severity of the dyspnea. For example, if dyspnea is persistent, then the person will require regular, around-the-clock opioids. If the dyspnea increases, the person will require an increase in the dose.

Pallium Canada and the End-of-Life Nursing Education Consortium (ELNEC) provide similar guidelines for managing dyspnea with opioids (ELNEC, 2015; Pallium Canada, 2013). The case studies on pages 152 and 153 provide examples of opioid orders for a person who has lung cancer who is receiving opioids but needs an increased dose, and for an opioid naive person with COPD.

Medications to manage dyspnea are usually administered orally. If the person is in distress, the subcutaneous delivery route results in quicker absorption. Remember to decrease the opioid dose by half when switching from oral to subcutaneous delivery.

Non-Opioid Medications

Phenothiazine, for example methotrimeprazine, can be used to manage the anxiety and agitation that often accompany shortness of breath. Phenothiazines should not be used for managing dyspnea unless used in combination with opioids.

Anxiolytics, such as lorazepam or alprazolam, can be used to treat anxiety that often accompanies the experience of dyspnea. The anxiolytic is not given routinely unless anxiety is a key issue.

Oxygen Therapy

Some people believe that oxygen is needed to relieve dyspnea. However, many people who experience breathlessness are actually able to take oxygen into their lungs and have sufficient oxygen in their blood (Fraser Health Authority, 2009). As discussed in the section on the pathophysiology of dyspnea, breathlessness is caused by many factors, and an insufficient amount of oxygen is only one. While practices may vary in different jurisdictions and health care settings, providing supplemental oxygen is primarily helpful for a hypoxic person experiencing shortness of breath, whose blood oxygen saturation is 88% to 90% or less. According to Cancer Care Ontario, "Supplemental oxygen is not recommended for non-hypoxic patients experiencing dyspnea" (Cancer Care Ontario, 2010).

Even when oxygen levels are low, proceed cautiously when using oxygen for people who retain carbon dioxide, such as people with COPD. In these people, oxygen may increase carbon dioxide retention, causing increased drowsiness, headaches, and, in severe cases, a lack of respiration, which may lead to death.

When a person is actively dying, introducing oxygen therapy with either a mask or nasal prongs may cause the person distress. Being present and explaining the normal changes in breathing to the family may be more helpful.

Palliative Sedation Therapy

When attempts to gain control over a person's dyspnea in an acceptable time frame for the person fail, and if the person is nearing death, palliative sedation may be an option, depending on the policies of the facility and setting. See Chapter 7, "Caring in the Last Days and Hours," for more information about palliative sedation therapy.

Case Studies

The following case studies highlight how the physician/nurse practitioner's order for opioids may differ depending on the diagnosis and whether or not the person is opioid naive. A care plan follows the two cases and illustrates the commonalities in the nursing care.

Case Study: Opioid Naive Person with Lung Cancer

Kaz is a 74-year-old man with lung cancer who has experienced increasing shortness of breath with exertion for the past three weeks. Today he rates his dyspnea at 2 to 3 out of 10 when he's at rest, and at 6 out of 10 with exertion. He struggles to provide personal care, and finds walking to the bathroom difficult. A thorough assessment is completed, and the physician/nurse practitioner is notified of Kaz's discomfort. In collaboration with Kaz, the physician/nurse practitioner adds opioids to the current medications and proceeds to investigate the cause of the increase in dyspnea. Kaz is opioid naive.

Orders

The physician/nurse practitioner orders the following:
1. Give morphine 2.5 mg PO q4h.
2. Give morphine 1.25 mg PO q1h PRN for BTD.

Case Study: Opioid Naive Person with COPD

Maggie is 74 years old and frail, has COPD, and has experienced increased shortness of breath over the past three weeks. She has no difficulty with shortness of breath at rest, but rates dyspnea at 2 to 3 out of 10 when doing any personal care, at 6 out of 10 when walking, and at 8 out of 10 if she is not able to stop and recover after short bursts of exertion.

Maggie has never taken opioids before. Until now she has been hesitant to take opioids because of concerns about the side effects. Today she is increasingly uncomfortable and has asked the physician/nurse practitioner for morphine.

The fact that she is frail, has COPD, is opioid naive, and is very concerned about taking opioids is reviewed again in a meeting with the physician/nurse practitioner and Maggie. She agrees to a trial of a very low dose of opioids, which will be increased very slowly and reassessed regularly. She is clear that she will keep taking the medication only if she does not experience side effects.

The physician/nurse practitioner follows the protocol from the Canadian Thoracic Society's practice guideline "Managing Dyspnea in Patients with Advanced Chronic Obstructive Pulmonary Disease" (Canadian Thoracic Society, 2011). This is a very cautious approach that is appropriate considering Maggie's disease process, her concerns, and her goals of care.

Orders

The physician/nurse practitioner orders the following:
- Give morphine 0.5 mg PO q12h for two days.
- Follow this by giving morphine 0.5 mg PO q4h when awake for four days, and then re-evaluate.
- Assess regularly, and monitor for side effects.

Care Planning for Both Case Studies

The care plan for the two preceding case studies is as follows:
1. Complete a thorough assessment and assist with investigations.
2. Integrate nonpharmacological comfort measures into care.
3. Reassess one hour and three hours after administering medication.
4. If dyspnea is not improved or if it recurs before the next dose, provide a breakthrough dose (if ordered) and notify the physician/nurse practitioner.
5. Monitor bowel patterns, follow bowel protocol, and prevent constipation.

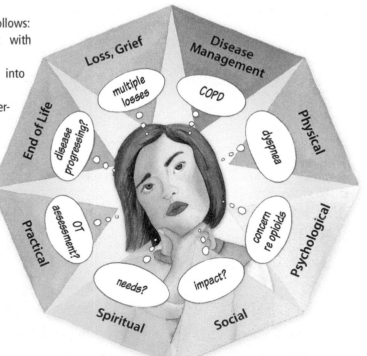

Ethics Touchstone

Provision 4

The nurse has authority, account-ability, and responsibility for nursing practice; makes decisions; and takes action consistent with the obligation to pro-mote health and to provide optimal care.

Code of Ethics for Nurses (ANA, 2015a)

What are your beliefs about using opioids to manage dyspnea? Do you have any fears or concerns?

What are the guidelines or protocols for managing dyspnea in your workplace?

What guidelines does your organization follow for managing dyspnea?

If you are afraid of administering a breakthrough dose of opioids to manage dyspnea, what are your options? Who could you consult with?

Given how distressing dyspnea can be for the person, it is important to evaluate to confirm the effectiveness of the comfort measures and pharmacological treatments being used. When the causes or triggers of dyspnea are being evaluated, it will be necessary to continue evaluating the frequency of dyspnea episodes to determine whether preventive measures are addressing the causes. Remember that dyspnea is a subjective experience and that it exists when the person says it does, regardless of any objective measurements (e.g., oxygen saturation).

Ethics Touchstone

Part I:D. Preserving Dignity, 4

Nurses question and intervene to address unsafe, non-compassionate, unethical or incompetent practice or conditions that interfere with their ability to provide safe, compassionate, competent and ethical care to those to whom they are providing care, and they support those who do the same.

Code of Ethics for Registered Nurses (CNA, 2008)

How might you address professional practices or conditions that interfere with a person's symptom relief and other goals of care?

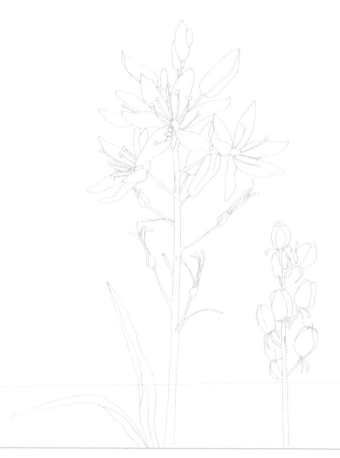

Fatigue

Energy is such a funny thing—it feels like it just drains right out of me. It is like I have just a tablespoon of energy, and when it is gone, instead of filling up quickly, it might take a day resting to recover. It is like the tap refueling me only refills a drop at a time.

Yetta Lees

What Is Fatigue?

Fatigue has been described as "feeling tired" or "having less energy than normal," and it affects a person's physical, emotional, and mental energies. As a symptom it varies in intensity depending on the illness, does not resolve with rest, and generally intensifies as the illness progresses and death nears (Ingleton and Larkin, 2015; O'Neil-Page, Anderson, and Dean, 2015). Because fatigue affects all aspects of living, it has a great effect on the person's quality of life (Yennurajalingam, 2016). However, because it is considered a non-urgent symptom, fatigue is often not reported or managed effectively (O'Neil-Page, Anderson, and Dean, 2015).

Prevalence

Early in a person's decline, fatigue is often the symptom that motivates a person to see their doctor. Among people receiving treatment for cancer, fatigue may partially resolve when treatments are successful. With chronic progressive illness, fatigue is one of the most common and most prevalent symptoms among people receiving hospice and palliative care (Yennurajalingam, 2016). It affects people with cancer (80%–90%), cardiac diagnoses (99%), COPD (96%), renal failure (82%), and HIV/AIDS (69%) (O'Neil-Page, Anderson, and Dean, 2015).

It's now 8 a.m. I've been asleep since nine o'clock last evening. I was used to getting up at 6 a.m. every morning. Now that I have the luxury of being able to sleep in later, you'd think I'd be happy. I'm not. Even though I have an easy sleep most nights, when I wake up I don't feel refreshed. In fact, I often lie there for several minutes wondering how I'll push myself out of bed. I'm finally able to get out of bed, but I need to drag myself into the kitchen to get a glass of juice then return to my nice comfortable bed. It seems to me that someone has drained all my energy from my body. But I push myself and manage to get dressed, although that leads to the need to take another period of rest."

(Dwyer, 2016)

Causes

Fatigue has many causes (Table 10) and is manifested in the body in many ways. In end-stage cancers, pro-inflammatory cytokines induced by illness or treatments cause neuro-hormonal changes, which in turn affect adrenal hormones and cause fatigue. Anemia initially may be a major contributor to fatigue, but its influence decreases as illness progresses, and disease processes, treatment factors, psychosocial factors, and personal factors contribute to the person's sense of fatigue. When asked, people identified unresolved pain, lack of sleep, and side effects of treatments as contributing to their fatigue.

Table 10. Causes of Fatigue

Disease Process	Psychosocial	Side Effects	Sleep	Personal Factors
• stage of illness • comorbidities • anemia • pain • dyspnea • anorexia • cachexia	• depression • fear • anxiety • distress • conflicts relating to family, culture, and ethnicity	• medication side effects • treatment side effects—surgical, chemotherapy, or radiation side effects	• disorders • disturbances resulting from illness	• age • marital issues • financial stress (e.g., lack of health insurance, lack of or difficulty with the support system)

Pathophysiology

An explanation of fatigue that fits all diseases and all stages of decline has not been defined. There are two theories—the depletion hypothesis and the accumulation hypothesis—that are equally valid for certain types of fatigue (O'Neil-Page, Anderson, and Dean, 2015). In the depletion hypothesis, essential ingredients for muscle activity are not available, resulting in fatigue. In the accumulation hypothesis, waste products are suggested to collect and exceed the body's capacity for disposal, resulting in fatigue. A third model, the central peripheral model, suggests an imbalance of control between the CNS and the reticular activating system, which would apply to illnesses such as multiple sclerosis. Still other research suggests dysregulation of the immune system and inflammatory cytokines as potential causes. It is possible that each of these models explains aspects of fatigue that are unique to specific diseases (O'Neil-Page, Anderson, and Dean, 2015).

Assessment

A person experiencing fatigue may present some or all of these characteristics:
- Be unable to complete activities of daily living (ADLs) and other tasks
- Spend increased time in bed
- Start a task but not be able to complete it
- Feel distressed with limited activities
- Withdraw
- Refuse visitors
- Lose interest in activities

Screen for Fatigue with the Edmonton Symptom Assessment Scale

When the ESAS returns a score greater than zero for fatigue, proceed by assessing the person for causes of fatigue.

Assess with the Symptom Assessment Tool Adapted for Fatigue

When fatigue is suspected, use the Symptom Assessment Tool adapted for fatigue (Table 11) to help identify causes and treatment options.

The most effective measure of the severity of fatigue is the verbal rating scale, whereby the person experiencing the fatigue assigns a value to the fatigue they are currently experiencing (O'Neil-Page, Anderson, and Dean, 2015).

Assess Frailty and Inform Goals-of-Care Conversations

Assess the person's frailty using the CSHA Clinical Frailty Scale or the PPS. Consider using the GSF PIG, the SPICT, or tools for prognosticating one-year mortality (see Chapter 4, "Using Standardized Tools") to inform goals-of-care conversations and determine whether investigations are appropriate.

Investigate to Identify or Confirm Causes

Reversible or treatable causes of fatigue may include:
1. Mood disorders (e.g., depression and anxiety)
2. Cognitive disorders (e.g., delirium)
3. Physical changes
   - Pain
   - Anemia
   - Infections
   - Metabolic disorders
   - Malnutrition
   - Sleep changes
   - Weight changes
   - Deconditioning

Investigate untreated pain as one cause of fatigue, as sleep changes and deconditioning would all be affected by pain. Blood tests may be able to rule out infections, anemia, and metabolic disorders. A dietary history may be able to determine whether malnutrition or weight changes are causing fatigue. Assessing psychosocial issues may also provide insight into a person's fatigue.

Table 11. Symptom Assessment Tool Adapted for Fatigue

		Symptom Assessment Tool Adapted for Fatigue
O	**Onset**	What changes in energy have you noticed? When did you first notice decreased energy?
P	**Provoking/Palliating**	What makes you more tired? What makes you feel less tired? What helps restore your energy? Is there anything that I can do to help you accomplish your priorities for today?
Q	**Quality**	How does fatigue affect what you do? How do you feel?
R	**Region/Radiating**	Are there any places in your body that feel more fatigued than others? If so, what are they?
S	**Severity**	If 0 is no fatigue and 10 is the worst fatigue you can imagine, how would you rate it right now?
T	**Treatment**	Has anything helped with fatigue in the past?
U	**Understanding**	What do you think is causing the fatigue?
V	**Values**	Are you concerned about being tired? What is your goal for this symptom? How can I help you today?
W	**What Else?**	• Physical exam as needed

Nonpharmacological Comfort Measures

Providing relief from fatigue may include strategies to reserve energy for highly desirable activities, and increasing comfort to enhance rest and sleep.

Preventing

Acknowledge fatigue as a valid symptom

Talk about fatigue with the person. Acknowledge that feeling so tired can be frustrating and can limit what one can do. You might explore how the person would like to use their energy, for example, by saying,

We are here to help so you can use your energy on things that are most important to you ... to provide support for activities of daily living to help conserve your energy.

Conserve the person's energy by planning

Encourage the person and their family to plan the day's activities in a manner that recognizes the person's energy levels. When the person finds it more difficult to restore their energy, conserving energy by planning activities will be the best method for reducing fatigue. Consider using these strategies:

• Plan the day's activities and treatments according to the person's energy needs and preferences. You might ask,

Do you want me to give you your bath in the morning or the evening?

Do you want to go out when you are more alert and energetic in the morning?

• Plan visiting hours for the time of day when the person's energy is at its best.
• Offer to limit visitors when the person appears fatigued.
• Postpone activities that are not important or critical.
• Help the person to listen to their body and learn when it is saying it needs to rest.

Trial mild exercise and physiotherapy

Exercise has been found to increase energy levels but is more likely to be helpful earlier in the disease process (O'Neil-Page, Anderson, and Dean, 2015). The person might be able to trial some gentle activity to find out if it is helpful or adds to the fatigue. Physiotherapy may relieve muscle or joint pain and reduce fatigue.

Distract the person and encourage restorative activities

Passive experiences such as listening to music, riding in the car, and sitting outdoors can distract a person from fatigue. Some people may find it restorative to be in nature, by going to a park or visiting the ocean or a lake. Participating in quiet, restorative activities such as prayer, yoga, and meditation may also help with fatigue. Remember to individualize distraction methods to meet the needs of the person.

Offer psychosocial interventions, as appropriate

Cognitive behavior therapy has been quite successful at reducing the person's report of fatigue and increasing their sense of vigor and vitality. Counseling and disease-specific group therapy have also been moderately successful at reducing the person's report of fatigue (Kangas, Bovbjerg, and Montgomery, 2008).

In the Moment

When a person is too tired to continue their planned activities, consider the following options:
- Reschedule treatments and activities.
- Offer to limit visitors.
- Offer a meal in bed so the person doesn't have to move to the table.
- Arrange for small snacks rather than a full meal.
- Offer to invite family members to help with ADLs if appropriate.

Be aware of the effects your energy has on the person. There are times when being positive and cheerful is helpful, and there are times when it may add to the person's distress with their lack of energy.

For the Family

Talk with the family about fatigue and how it will increase as the illness progresses. Listen to their concerns. The family may think that fatigue is caused by medications. If you hear concerns, record and share them with the health care team to help determine goals of care and adapt the care plan. Ask the family for ideas to assist the person when they feel fatigued.

If the family wants to be involved, and if appropriate, invite family members to participate in supporting the person in their ADLs. Discuss how to achieve a balance between assisting and doing for, as determined by the person's level of fatigue.

Help family members plan their visits and chats for times that the patient is more energetic.

As the nurse, you may share information about drowsiness that occurs when starting opioids and about the increasing fatigue, weakness, and sleeping that occur as death nears. You might say, for example,

> *It is normal for people to be drowsier for a few days after starting an opioid and for a few days after an increase in opioids. This side effect usually wears off in a few days.*

On Being with Mum When She Was So Weak

It was hard when I saw her sitting with her head dropping.
Was that really MY Mum?

It was good to help her walk.
Just letting her hold my elbow.

The day she wanted to go to the beach.
We helped her into the car and out of the car.
And she sat on the park bench looking at the water.
It was her last outing.

Bringing her tea.
Making her really comfortable with pillows. We did what we could.

We knew it was the end, the last Christmas, the last breakfasts, she wanted to teach us to make Bouillabaisse!
We did everything we could. We made a slide show,
Pictures of her family and friends
changed quietly on their own,
no effort to watch or to ... not watch.

Sitting giving her a foot rub.
And thinking
"What would she like?
What can I get for her?"
We did what we could.

And you were so good at lying down with her,
so that she did not feel alone.
We did what we could.

Barbara Lees

Pharmacological Measures

Managing fatigue is a combination of treating the causes and symptoms (Table 12). The majority of research on fatigue has focused on managing cancer-related fatigue. These treatments will be most useful early in the illness and may become less effective as the illness progresses.

Table 12. Pharmacological Measures for Treatable Causes of Fatigue

Treatable Cause	Treatment
Anemia	Transfusions or erythropoietin therapy
Deconditioning	Light exercise (e.g., yoga, walking with a small aerobic component)
Depression	Antidepressants (e.g., SSRI, especially if disrupted sleep is a contributing factor)
Infections	Antibiotics
Hypoxia	Oxygen therapy
Metabolic disorders	Replacement therapy (e.g., thyroid replacement for hypothyroidism)
Insomnia	Sleep training, trial of immediate-release hypnotics
Pain	NSAIDS

(Adapted from Yennurajalingam, 2016)

When a treatable cause has not been identified, fatigue may be relieved temporarily using these medications:
- Corticosteroids
- Emerging therapies such as thalidomide, methylphenidate or modafinil, melatonin, fish oil

Evaluating and Confirming

Managing fatigue will be an ongoing process that may require trialing different treatments as the person's illness progresses. Nurses will need to carefully evaluate each nonpharmacological and pharmacological strategy to help the person reduce their fatigue as much as possible through their illness. As each person is unique, the nurse will need to evaluate and confirm which strategies work best for each person.

Case Study

Mr. Jackson is lying on his bed. He is a quiet 79-year-old male, living in a small room in an assisted living home. He was accepted to the palliative care program two weeks ago. He tells the nurse,

No, I'm not tired—I had plenty of sleep. But I just don't have the strength to get out of bed this morning.

The nurse helped him sit up in his chair and brought him breakfast from the dining room.

When the nurse returned 15 minutes later, breakfast remained untouched and Mr. Jackson was lying on his bed beneath the blankets.

Information Sharing

Situation: I am with Mr. Jackson. Today he insisted that he was not tired but wanted to stay in bed due to no strength.

Background: He is a quiet 79-year-old male with advanced cancer with metastasis to the spine. His PPS is 50%.

Assessment

Onset: He says he woke with this feeling of extreme tiredness. He has no idea when it started.

Provoking: When I asked what brought on the tiredness, he said: "All I did was open my eyes and I was exhausted!"

Quality: N/A

Region/Radiating: N/A

Severity: Unable to rate. Mr. Jackson says, "I have nothing to compare it to."

Treatment: N/A

Understanding: Mr. Jackson says he has no understanding of this at all.

Values: Mr. Jackson says he would cry, but he is too tired. He does not know what is happening to him. He says he has never been this weak in all his life, but he does not feel he can do anything at all about it.

Request/Recommendation: Could you do some blood work to assess for possible causes of his fatigue?

Dry Sore Mouth

I asked if she had any pain. She replied, "No I don't have any pain, but I can't swallow because my mouth and throat are so sore."

Prevalence

Dry sore mouth affects between 30% and 50% of people receiving palliative care (Dahlin and Cohen, 2015) and can be a significant cause of pain. It is interesting that the person in the story above denied having any pain and yet had such a sore mouth and throat!

Causes

Dry sore mouth occurs when salivary secretions decrease. The dryness may be a side effect of medications (e.g., sedatives, antidepressants) or treatments (e.g., radiation, chemotherapy). The lack of moisture in the oral cavity causes cracks, sores, and open areas in the lips, corners of the mouth, tongue, throat, and esophagus. These can be a source of excruciating pain and may decrease a person's willingness to talk and eat.

Among causes to consider are:
- Poorly fitting dentures
- Dental caries (cavities)
- Contaminated toothbrush or dentures
- Toothbrush with hard bristles
- Side effects of many medications
- Dehydration
- Poor nutrition (associated with decreased intake)
- Spicy, salty, or citrus-based foods
- Anxiety and depression
- Compromised immune system leading to thrush

"Mucositis" refers specifically to a painful side effect of cancer-related chemotherapy and radiotherapy treatment wherein the mucous membranes anywhere along the GI tract become painfully inflamed and ulcerated. The term "oral mucositis" refers only to inflammation and ulceration present in the mouth.

Pathophysiology

Salivary secretions are essential for moistening the mucous membranes of the mouth, for helping mix food for swallowing, and for speaking. When salivary secretions are diminished or absent, the exposed tissues become dry and less flexible, and are prone to cracking and ulceration.

Assessment

Assess with the Symptom Assessment Tool Adapted for Dry Sore Mouth

Use the Symptom Assessment Tool adapted for dry sore mouth (Table 13) to assess for causes, selecting and adapting the questions to best suit the person.

Table 13. Symptom Assessment Tool Adapted for Dry Sore Mouth

		Symptom Assessment Tool Adapted for Dry Sore Mouth
O	*Onset*	When did you notice that your mouth was sore? Have you had this problem before?
P	*Provoking/Palliating*	Is there anything that makes the pain worse? Better? Does it hurt to eat? To drink? To brush your teeth?
Q	*Quality*	Can you describe the discomfort? How does this symptom affect you?
R	*Region/Radiating*	Where in your mouth and throat do you feel the pain? • Look for any changes, asymmetry, sounds, and areas that are sensitive to touch.
S	*Severity*	On a scale of 0 to 10 in which 0 is no pain and 10 is the worst pain imaginable, how would you rate your mouth pain?
T	*Treatment*	Have you ever taken medication for your mouth pain? Did it help? Is there anything else that helps?
U	*Understanding*	What do you think caused the sore mouth?
V	*Values*	What would you like done to help decrease the pain? What can I do to help you with this symptom?
W	*What Else?*	• Assess medications as possible causes of dry mouth.

Information Sharing

Share information with the person and their family about known causes of dry sore mouth as they pertain to the assessment, and about possible comfort measures and treatment options.

Nonpharmacological Comfort Measures

Providing mouth care regularly will help prevent mouth dryness and sores. The preventive mouth care strategies discussed below are useful for all people receiving supportive care and are especially important for those at high risk for developing thrush infections (e.g., during and after radiation or chemotherapy, and when receiving steroids). Focus on hydrating and lubricating the mouth in people at risk of experiencing dry mouth, such as those with limited intake or who are in their last days and hours.

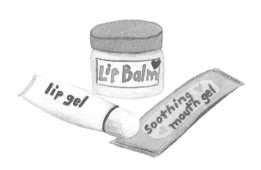

Preventive

These mouth care strategies can help prevent dryness that leads to sores, cracking, and bleeding:
* Provide mouth care before and after the person eats.
* Remove the person's dentures before providing mouth care.
* Gently brush or wipe the mucosa to remove plaque and debris.
* For people resisting mouth care, use creative strategies to complete the task (e.g., distract them with singing, talking, gently touching).
* If the person has a thrush infection, soak their dentures and toothbrushes in a vinegar or disinfectant solution to prevent spreading the infection.
* Use a soft toothbrush and, if necessary, a specialized toothpaste.

In the Moment

In addition to using the mouth care strategies listed above, if the person's mouth is dry, use these strategies to hydrate and lubricate:
* Offer water or other drinks frequently.
* Spray the inside of the person's mouth with cold water.
* Offer ice chips wrapped in a clean washcloth to moisten the mouth.
* Offer a slightly thawed frozen juice.
* Offer pineapple chunks, sour candies, or chewing gum, as tolerated, to help increase salivary secretions.

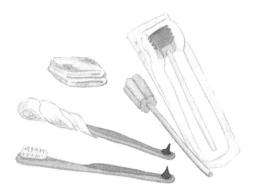

When a person cannot manage their own mouth care, use these strategies:

- Moisten their mouth mucosa gently using packaged or homemade mouth swabs.
- Offer liquids to rinse their mouth, such as water, salt water, diluted germicidal mouthwash, or soda water.
- Apply lubricant to the oral mucosa, using a swab, after the mouth has been cleaned and rinsed.
- Apply lip balm after applying the lubricant (use water-based products if the person is receiving oxygen).
- Use a humidifier in the room to moisten the person's dry airways.

With the Family

Invite the family to participate in mouth care as one way to support their loved one. Remind them to use gloves if the person has a thrush infection.

Pharmacological Measures

Medications may be necessary for pain relief, to prevent or treat infections, and to encourage healing. The delivery mode of topical treatments varies, depending on the medication; they may be of the "swish and swallow" or "swish and spit" type. Consult with the physician/nurse practitioner when a person is not able to swallow or spit. It may be necessary to "paint" medication on with mouth swabs or to squirt medication onto the inside of the person's cheeks using a syringe.

Medications that may help with mouth pain are:
- Oral gel containing a topical anesthetic suitable for internal use
- Acetaminophen
- Topical xylocaine or lidocaine for canker sores
- Anti-inflammatory medications for open mouth sores
- Prednisone for open mouth sores
- Nystatin for thrush

Evaluating and Confirming

A dry sore mouth can severely restrict the activities of the person and significantly affect their comfort. Remember the causes of mouth dryness and the fact that not all causes can be eliminated.

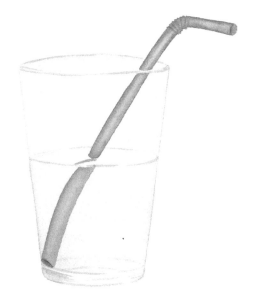

Nausea and Vomiting

As I was doing rounds for afternoon shift, I found Mrs. Lim at the side of her bed, vomiting partially digested food. She looked at me, gagged, and said, "Can you do something to stop this?"

What Are Nausea and Vomiting

People may describe nausea as queasiness in their stomach, an urge to vomit, or an uncomfortable sensation in the back of their throat. Vomiting is the observable forceful expelling of the person's stomach contents by the abdominal muscles and diaphragm. Following vomiting, the person may experience a lack of appetite and the bad taste of emesis in their mouth. A person may vomit without feeling nauseated and be nauseated without vomiting.

Nausea and vomiting are common symptoms that occur as a disease progresses and may accompany pain or anxiety. While nausea or vomiting may be ongoing, people report these symptoms as being slightly bothersome to profoundly distressing, overwhelming, or intolerable. For many people, nausea or vomiting may severely impair quality of life. Some people claim, "I would rather be in pain than be nauseated!"

Prevalence

Nausea and vomiting occur often in people with cancer, affecting 21–68%, depending on the type of cancer and comorbidities. Among people living with chronic illness, nausea occurred in 2–48% of the population, the percentage also depending on comorbidities. Nausea is much less prevalent in people living in residential care, affecting 1–8% of the population, increasing to 17% in the last two days of life. Nausea and vomiting are reported most often in people who are less than 65 years of age, female, and receiving medications, have a GI tract obstruction, or have cancer in the stomach, breast, or brain (Chow, Cogan, and Mun, 2015; Pallium Canada, 2013).

Causes

The most frequent causes of nausea and vomiting in hospice and palliative care situations are gastric irritation (often due to medications), intestinal obstruction, metabolic imbalance, infection, constipation, and brain metastases (Figure 8) (Fraser Health Authority, 2006). A person receiving hospice and palliative care may also be dealing with more than one cause of nausea and vomiting. Therefore, managing these symptoms may take considerable time, and resolving them may require more than one anti-emetic.

Pathophysiology

The brain contains a loose assembly of neurons called the integrative vomiting center. These neurons work together, receiving input from multiple body locations to determine when to initiate or stop nausea and vomiting. Stimulating or repressing neurons and receptors that provide input to the integrative vomiting center can cause or reduce nausea and vomiting (Chow, Cogan, and Mun, 2015; Fraser Health Authority, 2006).

There are four main causes of nausea and vomiting that are signalled through specific pathways to the integrative vomiting centre:

1. **Changes in cerebrospinal fluid and blood:** The chemoreceptor trigger zone (CTZ) in the brain detects and signals the integrative vomiting center about foreign chemicals (e.g., opioids), unusual metabolite levels, uremia, signs of infection, and radiation metabolites.
2. **GI tract issues:** Sympathetic nerves in the GI tract signal GI irritation, blockages, constipation, and so on to the integrated vomiting center.
3. **Changes in the vestibular apparatus:** Located in the inner ear, the vestibular apparatus sends signals about imbalance, labyrinth disorders, and cerebellar tumors. In vestibular disorders, nausea may occur when the body or the head moves (e.g., when the person rolls over, stands up, turns the head).
4. **Sensory input to the central nervous system (CNS) or CNS issues:** The cerebral cortex sends signals about previous experiences with nausea and vomiting and can be triggered by sights, odors, tastes, feelings, and emotions related to previous events. The cerebral cortex may also indicate the presence of CNS issues, such as increased intracranial pressure, and is also the origin of anticipatory nausea that can occur prior to therapy or appointments that cause the person discomfort.

In addition to the causes identified above, nausea and vomiting, especially in women, can be a sign of a heart attack. Remember this when assessing possible causes.

Figure 8. Causes of nausea and vomiting

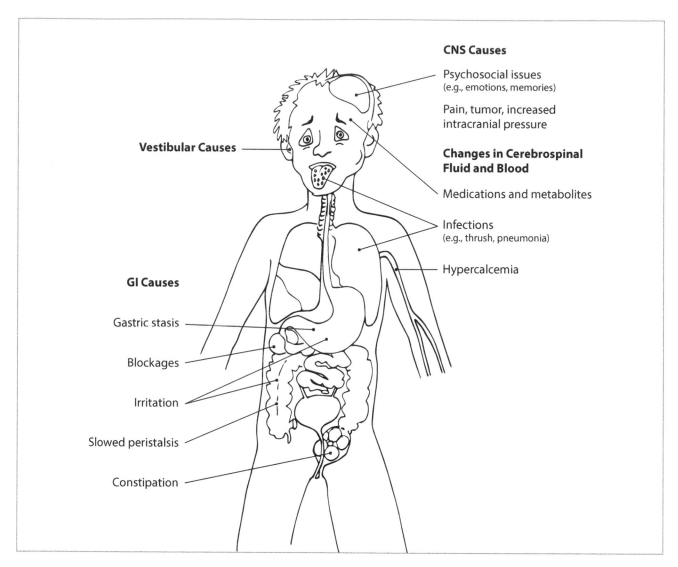

CNS Causes

Psychosocial issues
(e.g., emotions, memories)

Pain, tumor, increased
intracranial pressure

**Changes in Cerebrospinal
Fluid and Blood**

Medications and metabolites

Infections
(e.g., thrush, pneumonia)

Hypercalcemia

Vestibular Causes

GI Causes

Gastric stasis

Blockages

Irritation

Slowed peristalsis

Constipation

Assessment

Screen for nausea or vomiting using the ESAS when completing a thorough assessment. Follow up when a person says they are nauseated, or on any indications or reports of nausea or vomiting, as well as after an intervention.

Assess with the Symptom Assessment Tool Adapted for Nausea and Vomiting

Use the Symptom Assessment Tool adapted for nausea and vomiting (Table 14) to guide you through a thorough assessment and help you to identify possible causes. Choose a selection of questions from each section, and do not use questions that do not apply.

Assess Frailty and Inform Goals-of-Care Conversations

Assess the person's frailty using the CSHA Clinical Frailty Scale or the PPS. Consider using the GSF PIG, the SPICT, or tools for prognosticating one-year mortality (see Chapter 4, "Using Standardized Tools") to inform goals-of-care conversations and determine whether investigations are appropriate.

Table 14. Symptom Assessment Tool Adapted for Nausea and Vomiting

	Symptom Assessment Tool Adapted for Nausea and Vomiting	
O	**Onset**	When did you start feeling nauseated? When did you start vomiting? How long do the nausea and vomiting last?
P	**Provoking/Palliating**	What triggers the nausea and vomiting? How many times a day do nausea and vomiting occur? What decreases the nausea and vomiting? Is there a pattern to when they occur?
Q	**Quality**	Can you describe the vomiting (e.g., projectile, presence of nausea with emesis)? Can you describe the emesis, such as its odor (e.g., like fecal matter?), color (e.g., like fresh blood?), and consistency (e.g., like coffee grounds?)? Are there related problems? Are you able to eat or drink anything? When did you last eat? Drink? Are you belching or passing gas? Do you have any problems with swallowing? When was your last bowel movement (BM)? Have you used any laxatives recently? Can you describe your stool, the effort needed to have a BM, and its form and firmness?
R	**Region/Radiating**	Do you have pain associated with the nausea and vomiting (e.g., abdominal pain, discomfort, or tenderness)? • Check for bowel sounds (e.g., absent, hypoactive, hyperactive, high-pitched). • Palpate the abdomen and note any bulges or distention. • Observe for asymmetry.
S	**Severity**	Can you rate your nausea (or vomiting) on a scale of 0 to 10, with 0 being no nausea/vomiting and 10 being the worst nausea/vomiting you have experienced. You can also use the words "mild," "moderate," or "severe." • Check for signs of dehydration.
T	**Treatment**	Have you used any medications in the past or do you use them now to treat nausea or vomiting? Have you experienced any side effects from medications in the past? Have your medications been changed recently?
U	**Understanding**	What do you think is causing the nausea and vomiting? Can you describe how being nauseated feels to you? How do you feel when you vomit?
V	**Values**	What are your goals for the nausea and vomiting? On a scale of 0 to 10 measuring nausea and vomiting, where would you like the nausea and vomiting to be? Do you want to reflect on your goals of care overall? Do you have any changes in your hopes or expectations?
W	**What Else?**	• Physical assessment 　○ Assess rectum for stool. 　○ Assess person for changes in cognition. 　○ Inspect oral cavity—thrush? 　○ Check vital signs—any fever? 　○ Listen to lungs—signs of infection? • Other relevant findings 　○ Recent lab and diagnostic results—changes over the past days/weeks?

Tips for Identifying Possible Causes of Nausea and Vomiting

Specific causes will often produce characteristic types of nausea and vomiting. Consider each of these causes when the person presents these characteristic types of nausea and vomiting:

- **Response to new medications:** The person vomits within minutes or hours of starting a new medication.
- **Gastric stasis:** The person eats breakfast in the morning, eats a small amount of lunch at noon, and then vomits undigested breakfast and lunch a few hours later.
- **Constipation:** The person may have decreased intestinal motility due to constipation, leaving food sitting in the stomach, which may contribute to nausea.
- **"Squashed Stomach Syndrome":** This may be caused by a tumor pressing on the stomach, giving the person an immediate feeling of fullness. The person is able to eat only a few spoonfuls of food and then feels full.
- **Bowel obstruction:** The person may experience cramping, be unable to tolerate any food, and, depending on where the obstruction is, may vomit emesis that has a fecal odor.
- **Coughing:** After coughing, the person may experience a gag reflex, which can lead to vomiting.
- **Metabolic abnormalities:**
  - **Hypercalcemia:** The person experiences severe nausea and vomiting, accompanied by an altered level of consciousness, which may include confusion and/or drowsiness. Hypercalcemia is diagnosed by elevated corrected serum calcium levels.
  - **Renal failure:** The person's urinary output is decreased and the urine highly concentrated.
  - **Hepatic failure:** The person has a jaundiced appearance.
  - **Dehydration:** The person's intake is decreased, and the person is vomiting and has poor skin turgor, decreased urine output, and concentrated urine.
- **Anticipatory nausea:** The person becomes nauseated before an event (e.g., undergoing further chemotherapy, having visitors).
- **Psychological concerns:** The person may be anxious or fearful of events or symptoms.
- **Increased intracranial pressure:** The person feels a headache (due to a brain tumor, infection, or meningitis) and vomits without feeling nauseated.

Investigate to Identify or Confirm Causes

When symptoms of nausea and vomiting occur, the physician/nurse practitioner may order blood work (e.g., complete blood count, electrolytes, liver panel), X-rays, and medical imaging to further understand or confirm causes. For example, blood work can identify if the person has hypercalcemia, has fluid and electrolyte imbalances, or is experiencing kidney or liver failure. An abdominal X-ray may identify severe constipation, and medical imaging might identify a bowel obstruction.

Information Sharing

Share information with the person and the family about the process the health care team is following to identify causes of and manage nausea and vomiting.

Be sure to talk about medications commonly used to treat nausea and vomiting, and help the person and family understand that the person will need to take the medications regularly and around the clock. Explain that if the nausea and vomiting have more than one cause, controlling these symptoms may take a few days. Share with them that the initial focus will be to stop the vomiting, and then it will be to stop the nausea. Explain that the person will need to keep taking the medication as long as the cause of the symptom continues. However, if the person is experiencing nausea and vomiting as side effects of taking opioids, he or she may adapt to the medication and no longer need the anti-emetic.

Use the SBAR tool in Chapter 4, "Using Standardized Tools," to share the assessment with the care team.

If nausea and vomiting are new symptoms, the person's goals of care may need to be reviewed. If the cause of nausea is constipation, the discussion may focus on adjusting the laxatives to ensure regular bowel movements. However, if the person appears to have a bowel obstruction or hypercalcemia, the person and family will need to understand more about the possible causes, the investigations needed to determine causes, and treatment options available. With this information the person and family can review goals of care and, with the support of the care team, decide which investigations and treatments will best meet the person's goals.

Step-by-Step Approach to Managing Nausea and Vomiting
1. Stop the vomiting.
2. Stop the nausea.
3. Restart fluids.
4. Restart solids.

The care team will strive to identify the likely causes of nausea and vomiting, and select the appropriate interventions and medications that will target those causes. If the person is vomiting, the first priority will be to stop the vomiting, and then stop the nausea. The person may need to stop eating and decrease or stop their intake of fluids.

Nonpharmacological Comfort Measures

Preventing

Identify triggers of nausea and vomiting, and work with the person and their family to remove or avoid those triggers (Fraser Health Authority, 2006). Start with a basis of providing regular oral hygiene and keep the room odor free.

If the person has a history of being easily nauseated, be sure to record and report this to the care team, and suggest anti-emetics be started if or when opioids are initiated.

When a person is experiencing recurring nausea, reduce odors as soon as possible by providing:
- Fresh air—open the windows, turn on an exhaust fan, and clean the commode as soon as possible
- Fresh linens, a cold cloth, clean bedding and clothing as needed
- An emesis basin in case vomiting occurs

Monitor the input and output of liquids as a means of preventing dehydration if applicable.

In the Moment

When a person is nauseated:
- Coach the person in relaxation strategies, such as deep breathing, muscle relaxation, and guided imagery
- Distract the person with music, conversation, videos, and so on
- Offer frequent, small sips of chilled liquid
- Offer ice chips, or juice frozen into cubes or sticks to moisten the mouth
- Offer mints or hard, sugarless candies

When a person is vomiting:
- Provide privacy by closing doors and limiting visitors
- Prevent aspiration of emesis by assisting the person to an upright or side lying position, supporting with pillows as necessary
- Ensure safety by providing companionship and supervision

After a person has vomited:
- Provide mouth care or assist the person with mouth care.

When vomiting has settled and nausea is reduced:
- Slowly increase the person's fluid intake and if vomiting does not recur, offer semi-solid foods and then solid foods
- Offer small, frequent meals
- Provide bland foods such as crackers and dry toast
- Avoid spicy, fried, fatty foods or acidic foods (e.g., oranges, lemons, vinegar)

If nausea or vomiting recur:
- Return to offering sips of liquid, ice chips, or juice frozen into cubes or their sticks to moisten the mouth

With the Family

Share nonpharmacological comfort measures with the family, as above.

Explain the rationale for the regular and ongoing use of anti-emetics when these measures are necessary. Teach the family how to provide assistance and ensure that the person is safe when vomiting.

Many people have difficulty with the sight and smell of emesis. When this is the case, share the following tips to help the family support their loved one:
- Focus on the person.
- Breathe through the mouth rather than the nose.
- Use plastic bags inside brown paper bags as emesis containers to reduce the visual effect. Throw the bag away immediately.

With the Care Team

Consult with a clinical dietitian to provide dietary advice, as needed. Inform dietary staff about changes in the person's diet.

Follow up with the physician/nurse practitioner if vomiting does not settle or increases.

Principles for Using Medications to Manage Nausea and Vomiting

Follow the guidance in Part 1: Principles and Practices at the beginning of this chapter when using medications to manage symptoms. For managing nausea and vomiting, remember to do the following:
- Use the correct medication.
- Administer the correct dose on the appropriate schedule.
- Use a combination of medications to treat a symptom that has more than one cause.

Consider the following information when using medications to treat nausea and vomiting:
- Remember that medications can be started before the cause of vomiting is determined.
- Work with the care team to provide medications that address the most likely causes of nausea and vomiting for the person at the time.
- Advocate for the best medication route (e.g., change route from oral to subcutaneous or intravenous if needed) until the nausea and vomiting are controlled.
- When nausea is present, provide anti-emetics regularly. A PRN dose may be required to manage nausea and vomiting that occurs between regular doses of anti-emetics.

- Keep in mind that different causes of nausea and vomiting require different medication protocols. The person may need medications on an ongoing basis, or only temporarily until the cause of the nausea and vomiting is resolved.
- For people with sensitive stomachs, be proactive by starting a regular dose of anti-emetic when the person begins to receive pain medications.
- Be proactive by preventing constipation, which can lead to nausea. If the person is taking opioids or has reduced mobility, a bowel protocol should be considered.

Table 15 below provides lists of medications for palliating nausea and vomiting, based on the most likely cause of the symptom. You may notice different strategies being implemented to manage nausea and vomiting, depending on the needs of the person, the medications available, and the preferences of the care team.

Note: Metoclopramide is a gastro-kinetic medication, meaning it promotes intestinal motility. Because this medication increases not only the frequency but also the strength of the contractions in the small bowel, it is contraindicated in people who have a bowel obstruction or impending bowel obstruction and must be used cautiously for people who have a partial bowel obstruction.

Table 15. Medications for Managing Nausea and Vomiting, Based on Cause

Chemicals (Medications/Toxins)	Gastroenterological	Vestibular and Motion-Related	Central Nervous System	Cause Unknown
• haloperidol • prochlorperazine • methotrimeprazine • ondansetron • granisetron • olanzapine	Distension or lumen compression • metoclopramide • domperidone • methotrimeprazine Obstruction • haloperidol • octreotide Opioid-induced symptoms • metoclopramide • domperidone • methylnaltrexone Other vagal stimuli • methotrimeprazine • prochlorperazine • ondansetron	• dimenhydrinate • scopolamine	Emotional/anxiety-induced symptoms • lorazepam • nabilone Increased intracranial pressure • dexamethasone • dimenhydrinate	• haloperidol • methotrimeprazine • metoclopramide • olanzapine

(Adapted from Fraser Health Authority, 2006; Pallium Canada, 2013; and Chow, Cogan, and Mun, 2015)

Managing Dehydration Caused by Nausea and Vomiting

Dehydration occurs when more fluid is lost from the body than is taken in. It is common with reduced intake associated with anorexia, nausea, or GI obstruction, or by increased fluid loss associated with vomiting, diarrhea, fever, or side effects of medication such as diuretics.

When a person is dehydrated, they may have a dry mouth, decreased urine output, dry skin, headache, constipation, and/or dizziness. When a person is very dehydrated, they may have a very dry mouth, little or no urine output, sunken eyes, low blood pressure, and a fast heart rate. They may be extremely thirsty, irritable, and confused, and may experience delirium.

While it may be possible to rehydrate the person, it is more difficult to manage the symptom causing the dehydration, and it may be impossible to address the disease progression that is ultimately responsible. In deciding whether to try to hydrate a person with artificial hydration, the team, the dying person, and the family will need to consider the cause of the dehydration, the illness trajectory,

the pros and cons of hydration, and the person's goals of care (Bruera et al., 2013; Danis, 2015).

Strategies for supplying artificial hydration include using a central venous, intravenous, or subcutaneous route to deliver liquids.

The simplest method is hypodermoclysis, whereby the fluids are injected subcutaneously. In general, hypodermoclysis is appropriate for people who are mildly dehydrated. It is useful in situations when parenteral fluids are beneficial. Hypodermoclysis requires less technology than providing fluids by the intravenous route and may be preferred, especially when an intravenous administration is not available in the care setting. Hypodermoclysis is not indicated when the person has poor skin integrity, lymphedema, or edema, is severely dehydrated, and/or requires more than 3L in a 24-hour period.

Strategies for managing dehydration and comfort when the person is actively dying are discussed in Chapter 7, "Caring in the Last Days and Hours."

Ethics Touchstone

Use the IDEA framework to consider the ethical issues that might occur when a person is dehydrated as a result of nausea and vomiting. What strategies might help you support the person and the family to decide if they want to access artificial hydration?

Evaluating and Confirming

Ask the person questions like these to evaluate the treatment and confirm that it is having the desired effect:

- How are nausea and vomiting affecting your well-being now?
- Are your goals for managing your nausea and vomiting being met?
- Does the care plan need to be adapted or updated?
- Do you need any more information about nausea and vomiting, and the plan for controlling these symptoms in the coming days?

Case Study

The following case study illustrates the process of providing care from the nurse's perspective, beginning with assessment and information sharing, followed by care planning and confirming and evaluating.

As I was doing rounds for afternoon shift, I found Mrs. Lim at the side of her bed, vomiting partially digested food. She looked at me, gagged, and said, "Can you do something to stop this?"

Onset: The nausea began 3 or 4 days ago. The vomiting is a new symptom, as of this afternoon.

Provoking/Palliating: The nursing notes and medication record indicate that morphine for back pain was increased a week ago. Her last bowel movement was 3 days ago, despite taking sennosides 12 mg BID. Her stool was hard, and she needed to strain to defecate. She felt unable to evacuate all the stool.

She reported nausea twice, 3 days ago and 2 days ago, and was given metoclopramide 10 mg PO PRN both times. This reduced her nausea both times but was not given regularly. There was no ATC anti-emetic order.

Quality: The emesis is half-digested food. No fecal smell. Nausea is constant.

Region/Radiating: Abdomen is slightly tender in all four quadrants and is slightly distended. Bowel sounds are hypoactive. She is passing flatus.

Severity: Rates her current nausea at 6 on a scale of 0 to 10 and it is constant. No signs of dehydration.

Treatment: Mrs. Lim admits that she did not always report her nausea when she was experiencing it. She also stated that she had required anti-nausea medication for several weeks when her morphine was initiated months ago.

Understanding: Mrs. Lim believes that the pain medication (morphine) is causing the nausea. She states that she is "thinking about stopping the pain medication."

Values: Her goal is to stop the nausea as soon as possible so she can return home to her family.

In the Moment
Reassure the person by saying, for example,

I will speak with the care team and share the assessment and your goal to have the nausea and vomiting settled as soon as possible.

With the Team
The nurse informs the care team that Mrs. Lim is a private person who does not readily communicate how she is doing unless she is asked. Using the SBAR tool, the nurse discusses the clinical findings with the physician/nurse practitioner. Both agree that while Mrs. Lim's nausea could be due to the increase in her morphine dose and her constipation, the symptom could have many other causes. The admission notes indicate that Mrs. Lim's goal of care is full recovery and that she has no intention of dying.

The collaborative decision is this: given her goals of care, it is important to treat the symptom while also trying to identify its causes. The care team decided that it might be helpful to order blood work for Mrs. Lim to rule out hypercalcemia and check electrolytes.

With the Physician/Nurse Practitioner
Using the SBAR tool, the nurse prepared this report to give to the physician/nurse practitioner:

Situation: I am calling about Mrs. Lim, who has been nauseated for 3 to 4 days and then vomited this afternoon.

Background: Mrs. Lim is 56 years old and has cancer of the breast (diagnosed 3 years ago) with metastasis to the brain and lower spine. Her goal of care is for full recovery. She is being seen by the oncologist consultant next week. She wants to ask about further chemotherapy or radiation. She is a very private person and, according to her admission notes, has stated she has no intention of dying.

(continued on next page)

Assessment

Onset: The nausea began 3 or 4 days ago and the vomiting is new this afternoon.

Provoking/Palliating: The dose of morphine for her back pain was increased 7 days ago. Her last bowel movement was 3 days ago, despite her being on sennosides 12 mg PO BID. She reported being nauseated 3 days ago, and again 2 days ago. Metoclopramide 10 mg PO PRN was given both times when she reported nausea, which did decrease her nausea. It has not been given regularly. There is no regular ATC order. I just spoke with her, found out about the nausea, and discovered that she has vomited.

Quality: The emesis is half-digested food. No fecal smell. Nausea is constant. I would like to give her a dose of the PRN metoclopramide, but she cannot tolerate it orally.

Region/Radiating: Her abdomen is slightly tender in all four quadrants and is slightly distended. Bowel sounds are present, hypoactive. She is passing flatus.

Severity: Rates her current nausea at 6 out of 10 and it is constant. No signs of dehydration. Still able to tolerate fluids up until today. Today she vomited her lunch and has only had about 250 mL of fluid throughout the day.

Treatment: Mrs. Lim admits that she did not report being nauseated unless she was asked. She states that she had required anti-nausea medication for about a month after starting with opioids initially. She cannot remember the name of the medication. It helped stop the vomiting and the nausea.

Understanding: Mrs. Lim states that the pain medication (morphine) is causing her nausea and that she is "thinking about stopping the pain medication."

Value: The nausea is stopping Mrs. Lim from returning home to her family, which is her goal. As mentioned, she stated earlier that she has no intention of dying and hopes for a full recovery.

Request/Recommendation: Given her symptoms, and the finding that she does not always report her nausea and her goals of care, I am wondering if we can help to manage the nausea and vomiting and try to determine the cause.

Care Planning

The care team discussed goals of care, investigations, and treatment of symptoms. Discussion with the person and family followed, and a decision was made to investigate for causes. The physician/nurse practitioner ordered an ultrasound of Mrs. Lim's abdomen and blood work.

With the Person

I spoke with the care team and shared my assessment and your desire to have your vomiting controlled as soon as possible.

We spoke about possible causes. We agree with you that the nausea and the vomiting may be caused by the morphine. The physician/nurse practitioner recommends that you take the metoclopramide regularly. If the nausea is not settling, we do have an order to add another medication called haloperidol as needed to ensure your comfort.

To control the nausea, it is important that you take the anti-nausea medication regularly for the next days and weeks. It is possible that your body will get accustomed to the opioids and that you may be able to decrease the amount of medication at that time.

The physician/nurse practitioner also recommends that you increase the regular laxatives to help you have regular bowel movements. As long as you take opioids, it will be important to monitor your bowel movements. We can adjust the amount of laxative to meet your specific needs. And we encourage you to avoid solid foods today, and drink clear fluids until the vomiting is settled. If you cannot tolerate fluids, please let us know.

Do you have any questions? Any concerns?

Can I go ahead and start the regular anti-nausea medication now? Then you can start the laxative once your nausea is more settled in a few hours.

I recommend that you keep a journal and record when you are nauseated, how severe your nausea is, and when you vomit again, and we can also keep track of medications. Hopefully we will be able to see improvement.

How does that sound to you?

(continued on next page)

The physician/nurse practitioner gave these orders for Mrs. Lim:

1. Give metoclopramide 10 mg PO or SC QID.
2. Start haloperidol 0.5 mg to 1.0 mg PO or SC BID if nausea and vomiting do not stop within 24 hours.
3. Stop previous morphine order.
4. Start morphine 10 mg SC q4h regularly.
5. Give morphine 6 mg SC q1h PRN for BTP.
6. When vomiting stops and nausea settles, return to:
   a. Morphine 20 mg PO q4h regularly
   b. Morphine 12 mg PO q1h PRN for BTD.
7. Complete a rectal exam. If stool is present in the rectum, administer a bisacodyl suppository. If unsuccessful in emptying the rectum, follow with a sodium citrate/sodium lauryl sulphoacetate or sodium phosphate enema.
8. Increase sennosides 24 mg PO BID.
9. Complete the following tests:
   a. Ultrasound of abdomen
   b. Blood work: electrolytes, calcium, and albumin.
10. Update physician/nurse practitioner in 24 hours, or sooner if vomiting does not settle.

Confirming and Evaluating

The nurse will need to:

- Follow up one hour after medications are given, and re-assess to determine whether the vomiting has stopped, the nausea is more settled, and the pain is under control
- Complete a rectal exam (if appropriate), determine whether a suppository is required, and give an oral laxative when Mrs. Lim is able to tolerate it
- Discuss dietary needs with the dietitian and/or dietary staff

Pain

I cared for her over 30 years ago in a small-town hospital. Lying at the far end of the hall in a two-bed room, she would call out, "Nurse ... Nurse ... help me ... Nurse ..." and after a while, she would call out, "God, God, God ... help me God." When I look back all these years later, I can still recall her name, and can remember walking into her room, not knowing what to do or how to help. In retrospect, I think that she received two tabs of acetaminophen twice a day ... She was not assessed regularly for pain, she did not receive any additional acetaminophen when she called out. My memory of her still haunts me, and I regret not having known how to assess her pain and how to advocate for her.

What Is Pain?

Pain is the unpleasant sensory and emotional experiences of physical suffering and distress due to injury or illness. Pain can originate from a variety of diseases, for example, cancer, COPD, or arthritis, and for a variety of reasons, including physical and psychosocial issues (Pallium Canada, 2013). The way that people express their pain varies with different cultures (Carteret, 2011).

Margo McCaffery provides a straightforward way to look at pain that has become a classic in the field of pain management (McCaffery, 1968):

Pain is what the experiencing person says it is, and exists whenever the experiencing person says it does.

Dame Saunders and the Concept of Total Pain

Remember that pain, like death, is always experienced by the whole person, not just the physical body. Dame Cicely Saunders developed the concept of "total pain," which she defined as pain that includes physical, emotional, spiritual, and social dimensions of distress. The concept of total pain can remind you to look beyond the physical causes and see other factors that may affect and potentially increase a person's pain. The experience of physical pain may be greater when a person is afraid or concerned, such as when they are experiencing existential suffering, interpersonal conflict, financial challenges, family issues, and so on. Being aware that pain is experienced by the whole body and that issues affecting the body will affect the experience of pain will help you when providing care to increase physical comfort.

Prevalence

More than 80% of people with advanced cancer experience pain; 66% of these people will experience moderate to severe pain, and 60% will experience pain at more than one site. The prevalence of pain evaluated one month before death did not differ greatly by diagnosis: cancer—45%, heart disease—48%, frailty—50%, other diagnoses—47% (Smith et al., 2010). The actual prevalence of pain is probably higher, because some people do not report their pain.

The level and intensity of pain fluctuate as diseases progress and conditions decline. Regularly assessing pain and developing a plan of care focused on maintaining quality of life are essential steps to managing pain. Applying the basic principles of pain management will help manage pain in 85% of people experiencing pain due to advanced cancer (Pallium Canada, 2013).

These populations are at risk of having their pain undertreated:
- Children and the elderly
- People who are nonverbal or cognitively impaired
- People who deny pain, for personal reasons
- People who are unable to communicate their pain or have difficulty doing so due to a language barrier
- People who, because of their culture or traditions, are discouraged from talking about, expressing, or managing pain
- People with a history of addiction

Direct Causes

Disease-related causes of pain are illustrated in Figure 9. For example, a tumor invading the tissues or pressing on the bone or muscle accounts for approximately 75% of pain with cancer. In addition, spinal cord compressions, bone fractures, bowel obstructions, ischemia, infections, or abscesses can cause pain.

Indirect Causes

Indirect causes of pain include the following:
- Investigations (e.g., lumbar puncture), treatments (e.g., radiation, incisional pain), and side effects of medications (e.g. opioid-induced constipation)
- Effects of being ill and less mobile (e.g., constipation, muscle fatigue and aches)
- Pre-existing conditions (e.g., migraines, osteoporosis, past injuries, gout)

Figure 9. Causes of pain

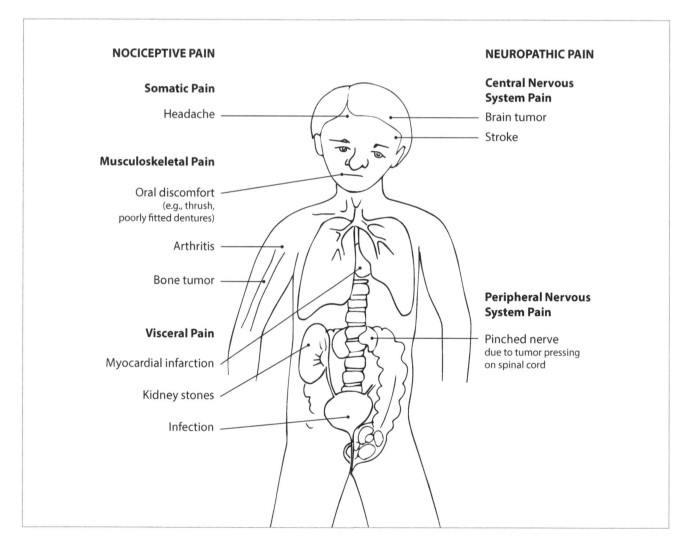

Pathophysiology

When tissues are damaged, signals are sent to the brain that communicate pain. The type of pain experienced will depend on the origin of the pain. Identifying the cause of pain will help to determine the best way to treat it.

Nociceptive and Neuropathic Pain

The origins and experiences of two types of pain, nociceptive and neuropathic, are identified in Table 16 and illustrated in Figure 9 (Pallium Canada, 2013; ELNEC, 2015).

Table 16. Origins and Characteristics of Nociceptive and Neuropathic Pain

Nociceptive Pain **Origin:** Damaged soft tissues and bones	Neuropathic Pain **Origin:** Abnormal signal processing in peripheral or central nervous system
Musculoskeletal Pain: • Originates in the bones and joints • Is experienced as a sharp or dull ache (e.g., bone tumor, arthritis) **Somatic Pain:** • Originates in skin, connective tissue, and muscle • Is experienced as sharp (e.g., mouth sore) or aching (e.g., muscle aches) **Visceral Pain:** • Originates in visceral organs (e.g., GI tract, pancreas, tumor that encapsulates an organ such as the liver, bowel obstruction that causes cramping) • Is experienced as a localized deep ache or cramping that may come and go	**Peripheral Nervous System Pain:** • Is experienced as burning, numbness, tingling • Is felt along either one or more peripheral nerves (and usually described as burning, numb-like, shock-like, or pins and needles) **Central Nervous System Pain:** Originates from stroke or brain tumor

Addressing pain is a nursing priority.

Listen carefully: pain is what the person says it is.

Assessment

Assess for pain regularly as part of your normal practice. Also assess for pain when the person's condition changes, if the person identifies pain, when their behavior suggests pain, when family members identify pain, and when medications for pain are initiated or adjusted.

Follow the person's lead and use their words when talking about pain. The person may use words such as "discomfort," "stress," "tightness," "soreness," or "ache" instead of using the word "pain." If pain is suspected, seek additional information to learn how the person has expressed pain in the past.

Consider the person's culture and how it may influence how pain is experienced or expressed. Remember the populations that are at risk of having undertreated pain. If language is a barrier to communication, invite a family member or translator to provide translations for words used in describing and rating pain.

Screen with the Edmonton Symptom Assessment System

Use the Edmonton System Assessment System (ESAS) to screen regularly for pain and whenever pain is suspected.

Assess with the Symptom Assessment Tool Adapted for Pain

Use the Symptom Assessment Tool adapted for pain (Table 17) to conduct a thorough assessment, including a physical assessment, and a review of the person's history and current relevant reports.

Assess Frailty and Inform Goals-of-Care Conversations

Assess the person's frailty using the CSHA Clinical Frailty Scale or the PPS. Consider using the GSF PIG, the SPICT, or tools for prognosticating one-year mortality (see Chapter 4, "Using Standardized Tools") to inform goals-of-care conversations and determine whether investigations are appropriate.

Table 17. Symptom Assessment Tool Adapted for Pain

	Symptom Assessment Tool Adapted for Pain	
O	**Onset**	When did you start experiencing pain? How long does the pain last?
P	**Provoking/Palliating**	What triggers your pain? How often do you feel the pain each day? What decreases your pain? Is there a pattern to when pain occurs? Does your pain increase the severity of other symptoms? Do other symptoms make your pain feel worse?
Q	**Quality**	Can you describe the pain, what it feels like?
R	**Region/Radiating**	Where are you feeling the pain? Any other areas? Are any of your pains radiating to other regions? Are any of your pains causing other symptoms?
S	**Severity**	Can you rate your pain (discomfort) on a scale of 0 to 10, with 0 being no pain and 10 being the worst pain you can imagine? Would you prefer to rate your pain with words such as "mild," "moderate," or "severe"?
T	**Treatment**	What medications have you used to control pain? What doses have you tried? What was effective? Did you experience any side effects when you took the medications? Have your medications for managing pain been changed recently?
U	**Understanding**	What do you think is causing the pain? How is this pain affecting your daily activities? Can you tell me how it is for you to be in pain?
V	**Values**	What are your goals for pain management? On a scale of 0 to 10, where would you like your pain to be? What is most important to you today?

W	**What Else?**	• Physical assessment
		   ○ Look for any changes, asymmetry, sounds, areas that are sensitive to touch or that feel warm.
		   ○ If pain involves the abdomen, auscultate, percuss, palpate, and notice any bulges or distention.
		 • Other relevant findings
		   ○ Medications
		   ○ Relevant lab and diagnostic results

Dr. Deb Braithwaite, a colleague and mentor, provided a list of questions that would help obtain the information physician/nurse practitioners need in order to identify the cause of pain.

When you call me to report that someone is having pain, I want to know:

What do you see *when you look at the person, and when you look at whatever part is experiencing pain?*
- *Are both sides of the body symmetrical?*
- *Are there any nodules, lumps, or bulges?*
- *Are there any discolored areas?*

What do you feel?
- *Any lumps or bumps?*
- *Any changes in temperature/body warmth?*

What do you hear?
- *Any sounds?*
- *What type of sounds?*
- *Are there any abnormal sounds?*

Screen for Pain in a Person Who Does Not Self-Report Pain

Culture, age, and personal expectations are reasons why a person may not self-report pain and may be at risk of having their pain untreated. In addition, people with limited ability to communicate may not be able to report their pain effectively. This includes people with aphasia, dementia, brain tumors, infections, and other disease processes that affect cognition and communication.

Screening and assessing for pain in people unable to communicate their pain requires nurses and HCPs to observe the person's behaviors and compare them to the person's normal behaviors. The American Geriatrics Society (American Geriatrics Society, 2002) grouped pain behavior indicators into six categories and Herr and colleagues evaluated the behaviors for their usefulness in indicating pain in people with dementia unable to self-report (Herr et al., 2006). These categories and behaviors are as follows:
- Facial expressions: frowning, sad, frightened, grimacing, distorted expression, tight or closed eyes, rapid blinking
- Verbalizations and vocalizations: sighing, moaning, groaning, grunting, chanting, calling out, noisy breathing, asking for help

- Body movements: rigid tense posture, guarding, fidgeting, pacing, rocking, restricted movements, gait or mobility changes
- Changes in interpersonal interactions: aggressive, combative, resistant to care, unwilling to interact with other people, socially inappropriate, disruptive, withdrawn, verbally abusive
- Changes in activity patterns: refusing food, appetite changes, increases in rest or sleeping, changes in rest, sudden halt to common routines, wandering
- Changes in mental status: crying or tears, increased confusion, distress or irritability

Draw on the experience of family members and others, including nursing assistants, personal support workers, and other frontline care providers, for their knowledge of the dying person's usual behaviors and their sense of any behaviors that may have changed.

Two tools, the Pain Assessment in Advanced Dementia (PAINAD) Scale and the Non-Communicative Patient's Pain Assessment Instrument (NOPPAIN), can be used to screen for pain in people unable to self-report. See pages 76 and 78 in Chapter 4, "Using Standardized Tools."

Using the PAINAD Scale
Nurses and nursing assistants/personal support workers can easily use the PAINAD scale (see Chapter 4, "Using Standardized Tools") to screen for pain in people with advanced dementia. Behaviors in three of the six American Geriatrics Society categories are observed and rated numerically (Warden, Hurley, and Volicer, 2003). Higher scores more strongly suggest that the person is experiencing pain; however, scores *do not* indicate the severity of pain. This tool must be used in concert with an assessment tool to determine the severity and location of pain.

	0	1	2	Score
Breathing Independent of vocalization	Normal	Occasional labored breathing. Short period of hyperventilation.	Noisy labored breathing. Long period of hyperventilation. Cheyne-Stokes respirations.	
Negative Vocalization	None	Occasional moan or groan. Low level speech with a negative or disapproving quality.	Repeated troubled calling out. Loud moaning or groaning. Crying.	
Facial Expression	Smiling, or inexpressive	Sad. Frightened. Frown.	Facial grimacing.	
Body Language	Relaxed	Tense. Distressed pacing. Fidgeting.	Rigid. Fists clenched, knees pulled up. Pulling or pushing away. Striking out.	
Consolability	No need to console	Distracted or reassured by voice or touch.	Unable to console, distract or reassure.	
			TOTAL	

Pain Assessment in Advanced Dementia (PAINAD) Scale

The benefit of the PAINAD scale is its ease of use. However, because it addresses only three categories of behaviors, the screening may miss other behaviors that indicate pain in some people. Familiarity with and knowledge of the person's normal behaviors could help in deciding whether this tool would detect pain behaviors common for this person.

The two most common indicators of pain are changes in behavior and resisting care. Use the PAINAD scale to screen regularly for pain if the person resists care or when their behaviors change.

Using the NOPPAIN tool

Nurses and other HCPs providing care for people with dementia can also use the Non-Communicative Patient's Pain Assessment Instrument (NOPPAIN) screening tool (Snow et al., 2004). The tool screens for pain behaviors in five of the six American Geriatrics Society categories, both when the person is resting and when active. The NOPPAIN tool includes a body map to use in locating the source of pain. (see Chapter 4, "Using Standardized Tools")

The benefit of this tool is that it screens for pain behaviors when the person is at rest and when active, and looks at five of six behavior categories. As when using the PAINAD scale, subtler behaviors that indicate pain may still be missed. Therefore, the family's and HCP's knowledge of the person's usual behaviors is invaluable.

Use the NOPPAIN tool to screen regularly for pain and whenever any behavior changes. Follow up with an appropriate pain assessment if the screening suggests pain is present.

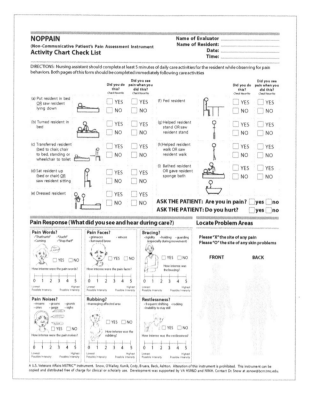

Non-Communicative Patient's Pain Assessment Instrument (NOPPAIN)

Assess with the Facial Grimace and Behaviour Assessment Tool When the Person Is Unable to Self-Report

The Facial Grimace and Behaviour Assessment Tool enables the observer to assess pain in a person who does not self-report pain or is unable to report pain (Brignell, 2009).

The nurse assigns a score to the person's facial expression and indicates the frequency of specific behaviors associated with pain. The activity level and dosing of medications are also recorded on the assessment sheet. Use this tool to assess the severity of pain and evaluate the effectiveness of pain management.

Pain assessment in a person who has difficulty reporting pain is challenging, yet it is not impossible, as is evident in the following story by Joe's wife.

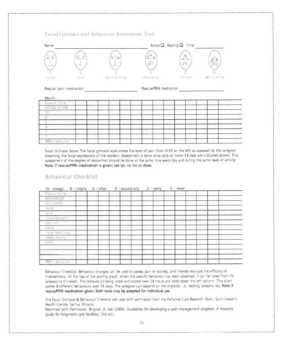

Facial Grimace and Behaviour Assessment Tool

Jenny, his nurse, noticed that Joe was grimacing, becoming rigid, and grabbing her sleeve during his morning wash. She asked me if this was normal for him. I told her he'd been like this all week—never wanting to be touched—then today, I noticed him stiffening up when they were transferring him to his chair.

"Perhaps he's having pain," she said. She asked us some more questions about what he was like at home, what he would have wanted if he was in pain. Then she spoke with the doctor about Joe, and they figured that

he might be in pain. The doctor ordered some medication to decrease the pain.

Jenny gave him the pills with a sip of his soup for lunch—she told me she would give it a chance to work before she moved him again, back to his bed. An hour later she moved him to bed. He did not tense up as much.

He's sleeping peacefully now, he's no longer fidgeting, and even his breathing is easier. It's good to see Joe comfortable.

Investigate to Identify or Confirm Causes

Identifying the causes of pain may require further investigations, such as blood work, X-Rays, CT scans, MRIs, colonoscopy, endoscopy, and gastroscopy. The type and extent of investigation will depend on the:
- Goals of care of the dying person and their family
- Person's position on their disease trajectory and prognosis
- Invasiveness of the investigation, for example, blood work versus a biopsy
- Availability of and access to investigative procedures
- Care setting

Use the SBAR tool to communicate the pain assessment to the physician/nurse practitioner and the team.

Information Sharing

When the assessment has been completed and recorded, consider what information the person and the family want and need to receive, and how you might best provide that information.

Explain that the goal of pain management is to focus on the dying person's goals of care. Generally speaking, this may include helping the person sleep better at night, helping the person become more comfortable at rest, and helping the person move with less or no pain. However, if the pain is severe, the goal may be to decrease the pain to a level that is more tolerable while investigations are completed to determine the cause of pain.

Case Study: A Person with Cancer

Robert, aged 65 years, has a primary diagnosis of prostate cancer, with bone metastasis. Today, Robert said his pain felt different to him. The nurse completed a focused assessment. Robert has been on the unit for five days. He has been slow in his movements and supports himself by holding furniture as he moves. Today, Robert had a Tylenol at 0800 for pain but found the pain continued to get worse as the day progressed. The nurse went in after breakfast to reassess his pain. He did not seem to be getting relief. She continued a focused assessment. Her notes are below.

Assessment

Onset: At 1000, aching in the morning and pain increased after shower.

Provoking/Palliating: Worse with movement, slight relief with rest.

Quality: Dull and aching.

Region/Radiating: Pain in left hip, radiates into left buttock.

Severity: 8/10, describes it as moderate pain.

Treatment: Historically Robert's pain has been well managed (rating it as a 2/10), with acetaminophen 650 mg, orally, every 4 hours, as required.

Understanding: Movement increased pain today but he has been finding the pain gets progressively worse. He knows the cancer is progressing and knows that is what is causing his pain.

Values: Manage pain so he is comfortable with doing basic daily activities. Wants to maintain independence and focus on his family rather than his pain.

Information Sharing

With the Physician/Nurse Practitioner
Using the SBAR tool, the nurse prepared this report to give to the physician/nurse practitioner:

Situation: I am calling about Robert in bed 43A. His pain has increased and is not well managed with his current order of acetaminophen, PRN. My assessment is BP 138/82, P 93, R 24 at rest. He is afebrile. His BP and pulse are elevated above baseline.

Background: The patient is alert and oriented, slightly anxious in discussing his increase in pain. He had an 0800 acetaminophen dose, which was ineffective. He has no allergies.

His skin is warm, he is slightly diaphoretic. He is not on oxygen, his oxygen saturation is at 96%, RA.

Assessment: His BP and pulse may be escalating due to the pain, as they were close to baseline at 0800. He has been getting slower in the last days and uses furniture and the walls to support himself as he moves. Is there something we can do to better manage his pain, as it is getting progressively worse?

Request/Recommendation: If we can start him on a regular analgesic, I can monitor his toleration. Would you like me to call you today to advise you of how he is doing?

Orders

The physician/nurse practitioner gave the following verbal order that the nurse transcribed:
- Morphine: 5 mg, orally, ATC, q4h
- Morphine: 2.5 mg, orally, PRN, q1h
- Dexamethasone: 4 mg, orally, at 0800
- Sennokot: two 8.6 mg tabs, orally, BID

After discussing the initiation of opioids with Robert, the nurse gave the first dose at 1200 and at this time his pain was 9/10. The nurse checked in after 45 mins to reassess Robert. His pain was 7/10, R 20, P 85, and BP 130/80. He was no longer diaphoretic. He said he felt a bit better but was not moving much. The nurse repositioned him with pillows, and he said he will try to rest.

At 1315, the nurse checked in with Robert. He reported his pain as 6/10 and was still visibly uncomfortable. After discussion, Robert decided he would like to try a breakthrough dose.

At 1330, a breakthrough dose was given.

The nurse reassessed Robert at 1355. He reported his pain to be 3/10 and he was able to move himself in bed. His vital signs are P 76, BP 124/80, R 18. He said he was feeling much better.

The nurse called the physician/nurse practitioner to discuss the assessment findings.

Remember that the goals of pain management must always reflect the goals of the person.

Nonpharmacological Comfort Measures

Share information with the person and family about nonpharmacological measures that may provide immediate comfort. Consider using comfort basket items, integrating what you know about the person to individualize the comfort measures to best meet their needs. Information that you gather when a person is comfortable may help you know how best to provide comfort when they are in pain.

Communicate the steps the health care team is taking to address the person's pain. Remember the concept of total pain, and consider whether a member of the interdisciplinary health care team might be able to support the person in addressing nonphysical sources of pain.

A treatment or comfort measure that works one day may not work another day.

Respect the individual and individualize the care.

Preventing

It is easier to prevent pain than to treat pain. The nonpharmacological comfort measures discussed below may help to prevent pain or prevent the escalation of pain.

Create a relaxing pace for daily activities
A person's sensation of pain can increase with stress. If changes in activities or plans are stressful, create a plan that encourages an unhurried approach. Plan activities for times when the pain medication is most effective.

Position for comfort
Prevent skin breakdown and ulceration by ensuring a smooth, clean, dry, and wrinkle-free surface wherever the person is sitting or lying down. This is especially important for people who are less mobile and are unable to reposition themselves.

Turn a person in stages through the night
Over the course of a night, you can gradually move a person from one side to their other side in small increments every few hours (Figure 10). Repositioning every few hours reduces the risk of pressure ulcers but does not wake the person fully or interfere with sleep.

Figure 10. Turning a person in stages through the night

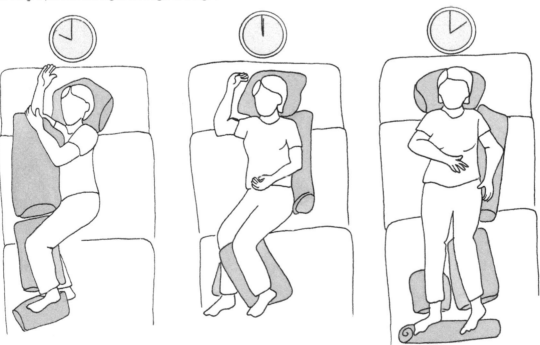

Protect the skin before turning the person

Before turning a person, gently stroke or massage the skin on the side they will be lying on. Light massage will improve blood flow and reduce skin breakdown. After turning the person, do not touch or massage the newly exposed skin on which they have lain. The oxygen-deprived tissues are very susceptible to damage.

Position and reposition the person for comfort. Bed-bound and mobility-limited people are at high risk for pressure ulcers. Reposition the person every two to four hours to reduce the risk of pressure ulcers (see Figure 10).

Check mobility aids for safety

Ensure that mobility aids are safe by checking the following:
- The fit of the wheelchair: Ensure that it does not put pressure on the person's arms, hips, heels, and calves, and that the person can use the footrests comfortably.
- The comfort of the seat: Ensure that the cushion is properly inflated and positioned.

It may be helpful to have a physiotherapist or occupational therapist consult about what seating would be best for the person. Consider suggesting a consult if the person:
- Squirms constantly in the wheelchair
- Needs repositioning every 30 minutes
- Has a pressure ulcer

In the Moment

Distract the person for comfort

Distracting a person can decrease their pain for a short time. A person can be distracted by chatting while visiting, having stories told to them, reminiscing, laughing, being with a pet, watching TV or videos, reading, or breathing fresh air. Explore which distractions might work best for the person in your care. Individualize the care—what might distract one person from their pain might cause another person to feel more pain! Consider this strategy when a person is waiting for a pain medication to take effect or is in the midst of a painful procedure.

Encourage relaxation for comfort

Relaxation strategies such as massage, guided imagery, breathing exercises, and music care can decrease the sensation of pain, as well as improve the effectiveness of medications. Guided imagery can help a person relax until the regular dose or breakthrough dose of medication takes effect. Similar to distraction, relaxation measures are excellent short-term comfort measures

Stimulate for comfort

Warm flannels, heated beanbags, cool cloths, frozen compresses, or creamy lotions applied with a gentle but firm touch can stimulate the senses and help the mind focus on something other than pain. Sometimes gentle stimulation in one area can decrease the sensation of pain in another. Remember that gentle massage may be soothing, but touching or massaging sensitive or painful areas should be avoided.

With the Family

Invite the family to participate in providing comfort. Care provided by family members can be particularly effective at soothing a person. It may also comfort the family members who provide care because they feel helpful and involved. Some family members may feel completely comfortable participating in the person's care, while others may need support to get started.

Provide wheelchair massage

People with normal mobility maintain their comfort by constantly changing their posture and position in multiple little ways. People with limited mobility cannot make these little adjustments and may become uncomfortable as time passes. Wheelchair massage may be a wonderful comfort measure that the HCPs or the family can provide. Provide simple directions for giving the massage:
- Slip your hands between the person's body and the chair.
- While resting the back of the hand against the chair, apply gentle pressure with curved fingers and massage or press on the back, under the legs, under the hips.

Hold and snuggle

The person may enjoy and be comforted by being held and snuggled. Discuss with the person and the family how they might be able to hold their loved one in a way that facilitates closeness and comfort. Provide opportunities and privacy for people to be close.

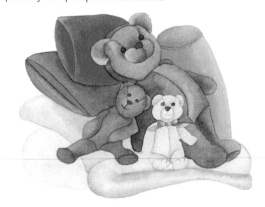

Pharmacological Measures

Pharmacological measures aim to use the medication with the best chance of providing relief and the least side effects. Pharmacological adjuvants and non-opioid analgesics work for mild to moderate pain. Opioids are used for moderate to severe pain. Remember that pain is what the person says it is. Review the principles for symptom management when using medications and strategies for using opioids to manage symptoms (see Part 1: Principles and Practices at the beginning of this chapter).

Principles for using medications:
- Respect and follow the person's goals of care.
- Use the oral route if possible.
- Titrate to the effective dose.
- Provide medications regularly, around the clock, at the dose needed to manage pain.
- Provide breakthrough doses as needed.
- Use a combination of medications as needed.

If pain is suspected in a person who cannot self-report, consider a time-limited trial of an appropriate type and dose of an analgesic, and, as with any care plan, evaluate the pain-related behaviors after administering the analgesic.

(Horgas, Yoon, and Grall, 2013;
Warden, Hurley, and Volicer, 2003)

Non-Opioid Analgesics

Analgesics are medications whose primary actions are to relieve pain. Acetaminophen is a common analgesic and is often the first-line analgesic used for pain. Regular use of acetaminophen may be sufficient to relieve mild pain, but it provides exceptional pain relief when used in conjunction with an opioid. Use non-opioid analgesics with caution and ensure that the person does not take more than the maximum daily dose.

Adjuvants

Pharmacological adjuvants are medications that assist with pain management, and they usually have a different primary purpose than treating pain. Some adjuvant medications are used alone, while others augment the effect of opioids or other analgesics.

Non-steroidal anti-inflammatory drugs (NSAIDs)—first-line adjuvant analgesic for nociceptive pain (bone pain)

Anti-inflammatory medications decrease pain by reducing inflammation at the source of the pain. Examples of NSAIDs include acetylsalicylic acid, ibuprofen, and naprosyn. Side effects from these medications may limit the amount taken and restrict who may be able to use them.

Tricyclic antidepressants (TCAs)—first-line adjuvant analgesic for neuropathic pain

Use low doses of tricyclic antidepressants to help decrease neuropathic pain by blocking neural signaling. Examples of TCAs are amitriptyline, desipramine, nortriptyline, and imipramine.

Anticonvulsants

While these medications are normally used to help control seizures, anticonvulsants work to reduce neuropathic pain by decreasing the excitability of nerves and thus decreasing the pain impulses transferred to the brain. Side effects must be monitored carefully, as sedation is common. Examples of anticonvulsants are gabapentin and pregabalin.

Antimicrobials—first-line adjuvant for infections

Antifungal and antibiotic medications treat infections, thereby reducing pain related to the infection. For example, people who have a compromised immune system and are receiving chemotherapy or radiation treatments will commonly develop a fungal infection known as thrush. Thrush infections can cause considerable discomfort when swallowing. Nystatin is an antifungal medication that kills the fungus, thereby decreasing the pain of swallowing. Antibiotics can treat bladder infections and decrease the pain associated with voiding.

Antispasmodics

This type of medication decreases painful muscle spasms that may occur in the bladder or intestines. An example is hyoscine.

Anxiolytics

Anti-anxiety medications may decrease the anxiety associated with anticipated pain, actual pain, and total pain. An example is lorazepam.

Opioid Analgesics

Opioids are crucial to pain management in hospice and palliative care and are being used earlier in the disease process than was the case in previous decades. It is important for nurses to become familiar and comfortable with opioids when working in hospice and palliative care, because of the incredible ability of these medications to relieve even the most severe pain. Review the section on how to use opioids in Part 1: Principles and Practices at the beginning of this chapter. Remember to:

- Follow the principles for using opioids in addition to the principles for using medications to manage symptoms
- Address fears and concerns of the person, the family, and the HCPs

Adjuvant Therapies

Many adjuvant therapies, with varying levels of invasiveness, are available for treating pain. Non-invasive therapies such as massage, relaxation, and distraction have already been discussed. Others to consider are:

- Transcutaneous electrical nerve stimulation (TENS)
- Acupuncture
- Heat or cold
- Exercise, if possible

Invasive or aggressive adjuvant therapies need to be discussed with the person and family, and the benefits weighed against the burden of treatment and whether the treatment aligns with the person's goals of care. Some therapies to consider are discussed below.

Palliative radiation

Neuropathic pain is often associated with cancer (Pallium Canada, 2013). Palliative radiation treatments can address neuropathic pain associated with spinal cord compression.

Nociceptive bone pain may also be treated with palliative radiation (Pallium Canada, 2013). It is helpful to remember that radiation often causes inflammation initially, which can increase the discomfort until the swelling subsides. Pain relief occurs within 5 to 10 days after treatment, reaches peak effectiveness at six weeks, and may last for months (Pallium Canada, 2013).

Nerve blocks

People with chronic pain may benefit from nerve blocks. Epidural or intrathecal administration of medication can be very helpful in controlling pain, especially lower limb or pelvic pain.

Surgery

Surgery is an adjuvant therapy that may provide only short-term benefits but is often worthwhile because it increases the person's quality of life. Examples include pinning a fracture for pain management, vertebroplasty, or laminectomy.

Evaluating and Confirming

Evaluating the effects of treatments in light of the person's goals of care is intrinsic to the process of enhancing physical comfort. Remember these key points:

- The person determines the goal.
- It is easier to prevent pain than to treat escalating pain.
- Regular, around-the-clock medication is needed to manage ongoing pain.
- Breakthrough doses should be available.
- A combination of medications may be needed.
- Doses of medication need to be adjusted to meet the needs of the person.

When Pain Management Goals Are Not Met

There are many reasons why pain may be difficult to manage and the person's goals for pain management may not be met. When this arises, consider these questions:

1. What has been working?
2. What hasn't been working?
3. Did the care team, the person, and the family follow the care plan?
4. Has the pain changed? For example, is there:
   - Pain due to disease progression?
   - Pain unrelated to the disease?
   - A palliative emergency (spinal cord compression)?
   - Altered cognition that makes pain more difficult to assess and treat?
   - A sudden complication of the disease, for example, a fractured bone?
   - Total pain?
5. Is there any other new pain that you have not identified?
6. Is the dose of the medication titrated well enough, and is the delivery route the best choice?

Whatever is important in the life of the dying person and the family at this time will guide the level of intervention required, while managing the symptom of pain as quickly as possible. Reflect on these questions as you consider ways to increase physical comfort for this person while considering their goals of care:

- Is the person's pain being managed in an acceptable time frame, given their prognosis?
- Are the right resources and HCPs with the right expertise in place to manage this pain (Pallium Canada, 2013; Downing and Wainwright, 2006)?
- Would it be helpful to consult the palliative care specialty team to help manage pain in the timeliest manner?

Case Study: A Person with Advanced Dementia

Sarah is a frail, 90-year-old woman with osteoarthritis and advanced Alzheimer's disease. Over the past month her condition has deteriorated from PPS 30% to PPS 20%, she is in bed all the time, is not able to speak, and over the past week she has been pushing people away when they attempt to provide personal hygiene or reposition her. She often refuses food. Sarah's adult children visit weekly. They want her to be comfortable.

At 0830 the health care worker reports, "This morning Sarah was crying, groaning, frowning, and breathing rapidly. She pushed me away and was not comforted with a warm flannel blanket. With the PAINAD tool, I rate her at an 8/10."

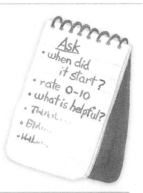

Ask
• when did it start?
• rate 0–10
• what is helpful?
• Th/H il...
• BIA....
• 14L...

Assessment

The nurse and the health care worker complete the Symptom Assessment Tool together. The nurse phones the daughter who is the Substitute Decision Maker, updates her on Sarah's condition, clarifies goals of care, and uses the SBAR communication tool to report to the physician/nurse practitioner.

Information Sharing

Phone report to the physician/nurse practitioner at 0930

Situation: I am calling about Sarah ... She has declined over the past month from a PPS of 30% to 20%. In the past week she has been pushing away those who try to provide personal hygiene or attempt to reposition her. Her vitals are: P 60 and thready; R 16 with periods of hyperventilation; she is afebrile and her skin is cool and dry. Using the PAINAD tool we rate her at an 8/10.

Background: Sarah receives acetaminophen @ 650 mg po TID; today she was unable to swallow her pills. Sarah has no allergies. I spoke with her daughter and clarified that the goal of care is to help Sarah be comfortable. The daughter is aware that Sarah is declining, has been refusing care and often refuses food, and she is concerned that Sarah is in pain

Assessment

　Onset: This morning Sarah appears to be in pain.

　Provoking/Palliating: Sarah refuses personal care, repositioning and food. In the past she was sometimes comforted with a warm flannel, quiet music and family companioning. Today the warm flannels are not helping.

　Quality: Unable to describe pain.

　Region/Radiating: Unclear, though she does prefer to lie on her left side.

　Severity: Using the PAINAD tool, we score Sarah at an 8/10.

　Treatment: Acetaminophen, 650 mg TID for three months. Unable or unwilling to swallow pills today. It is unclear if the acetaminophen has been helpful over the past weeks.

　Understanding: Sarah's daughter is concerned that Sarah is in pain.

　Values: The daughter wants Sarah to be comfortable, remain here, and receive comfort measures. She does not want her to receive CPR.

　Request/Recommendation: Sarah's behaviours are typical of a person with advanced dementia who is experiencing pain. Nonpharmacological measures have been tried with no apparent relief. She may require additional analgesia for pain management. How soon do you think you can come and see Sarah to assess for further analgesia and review other medications? Are you able to order any additional analgesia now? When might you be able to talk with the family, and help prepare family for the possibility of further decline?

(continued on next page)

Chapter 5: Enhancing Physical Comfort   185

After discussion, the physician/nurse practitioner provided the following order:

- Hold acetaminophen when Sarah is unable to take oral medication.
- Begin with a regular dose of hydromorphone, 0.5 mg, SC, q4h
- Use a Breaththrough dose of 0.25 mg, SC, q1h PRN.

Care Planning

This care plan was developed in collaboration with the family:

- Begin hydromorphone as per Orders.
- Postpone personal care and hygiene for at least one hour after the hydromorphone is administered.
- Reassess prior to and one hour following medication being administered to ensure medication has been effective.
- Provide Sarah with a warm flannel blanket and other comfort measures as needed.
- Update the physician/nurse practitioner within 24 hours or if there is any change or increase need before then.

Further topics to discuss with the family:

- Review declining condition, mention changes over the past months, weeks, days.
- Review goals of care.
- Discuss what to anticipate with regards to general decline, possibility of death nearing.
- Explore ways to best support Sarah and her family.
- Explain the use of Breakthrough Doses to help manage pain. For example you could say, "We will give Sarah breakthrough doses when needed to help Sarah become more comfortable. Tomorrow we will talk with the physician/nurse practitioner, will reevaluate her medications and if needed the pain medication can be increased."

Confirming and Evaluating

Documentation:

0300 One hour post medication: Briefs changed and Sarah was repositioned. Did not resist care, no moaning when repositioned.

0800 Sarah is sleeping, no facial grimacing, respirations regular, not labored, body appears relaxed ... she did not resist care during personal hygiene but was tense and called out when repositioned. She settled with a warm flannel. Using the PAINAD tool Sarah was scored at 4/10.

1000 Sarah is awake, appears sad but is not grimacing, took sips of water, few spoons of fruit sauce. Phone call to update the daughter and the physician/nurse practitioner.

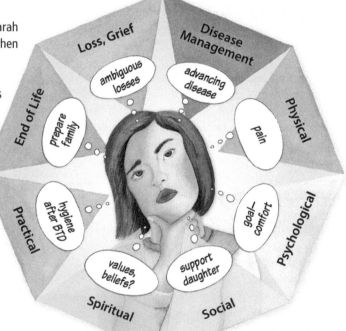

Best Practice in Providing Care for a Person with Late Stage Dementia

What is known about people dying with dementia?

The person's overall trajectory will decline.
- There may be "ups and downs" but overall, their health declines.
- A person with Alzheimer's type dementia will first lose skills associated with higher-level functioning, such a balancing a bank account or following a recipe. Eventually the person will lose basic skills, including doing self-care, dressing, and walking. Eventually people with this type of dementia will not be able to feed themselves, and if they live long enough, they will lose the ability to swallow, one of the most basic reflexive behaviours.

Death is certain to occur.
- It is easy to forget this reality when a person has declined slowly over so many years, when the person has improved in the past when they seemed to be dying, and when the person seems relatively stable now.

Comorbidities will affect the trajectory.
- If a person is healthy other than having whatever is causing the dementia, they might live longer than a person who has a history of strokes, diabetes, cancer of a vital organ, and so on.

Specific interventions, (identified below) are not effective in late-stage dementia.
- Cardiopulmonary resuscitation.
- Gastric tube feedings, which are not able to prolong survival, reduce the risk of infection, prevent aspirations, improve functional status or improve comfort.
- Intravenous antibiotics requiring transfers to hospital.
  IV antibiotics are no more effective than oral antibiotics for repeat infections in late-stage dementia. The body requires a functioning immune system for antibiotics to be effective. Antibiotics are not essential for comfort in the last days.

Indicators that may precede active dying in people dying with dementia

In the period before death, a person dying with dementia may
- Experience repeated infections
- Develop skin ulcers that do not heal
- Experience a significant decline in intake
- Be unable to swallow
- Increase the amount of time that they sleep, and withdraw from others.

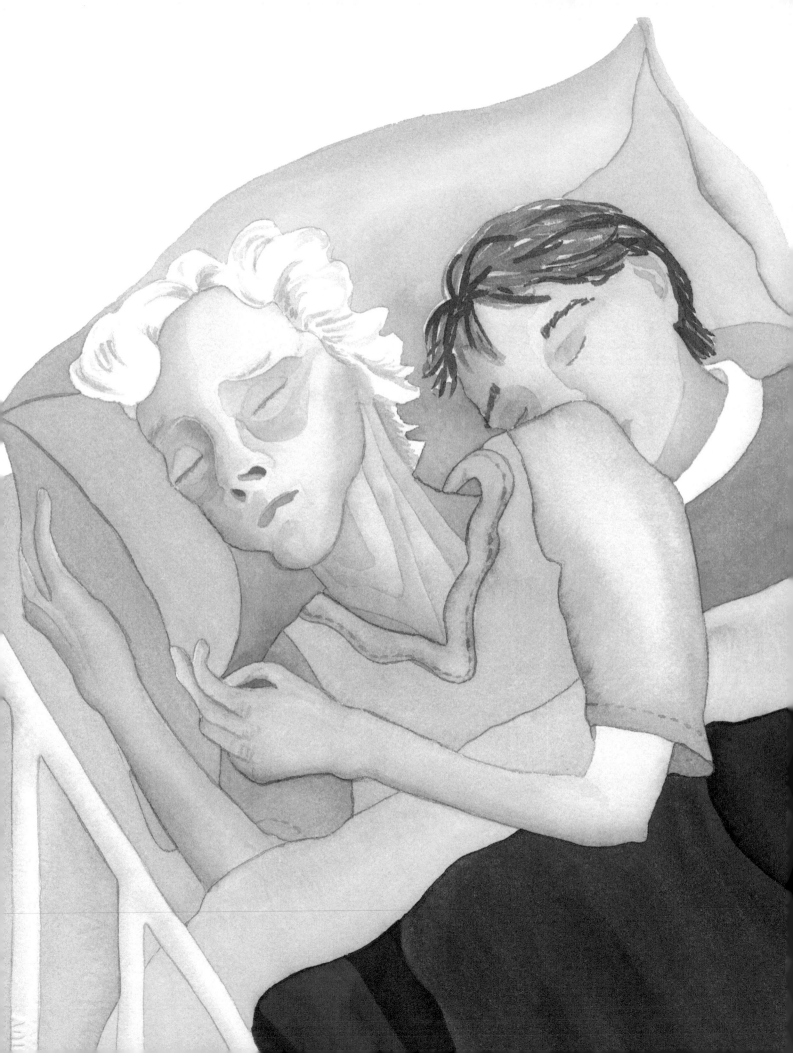

Providing Psychosocial Care

What Is Psychosocial Care?

The word "psychosocial" refers to the emotional, intellectual, spiritual, interpersonal, and cultural aspects of a person. Simply said, it means "everything except the physical." In this text, physical symptoms and psychosocial issues are addressed in separate chapters. However, it is important to remember that people do not experience life in an unconnected or compartmentalized way. Human beings are whole persons and are holistic. Care that is holistic recognizes that a person's whole being is involved in their care. It involves how they are emotionally, spiritually, cognitively, socially, and physically. It is recognized that physical symptoms can have emotional effects, and that emotions can have physical effects. Hospice and palliative care includes a holistic approach that sees the person as more than their illness, more than the sum of their body parts, and more than their emotional reactions to death, dying, loss, and grief.

This chapter focuses on ways to provide psychosocial support for the person and family experiencing transitions, uncertainty, loss, and grief. Having difficult conversations about advance care planning, for example, is discussed as a way to help people identify their priorities, concerns, hopes, and fears so that their wishes can be honored when they are unable to speak for themselves.

Use the Psychosocial Assessment Form (see pages 83 to 88 in Chapter 4, "Using Standardized Tools") to help understand the person, their goals of care, their family, and their support needs, and to inform goals-of-care conversations.

Common Psychosocial Responses to the Diagnosis of Life-Limiting Illness

Advances in disease diagnostics and treatments have increased the length of life for most people. However, the combined effects of multiple diagnoses that the majority of dying people now experience severely affect their quality of life. While the diagnosis of diseases and the integration of hospice and palliative care are currently moving upstream, management of psychosocial issues must now also move upstream to support people and their families through multiple changes in their health and psychosocial transitions (Pasacreta et al., 2015).

People vary in their responses to a diagnosis, depending on the illness, their personal experiences, and the ways that they process information (Pallium Canada, 2013). Emotional responses may include feelings of shock, disbelief, anxiety, depression, denial, irritability, and turmoil. These responses may present as physical symptoms, such as sleep loss and changes in appetite, as well as difficulties with concentrating and performing normal tasks (Pasacreta et al., 2015). Responses may last only days for some people and may extend into weeks or months for others. Ideally, reactions diminish when the person knows the treatment plan and comes to terms with the expected outcomes. Some people may require medication to help settle their reactions.

Of particular concern is the assessment and support of people experiencing anxiety and depression in response to an initial diagnosis and during transitions. Anxiety and depression are natural reactions in people with chronic illness. However, physicians/nurse practitioners may not treat these reactions, considering them to be organic, appropriate to the situation, or not severe enough to warrant treatment. Sometimes this can lead to extended unhappiness, increased family conflict and worry, non-compliance with treatment, and suicidal thoughts (Pasacreta et al., 2015). HCPs can support ill people and their families who are coping with anxiety and depression by offering cognitive behavioral therapy and, for some people, medications. Cognitive behavioral therapy has been successful in helping people cope with their anxiety and depression and is more desirable in some cases because it does not involve medication.

HCPs, specifically nurses, can help by being aware of the signs and symptoms of depression and anxiety that may occur alongside, but independent of, the progressing disease. When distress is noticed, HCPs need to review all potential sources, including unmanaged symptoms. Nurses can support a person experiencing anxiety and depression by providing a caring presence, referring for counseling and alternative therapies, and, for some people, suggesting treatment through medications.

Myths about Depression in People Diagnosed with Life-Limiting Illness

1. All people receiving hospice and palliative care are depressed. *FALSE*

TRUE: Many people experience acute stress at diagnosis and at transitions. Some people may be at high risk for developing a major depression, depending on their life experiences, mental health history, social support network, and psychological coping strategies.

2. Depression and anxiety do not need to be treated. *FALSE*

TRUE: While depression and anxiety are normal responses, the decision to seek treatment will de-

pend on the person and the severity of their symptoms. HCPs, the family, and the person should be made aware of potential coping strategies and treatment options that may be effective.

3. Depression and anxiety do not respond to treatment. *FALSE*

TRUE: Treatments need to be individualized to the person and may include counseling, spiritual support, medications, strategies for managing anxiety, and so on.

(Pallium Canada, 2013; Pasacreta et al., 2015)

Supporting People through Times of Transitions

In psychosocial terms, a transition is a period of substantial change in a person's life as they grow and adapt to a new reality, for example, marriage, graduation, job layoffs, and illness. Transitions at any time of life can be complex and difficult; transitions that include illness, discomfort, decline in functioning and health, uncertainty, and lack of control may be especially challenging experiences. Supportive care during transitions can ease the process of changes for the person and family. Providing information, validating, and listening are ways to be supportive.

When people are living with life-limiting illness, psychosocial issues commonly occur at key times of transition in their disease progress. These key transitions, identified here using the Palliative Performance Scale (PPS) (see Chapter 4, "Using Standardized Tools"), begin as early as diagnosis (Victoria Hospice Society, Wainwright, W., and Thompson, M., 2016; Downing and Wainwright, 2006).

Key Transitions in Dying

PPS 100–90%

A PPS score may be between 100% and 90% when the person is first diagnosed. At this time, the person and their family may experience acute stress as they struggle to understand the illness and make decisions about treatment.

Following treatment, the person may recover and return to their previous activities of daily life (Pasacreta et al., 2015).

As a nurse you can help ensure that the person receives information they need, in a format they understand, in a timely manner before they are required to make decisions about treatment options. They may need to have the same information repeated many times as they work through the new language of diagnosis and treatment options. The person and family may have many questions that you can answer. You can support decision making as you listen to fears and concerns, and answer questions about the disease and possible treatments. You can empathize with how difficult it can be to make decisions, and you can remind the person and family how to access the health care team to request support.

You may have the role of liaison, helping the person and family learn to navigate the health care system. You can advocate on behalf of the person and family when you hear them express questions or fears, and you can request referrals for them to see other team members as appropriate. Finally, you can support the person's decisions once they have been made.

PPS 80–70%

This transition can be very difficult for the person and family, as it usually indicates that the illness is not responding to treatment and may indicate disease progression. For some people, this is the most emotionally distressing time (Pasacreta et al., 2015). The person may have hoped for a cure but must now deal with the continued presence of disease. In the book *Transitions in Dying and Bereavement: A Psychosocial Guide for Hospice and Palliative Care,* this is called "the path not chosen." And so it is. The person is in a state of limbo, because they are neither healthy nor imminently dying and as such may feel disconnected from others. The person may experience significant psychosocial issues; depression is more likely to appear at this time as the person faces a very different future (Pasacreta et al., 2015).

Nurses can provide support by sharing information about this stage of illness, answering questions about treatment options, opening the door to advance care planning, and engaging in goals-of-care conversations. You support by listening to fears and grief about this new phase of their illness and the implications it has for their future. You also support by communicating what you hear to other team members and by suggesting, if appropriate, a referral to a doctor, counselor, other team member.

PPS 60–50%

For a person whose PPS score is 60%, their disease is now extensive and advanced; a cure is not possible. The person can no longer ignore the illness. Fatigue and weakness often mean that the person is no longer able to work or participate in hobbies, and they may spend most of their time sitting or lying down. The person may become concerned about being a "burden" to family members who are caring for them. The dying person may feel cut off from the rest of life. This can be a time of loneliness and isolation, and the person may feel that their life no longer has meaning or purpose. Family members may feel overwhelmed with the demands of care and the losses, such as having limited time for themselves, that caregiving brings to their own lives.

This is an appropriate time to ask the Dignity Question (see page 36) and provide care that reflects the dying person's preferences. If the person is interested, provide options for discussing spiritual and religious concerns they may have. As physical care needs increase, you can offer attentive and responsive care, as well as a listening ear. You can encourage family members to continue interacting with the person who is dying, to help combat loneliness and isolation. It may be appropriate for you to open a discussion between the dying person and family members about the notion of being a burden. Continue to as-

sess and update other team members, and encourage the dying person and family to have conversations with other health professionals if appropriate.

PPS 40–30%

A person with a PPS score between 40% and 30% is weaker and often very tired, and becomes unable to provide self-care. Initially the person may still want to get out of bed, and if the person has delirium or is restless, this period can be one of intense caregiving, with a focus on preventing falls and injuries, and supporting the family. Once the person is in bed full-time, the work of caregiving may be a bit less stressful. However, this may be a difficult time for the dying person, who is no longer independent. When the person is at home, this may be when health care workers, (e.g., personal support workers or nursing assistants) become involved and provide ongoing care and support for the family.

As a nurse, your role as a mentor for the health care workers is valuable. Assist them in meeting and learning about the person and family. Develop and communicate a clear care plan that includes the preferences and needs of the person and family. Respond to any questions and concerns health care workers may have.

This is a time when silence can become a powerful way of connecting with the dying person. They may not want or have the energy to do a lot of talking, but someone who is willing to offer a quiet presence can be very meaningful to them.

PPS 20–10%

When the person's score on the PPS descends to between 20% and 10%, the person becomes less alert, is less responsive, and often appears to disconnect from the world around them.

As a nurse you can provide psychosocial support for the dying person by explaining procedures that are being done, talking as though the person can still hear you, and continuing to provide care that follows the dying person's advance care plan and aligns with recent goals-of-care conversations. You can also support family members as they shift from "doing" to "being" with the person who is dying. Model ways of being with the dying person and encourage continued interaction. Be willing to listen to and answer any questions family may have about the time of death and the events that follow. Be present for their grief as the reality of losing their loved one comes closer for them.

PPS 0%

When a person's PPS score is 0%, they have died. Chapter 7, "Caring in the Last Days and Hours," discusses how to provide care at the time of death, knowing when death has occurred, and preparing the body after death.

Ethics Touchstone
Caregiving includes bearing witness and validating a person's worth as they die.

How would you want to die?

What would be meaningful for you in the dying process?

Experiencing Multiple Losses Due to Progressive Life-Limiting Illness

A person experiences loss when they are deprived of someone or something important to them. Examples are children who experience loss when they go to kindergarten and leave parents at home, and adults who experience many different losses when they move to a different city to start a new job. Some losses in life are tangible, such as the death of a person or pet, and some are symbolic, such as the loss of a dream.

A person experiences losses as soon as they are diagnosed with a life-limiting illness, such as the loss of their ideal future. As the person's health continues to decline with illness progession, they experience multiple ongoing losses. Their losses may include loss of activities and work they enjoyed, or loss of independence and control over much of their daily routine. People often struggle with losing their role in the family—for example, as the provider, as the parent, or as the partner. Many people struggle with losing their independence (Pasacreta et al., 2015). When a person loses independence and requires help to accomplish daily tasks, they may feel sad, frustrated, and angry because they can no longer do these things for themselves. Some will fear becoming a burden.

The family and the dying person suffer losses when the person's abilities decline, mutual activities disappear, and the relationship changes. Family members also experience losses when their relationship changes because they provide care for their dying loved one. They experience further loss when caregiving transitions from "doing for" to "being with."

When people experience repeated losses, one after another, they may feel that they are losing their quality of life. People often define themselves by what they do, so they may lose their sense of self when they can no longer participate in their daily activities.

A palliative approach supports the dying person and family from the time of diagnosis through the dying process and care of their body following death, and, for the family, through losses and grieving. You can support people experiencing losses by listening to how the losses are affecting them and by remembering that each loss will have unique meaning for each person. What one person considers a major loss may be a minor loss to someone else.

Sharing information about loss with the person and the family may be helpful, and sharing information with the team about the person's experience with loss may also be helpful.

It all began when Len woke up one day and his speech was slurred. The kids and I laughed at him. Then he began tripping over things and having trouble using his hands. By the time he was diagnosed with ALS, we stopped laughing. It seemed that every day he experienced one more loss. He became frustrated. Sometimes he yelled at me. Going for our daily walk, having a pleasant drive, playing cards, watching TV, entertaining our friends—all these usual activities became impossible. All the things that gave our life meaning and happiness disappeared one by one. After a while he could do nothing for himself. Our relationship became that of patient and caregiver. Life as we had known it was gone forever. Some days I would lie on my bed and sob. One time I was interrupted in my crying by the sound of him crying in the other room. It just broke my heart. I realized then that grief begins long before a person dies.

The Difficulty of Ambiguous Losses

Some losses are ambiguous—difficult to identify—such as the gradual loss of cognitive functioning with dementia and the accompanying losses. The person is still alive but is not the same as they once were. Because the losses are often not tangible and may be difficult to identify, these losses may be more challenging for the family.

When Mom could no longer care for herself and had to be placed in a facility, I had to be like the mother advocating for my "child." I still loved her, but it was different and my emotions were all mixed up. Sometimes I felt sad, but I was also angry and scared. I lost the mom I knew long before she died. But I couldn't really grieve the loss like I could have if she had died, because she was still alive. It was a difficult time and very few people understood what I was feeling.

Preparing for Expected Losses

Some losses are expected or "certain," while others are unexpected. In general, unexpected losses are more difficult experiences because the person cannot prepare for them mentally or emotionally. Finding ways to help the dying person and their family prepare for expected losses may help them to adapt to the losses.

Preparing for a loss may include opening a conversation with the person on what the loss might mean to them. As a nurse, you might ask the person about losses with questions like these:

You have lived in your home for a long time on your own. How are you feeling about the move to assisted living?

I've noticed that it seems harder for you to get around without your walker lately. How is that for you?

Your family seems happy to prepare meals for you, but you have told me that you love to cook. How are you feeling about handing that task off to someone else?

Basic Truths about Loss and Grief

These basic truths about loss and grief can help the health care team understand the needs of people dealing with loss:

- Loss is natural. Everyone experiences loss as part of being alive.
- People whose health is declining and who are dying experience multiple losses.
- Grief is a natural, healthy response to loss that helps people adapt to living in a changed world.
- Grief is a whole person experience.
- People grieve differently over time.
- People grieve in different and unique ways.
- Denial can be an effective way to cope with overwhelming loss and grief.
- Hope is a wish for something that is important to the person.

Grief—an Adaptive Response to Loss

Grief is a healthy and natural adaptive response to loss. It is a natural, subjective, and complex reaction. People grieve when they lose someone or something that is important to them. Grieving is the process of adapting to the loss in the changed environment. Grieving is a whole person experience that includes the sorrow and suffering caused by the loss, as well as the personal growth and insight that people may experience after a loss.

The word "grieve" comes from the Latin and Old French words meaning "heavy" and "burden," respectively. Grieving people frequently describe feeling weighed down or burdened.

Bereavement

While definitions of loss and grief appear to be universal, definitions of bereavement are not clear. Rando defines bereavement as "the state of having suffered a loss" (Rando, 1984). Hyslop Christ says: "bereavement is an umbrella term that includes overall adaptation to the death" (Hyslop Christ, 2000). Silverman calls bereavement "a time of changing relationships and transitions" (Silverman, 2000). Due to the lack of clarity about what "bereavement" means, this text uses the terms grief, loss, and illness to indicate that these are a natural part of life.

Theories of Grief

Theories and beliefs about what constitutes a healthy grief process have evolved over time.

Freud

Early writings by Freud regarding grief and mourning are considered the historical starting point for theories on grief and loss (Klass, Silverman, and Nickman, 1996). In fact, Freud was describing the loss of attachment to a parent that a child experiences through development, rather than the loss experienced following the death of someone significant. The thrust of the theory was that once the attachment was severed, the child was free and uninhibited, and the work of mourning complete. Psychoanalysts who followed Freud further supported the interpretation that mourning was not complete until the attachment to the

person who had died was completely severed. So began a time of confusion for people who were grieving the loss of someone significant to them and who did not want to completely sever that relationship.

Bowlby

Bowlby was the next major theorist to create a model of grief. Bowlby's theory also centered on attachment. However, he studied children who were deprived of their mothers under traumatic curcumstances. Others applied his theory to help understand people grieving the death of someone significant to them. Bowlby also supported the notion that mourning was complete when a relationship was severed. The word he used to describe this separation was "detachment."

Kübler-Ross

Over 50 years ago Elizabeth Kübler-Ross pioneered work on loss and grief by asking dying people and their loved ones what they were going through and what they needed from professionals. She was valuable for prompting people to talk about death, dying, loss, and grief, and proposed what she called the "stages of grief." Kübler-Ross identified shock and disbelief, anger, bargaining, depression, and acceptance as the stages of grief people experience when they face death. The stages seemed to resonate with many people, possibly because the stages made the variety of emotions of grief seem normal.

An incorrect understanding evolved, however, that grieving people were thought to move sequentially through each grief stage, resolving the emotions of each stage before proceeding. This was not Kübler-Ross's intent. People also mistakenly thought that the goal was for people to "accept" their illness and their death. We know now that many people do not want to accept death or the loss of a loved one. They do not want to "let go and move on."

Grief specialists now teach that people grieve following their own individual pathway (ELNEC, 2015). Such specialists teach that the goal of the grieving process is to accept the loss or find closure. While people who lose a loved one usually find ways to adapt to the loss and experience joy again, it is also true that grief often "walks with them" for the rest of their lives. This is an important perspective, because the goal shifts then to supporting people to find their way on their very personal and unique journey.

Parkes

Colin Murray Parkes, a British psychiatrist and grief specialist, reported on his research of widows in London, and supported the idea that healthy grieving included the person changing their worldview and the way they have dealt with life previously (Parkes and Prigerson, 2013; Hadad, 2009). Parkes did find evidence that the widows continued their relationship with their deceased husband, but he promoted the idea that this happened in early grief and stopped in later phases of grief (Klass, Silverman, and Nickman, 1996). For many decades grief and loss professionals held the belief that in order for a person to complete their mourning, all ties to the deceased needed to be broken. Meanwhile, people who were actually grieving were going underground with their experiences—finding ways for their relationship with the deceased person to continue—out of concern that they would be judged as unhealthy or "crazy."

Klass, Silverman, and Nickman

Klass, Silverman, and Nickman developed the concept of "continuing bonds" in grief and loss (Klass, Silverman, and Nickman, 1996). Their phrase expresses how people "hold the deceased in loving memory for long periods, often forever, ... maintaining an inner representation of the deceased is normal rather than abnormal"(Klass, Silverman, and Nickman, 1996). The concept of continuing bonds reflects the ongoing relationship that a bereaved person has with the person who has died. Though that person is no longer physically present in the bereaved person's life, a relationship continues with the deceased, and this is normal and healthy. Bereaved people responded very positively to this shift in thinking about grief and loss due to a person's death, probably because it matched the experiences they were having.

Continuing bonds occur in many forms. Ways that people continue their relationship with someone who has died include:

- Having two-way inner conversations with the person who has died
- Having one-way conversations with the person who has died
- Feeling visited by the person who has died
- Dreaming of and remembering the person who has died
- Keeping cherished objects that are reminders of the person who has died

(Klass, Silverman, and Nickman, 1996)

Perhaps the most important lessons to be learned from the continuing bonds model are recognizing that grief is an individual and unique experience, and that continuing to relate to the person who has died is an important way for people to continue to have room for happiness and health in their lives. As the authors of *Continuing Bonds: New Understandings of Grief* say, "We need to allow individuals room to make their own meaning and their own peace" (Klass, Silverman, and Nickman, 1996).

Grief as a Whole Person Experience

Parkes also says that grief is the price we pay for love (Parkes and Prigerson, 2013). If we ignore this truth, we will be unprepared to experience loss in our life or support other people in their grief. Grief is a "whole person" experience that affects every area of a grieving person's life—physical, social, emotional, spiritual, and mental. Human beings experience and express grief in many different ways. People who like to draw as a way to reflect on their loss may find using a body map helpful to understand their whole person experience of grief (Parkes and Prigerson, 2013).

Expressions of Grief

Physical

Grief can be felt as an aching in the stomach, head, or chest, or as fatigue, restlessness, or listlessness. Sleeping can be difficult, even when the grieving person is exhausted. Fatigue can be overwhelming. Some people who are grieving have no appetite, while others take comfort in eating.

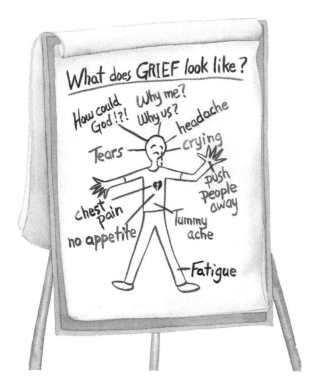

Social

Some grieving people find it impossible to be with friends and family, because conversations that are not about grief seem trivial, yet if they do talk about their grief, they feel vulnerable and exposed. Others find that they need family and friends to distract them from their emotions, and may feel frightened, lonely, and even resentful when family and friends leave. Still others worry that they will upset other people if they speak of their grief and so prefer to be silent.

Emotional

The emotions of grief can feel overwhelming. Sadness is a common emotion of grief, as are anger, depression, irritability, annoyance, intolerance, and frustration. A person's feelings can be more intense with sleep deprivation, ongoing decline in functioning, the fear of being a burden, the fear of separation, and the challenges of facing the unknown. While some people readily express emotion through tears or angry outbursts, others may be more comfortable keeping their emotions to themselves.

Spiritual

It is common for people who are grieving to question their beliefs and long-held worldview as they try to adjust to their new reality and find meaning in the loss and the situation. This may be particularly painful and surprising for those who have held strong beliefs and found comfort in those beliefs.

Mental

A grieving person may have difficulty thinking clearly. For some people, their mind is busy, going over and over the course of events, trying to recall or understand what happened. Others have trouble concentrating and may be forgetful, have difficulty doing things that were formerly easy, or have difficulty learning new things. The person may become easily confused and feel mentally exhausted even after sleeping, or may forget simple things, such as how to get to the store or how to cook a basic meal. Some people fear they are going crazy.

Factors Influencing a Person's Grief

In your caregiving, you will care for people who grieve in a variety of ways. The intensity of a person's grief is influenced by the timing of the loss, the nature of the loss, what the loss means in terms of the progression of their illness, and how the loss affects the person's ability to maintain hope. A dying person's perception of a loss and its effect on quality of life are the most significant influences on their grief. Consider these three losses:

- The loss of independent living when moving into an assisted living facility
- The loss of independence when help is required for daily activities
- The loss of privacy when a person needs total care

While these losses commonly occur as illness progresses, the meaning of each loss will be different for the person experiencing the loss. For example, while one person may grieve the loss of the ability or opportunity to cook, another may be relieved that someone else is now responsible for doing the grocery shopping and making meals. Understanding the meaning of the loss to the person at the time will be important to understanding their grief.

Changes in Grief Over Time

One of the truths about grief is that grief does not end. The intensity and energy of grief usually decrease over time but are woven into the fabric of a person's life in some form.

Initially I was completely wiped out. I dragged myself through each day. I could not think clearly to make decisions. I had to rely on others to help me sort out the big stuff. I was unable to eat. The first year after my husband died in the accident, I was a mess. People were kind. They brought meals. They drove the kids to school. They put snow tires on the car. They winterized the house. I don't know where I was, but I know I did not function well. Now, the kids and I are managing better. We still miss him. I think of him every day. I miss him especially at special times for the kids. But, it does not hurt so much anymore. And I don't cry as much as I used to cry. It is easier. The blanket of grief is not as heavy. There are holes in it, and it is more a part of my life.

Worden's Model of Grief

Models of grief have been developed over the past centuries as ways to help people understand and support others who are grieving. A model of grief creates a framework that puts the theory into practice and provides guidance on how to support grieving people.

J. William Worden is a researcher and practitioner who developed a model of grief that presented a set of four tasks that people move through in a healthy grieving process (Worden, 1991). These tasks are as follows:

1. **To begin to move from denial to acceptance or cognitive understanding that the death has really occurred.** In early grief, people move in and out of the reality that the death has occurred. Some days it feels very real, and other days it feels like it could not have happened. At some point people begin to understand that the person who has died is not coming back. Before this realization, some part of the grieving person is waiting for the deceased to return. After this point the reality that the person who died is not coming back sinks in. There is often a strong upsurge of emotion when this understanding occurs.

2. **To acknowledge, experience, and work through feelings that arise.** A grieving person experiences a myriad of reactions to the loss: some are emotional and include a wide variety of different feelings; some are physical, such as changes in sleep, appetite, and energy. Further reactions happen on the cognitive level: people struggle to focus, remember things, or express their thoughts. Social reactions also occur: people withdraw from activities or need to be out and about a lot. Finally, spirituality is affected. People may go on a quest to answer big questions that they have about life and why things happen, or they may find their beliefs challenged by the death. People often experience their grief as unpredictable at this time. They feel like they are riding the waves of reactions.

3. **To adjust to life without the person who has died.** During this task people feel energy returning and may start reinvesting it in new ways. Some may go back to doing exactly what they had done before, but with a greater sense of peace within themselves. Others experience a shift in priorities. What once felt important no longer feels important; something new may emerge. These people reinvest their energy in the new priorities, sometimes significantly changing their lives.

4. **To emotionally relocate the deceased and move on with life.** Initially Worden's work did not support the concept of continuing bonds, but eventually he found that the continued relationship with the deceased person was an important part of healthy grieving. He adjusted his final task of grieving accordingly. The grieving person successfully creates a new relationship with the deceased person that allows it to continue even though the deceased is no longer able to physically maintain the relationship. The relationship continues through memories, conversations, and objects belonging to the person who has died that create the feeling that the deceased is close by. To move on with life means to continue to be connected with the person who has died and begin to move forward with living a life that the grieving person finds pleasurable. Grief continues to be a part of the grieving person's life but shows up as upsurges of grief, often around special occasions that mark events in the family's life (e.g., high school graduation, wedding, birth of grandchildren). The upsurges tend not to be so overwhelming to the bereaved and are likely to settle down again after a short period of time.

Types of Grief

Specific types of losses may create different types of grief responses.

Anticipatory Grief

Anticipatory grief is an emotional response to future losses and may, in part, be based on the dying person's or the family's experience with previous losses. When a dying person is told that curative treatments or acute interventions are no longer helpful, the person may become aware for the first time that dying sooner than later is a more certain possibility. They may grieve the loss of a long retirement or the loss of freedom to travel far or nearby. Any unfinished losses in their life may resurface with the new losses that are experienced when a life-limiting illness is diagnosed. Common examples of past losses include miscarriages, estrangements, and unfinished goals, (e.g., high school graduation). Family members also grieve past, present, and future losses when they learn that someone they care for is now receiving palliative care. They may grieve, for example, their role change from partner to caregiver, the loss of a fully functioning parent, or the loss of a cherished grandfather who is able to build things with them. Anticipatory grief is expressed with the same level of unpredictability as all other grief. This may mean that family members experience their grief at times unique to each of them. Either way, it is challenging for them to have the energy to be understanding of one another, or they may choose to protect one another from their pain so that it remains unshared. The results can be misunderstandings or people feeling isolated and alone with their sorrow.

As a nurse you can support the dying person and family by acknowledging the grief that each may be experiencing, providing them someone to safely share their pain with, and encouraging them to talk with one another about how they are feeling. This may assist the dying person and family to feel more comfortable with communicating more openly with one another and sharing the experience of the dying process.

Disenfranchised Grief

Disenfranchised grief is grief that is unacknowledged, invisible, or socially unacceptable to others. It is often experienced by people who are marginalized, such as people who are elderly, homeless, or suffering from addictions, people with dementia, and people who are part of a same-sex couple. Disenfranchised grief leaves the grieving person feeling isolated. At times their grief goes underground and does not get expressed, leaving them vulnerable to a difficult grief journey later on.

As a nurse you are in a positon to identify people who are either currently experiencing disenfranchised grief or at risk of experiencing it later. When you encounter such people, you can provide support by recognizing their loss with them and listening as they speak of it. Your willingness to talk and listen to their pain may help remove some of the loneliness and isolation they are probably experiencing. If you assess that someone is at risk of experiencing disenfranchised grief following the death of someone they care about, you can encourage them to seek support after the death has occurred and refer them to an appropriate community resource.

Pat had been a vibrant, active wife, mother, and teacher. Eighteen months ago she was diagnosed with dementia. Now she struggles daily to remember where to find things in the house and gets lost when she goes out. She feels devastated by her loss of independence. Her family doesn't share their grief with her—they want to focus on being positive. Pat felt she could not share her grief about what was happening to her mind with anyone, as no one seemed willing to hear it.

Melanie had been a full-time HCP for Joan, who had ALS, for six years when Joan died. At first, Joan could talk and the two women shared stories about their lives and families. Over time Melanie often felt like she was looking after a friend and gave Joan the loving care she would have given a family member. When Joan quietly died, Melanie felt bereft. She had lost someone she had seen almost daily for six years and whom she had grown to care about. Melanie also lost contact with Joan's family, whom she had grown to know. Melanie felt that she had no one to share her grief with, because everyone else thought this was just her "job" and that she would be happy for a change.

Harry and George were in a loving, committed relationship for 25 years when George was diagnosed with pancreatic cancer. He died three months later. Harry found that his gay friends were very supportive of his grief, but family and co-workers did not acknowledge the huge loss Harry was experiencing. Harry felt he couldn't talk to them about it, and felt very angry that people he cared about and he believed cared about him did not understand his grief about George's death.

Complicated Grief

"Complicated grief is an intense and long-lasting form of grief that takes over a person's life" (Columbia School of Social Work, 2016). In complicated grief, the loss remains at the forefront of life rather than receding into the background. Early in the grief process, intense feelings, thoughts, and physical reactions are healthy parts of the grief process. People eventually experience a shift in which there is some resolution to the loss and they are able to move forward with living. In complicated grief, the feelings, thoughts, and physical reactions remain intense, and the shift toward resolution does not happen. It is important to note that grief is not considered "complicated" until a minimum of six months after the death. The key points are that grief has remained *intense* at six months or even longer after the death has occurred. Many factors are involved in the genesis of complicated grief. The nurse might suspect complicated grief in a person who:

- Attempts to keep the relationship with the person who has died in the physical realm
- Yearns or longs for the person who has died
- Thinks so much about the person who died that this preoccupation interferes with other relationships
- Shows signs of not fully understanding or comprehending that death has occurred, for example:
  - Experiences ongoing feelings of shock and numbness
  - Avoids places, people, or things that are reminders of the loss
  - Experiences emotional or physical distress when confronted with reminders of the loss
  - Experiences a strong urge to see, touch, hear, or smell things to feel close to the person who has died
- Feels that meaning in life is missing, because they
  - Feel lonely even when others are around
  - Feel angry and bitter in relation to the death
  - Believe life is meaningless without the person who has died
  - Find it hard to care about or trust other people
    (Columbia School of Social Work, 2016)

Complicated grief is treatable and, with help, people are able to move forward to a healthy place in their lives. Complicated grief does require counseling support, and as a nurse you can help someone experiencing complicated grief by doing a thorough assessment based on the above factors and then referring appropriately. Remember, it is not your role to diagnose complicated grief. It is your role to consider the length of time following the death, and if it is six months or more and you are aware that the factors listed above are present, then consider referring the person for additional support.

Intuitive versus Instrumental Styles of Grieving

Grief is an individual experience, and people find their own ways of grieving. Grieving styles are on a continuum, from intuitive grieving at one end to instrumental grieving at the other end (Table 1). It is important to understand that this model of grieving styles does not indicate that a person is either intuitive or instrumental. Instead, people present along a continuum of the two styles, tending to gravitate toward one style more than another, but at any time in their grief process they may move toward the other style because of their needs and desires (Doka and Martin, 2010).

As a nurse, it is important to be aware of your own grieving style as well, so that you are not judgmental toward a dying person's or family member's way of coping with their grief. There is no "one size fits all" with grief. HCPs need to be aware of their own style so that they can accept and be comfortable with another person's different style.

Table 1. Characteristics of Intuitive Versus Instrumental Grieving Styles (Doka and Martin, 2010)

	Intuitive Grieving	Instrumental Grieving
Experience of Grief	Emotional	Cognitive, physical
Expression of Grief	Outward mirroring of inner experience Shared feelings Low physical activity Depression	Planned tasks and projects Shared activities High physical arousal Anxiety
Coping Strategies	Take time to grieve, adjust slowly Share feelings	Readjust and restore normal routines Solve problems related to loss

Continuum

Considering a person's grieving style will help you understand how to support them. For people who lean more toward intuitive grieving, providing opportunities to talk about a loss can be very helpful. Emotional expression and connecting with others are the keys to support. Listening, responding gently, and respecting how the person describes the experience of the loss provide an outlet for their emotions associated with the loss. Providing information about available support groups can also help, as intuitive grievers appreciate exploring, expressing their feelings, and being able to connect with others having a similar experience (Downing and Wainwright, 2006). Groups such as a breast cancer support group and family caregivers networks may meet the person's need for sharing.

For people who lean toward a more instrumental style of grieving, information and action are the keys to support. They may respond best to concrete information about grief. These people may benefit from having projects and assignments to address the needs of the people involved. Providing pamphlets, books, and web resources about grief may be appreciated. Similarly, providing information about fundraising campaigns (e.g., Run for the Cure), may help instrumental grievers.

Greta and Jack cared for their adult son for months when he was dying. Greta attended to his every need. After his death her days seemed endless and her grief was overwhelming. She sobbed for hours at a time. She talked with others who understood and who allowed her to cry. Jack was dry eyed. He arranged the funeral, found hotels for out-of-town relatives who came to the funeral, gave a brilliant eulogy, and later made a bench with a plaque dedicated to his son. He applied to the city to design and build a small memorial garden in a local park where the bench would be placed.

The story of Greta and Jack shows her to be an intuitive griever. Greta's emotions are easily accessible. In her grief, she cries frequently and sometimes feels like she lacks control. She finds support in being with other people. At times, the intensity of her feelings is frightening to her, and she is often fatigued. Her focus is on her feelings, not on accomplishing tasks.

Jack is an instrumental griever. He stays busy attending to tasks, focuses on caring for others, and appears to be coping with daily activities. He makes meaning of his son's death by memorializing him and preparing a park bench to celebrate his life. Jack struggles to maintain control while he feels deep pain, turmoil, and anxiety. He copes with the loss in the same manner that he copes with other problems that he needs to solve. He appreciates privacy. He does not welcome questions that address feelings but may accept help with his projects.

Greta and Jack grieve in different ways. Both Greta and Jack are adapting to the world without their son. Neither way is right or wrong. The two stories above illustrate different grieving styles. Knowing a person's grieving style makes it less likely that you will judge, evaluate, or label their behavior. Knowing their grieving style makes is easier to support them in their grieving.

For example, Greta might appreciate attending a support group as she grieves, while Jack might prefer to work with the community to establish the memorial garden.

Caregivers need to refrain from judging or labeling the behavior of grieving people. Instead, you can support them by letting them know that their grief and ways of expressing grief are normal, and by helping them identify their own strengths in coping and accept the way others are grieving. When you give people the chance to identify what is helpful to them, you can better support them.

Denial—an Effective Coping Strategy of Grieving

People may use denial to cope with overwhelming emotions (Victoria Hospice Society, Wainwright, W., and Thompson, M., 2016). Every person has a unique response to bad news, grief, and loss. While some people ask questions, take notes, and read as much as they can to understand what is happening, others appear to withdraw and reject the information and its implications. When a person appears to ignore the reality of a diagnosis, prognosis, or suggestion (e.g., that they need to use a walker), they may be labeled as "in denial."

Denial may be misunderstood by the health care team, which may view someone who is in denial of their illness as someone who is not accepting it. In fact, denial is a coping strategy. It is used when a situation or information is too much for a person to absorb all at once. Someone who is overwhelmed by the situation or information may choose to acknowledge pieces of it, the pieces that person can bear emotionally at the time. This is often unconsciously done, but it is a strategy that helps that person ward off feelings that may be unbearable. When someone is using denial as a form of self-protection, the care team must respect that boundary. Trying to push the dying person beyond the boundary they have set can lead that person to mistrust the care team or be in a state that feels unbearable to them.

It may be helpful to consider that people use denial as a way to reduce the flow of bad news, allowing only as much information in as they can comfortably tolerate. This situation is not unlike that of the farmer who builds a floodgate to manage the flow of water onto his land. The floodgate limits the amount of water coming in and preserves the land. In this analogy, the water is the flow of bad news, and closing the floodgate (denial) is the person's way to limit the flow of information. Each person has a unique capacity to process information, and some people create an internal floodgate to control the flow of bad news as a means of self-preservation. Denial is one method people use to control the flow of difficult information so that they can deal with it in smaller amounts. It is another way of saying, "I'm just not ready for that information yet. I need more time to take it all in."

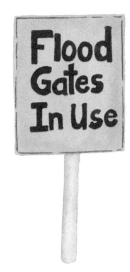

It's important to remember that each person will respond differently to bad news and will absorb the information as they are able. You can acknowledge to the person and their family that it is normal for people to take in information at different rates. This may help family members be less judgmental with one another.

You may support the person by saying, for example,

Sometimes it takes people a bit of time to adapt to all this information. That is all right.

You can encourage the person to ask questions as they arise for them. You could say,

People often need time to absorb what they have heard. If you find that you have more questions after you have had some time to consider this news, know that your questions are welcome at any time.

It can be helpful to talk with the family about how everyone absorbs information at a different rate and therefore not to expect that everyone will be at the same place at the same time. You could say,

People understand or want information at different rates. That is true even when you are in the same family. You will each have your own pace, and that is okay. Just know that things can become confusing and everyone has a different pace, and what helps the confusion is to talk about it.

Supporting Hope

Hope is both fragile and resilient. Hope is not rational; it does not depend on statistics or facts. A person who receives a diagnosis of a life-threatening illness may hope that the illness will not significantly affect their quality of life, that it will be curable, and that it will not cause their death. When the same person is told, "There is no cure and no further treatments available," they may maintain hope for a long life, even when they recognize that having a long life would require a miracle. And when a person no longer hopes for a cure, they may hope to see the next grandchild born, or hope for a pain-free death, or hope their family will be well supported following death.

Hope can help sustain a person's emotional well-being by allowing them to look forward to good things in the future. A dying person may say, "I hope I can go fishing next summer like I have done for 55 years!" even when they know they may not live through the next month.

It is not helpful to confront a person with the reality that they are dying. It would not be supportive to say, "Don't you understand? You will never be able to go fishing again." Neither would it be helpful to say, "Of course you'll be able to go fishing next summer. Just set your mind to it and think positive thoughts."

You may be able to support the person and their hope when you:

* Respond from a genuine but neutral place

Wouldn't that be wonderful? I hope you get your wish. What else do you hope for?

* Respond to the feelings behind the hope

It sounds like you loved fishing. Where was your favorite fishing hole? What is your favorite fishing story?

It is helpful to remember that hope is always possible and that hope can change.

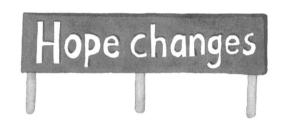

Post-traumatic Growth

Richard Tedeschi and Lawrence Calhoun introduced the concept of post-traumatic growth, which emerged from the field of positive psychology. Post-traumatic growth is defined as the "experience of an individual whose development at least in some areas has surpassed what was present before the struggle with crises occurred. The individual has not only survived but has experienced changes that are viewed as important, and go beyond the status quo" (Tedeschi and Calhoun, 2004). Stephen Joseph's research on post-traumatic growth suggests that people report three different ways that their psychological functioning improved following traumatic experiences (Joseph, 2013):

1. Relationships are enhanced. For example, people value friends and family more and experience increased compassion for others.
2. People change their view of themselves in some way, for example, developing in wisdom, personal strength, and gratitude, sometimes coupled with greater acceptance of vulnerabilities and limitations.
3. People describe changes in life philosophy. Their understanding of what really matters in life shifts, and they are more able to live in the present and are less materialistic (Joseph, 2014).

As someone who works closely with the dying and grieving, you may recognize some of these changes identified in the post-traumatic growth research. Often grieving people will describe themselves as having more compassion for others following their loss experience. They describe shifts in their priorities; what felt important before the loss no longer feels important after the loss. It is very possible that despite the pain and disorientation following loss, positive growth can occur.

Supporting a Grieving Person

There are many ways that you can support a grieving person. The most important tool, however, is your relationship. In a caregiving relationship, an outside person enters into a family in a unique role. Getting to know the person that you are caring for as an individual with unique experiences and needs builds the foundation for trust that can then allow space for a person's grief. Once the caregiving relationship has been established, a number of supportive strategies can be used. These include acknowledging the many emotions involved in the loss, assessing the loss, individualizing care, making room for tears, and remembering the whole picture.

Acknowledging Loss

Mixed emotions are common in people who experience losses. Family members feel sadness about the impending loss of a loved one and at the same time may feel guilty for being well, for wanting time for themselves, or for being frustrated and angry at having to take time away from work to be a caregiver. The dying person may feel grateful that you prepare the meals and help with personal care and at the same time resent needing your help. After a loved one dies, a family member may express both relief and grief, especially if they have had to cope with many losses during a long and slow dying process. These are all examples of mixed emotions and a range of emotions. There are no good or bad emotions in the grieving process, just as there is no right or wrong way to grieve.

It may be helpful to acknowledge that emotions, like relationships, are complicated, and to acknowledge the loss, grief, and mixed emotions the person is experiencing. You might say,

You have had many changes in the last few months. How has that been for you?

This seems really hard for you. I hear the pain in your voice.

You can support a person who is expressing mixed emotions by acknowledging that relationships are complicated, that both caregiving and being sick are difficult, and that having mixed feelings is normal.

Assessing Loss

While grief is a healthy process, there are times when a grieving person may benefit from more specialized support. Some people need additional support when grieving after the death of a loved one. In some cases, this is because the death was sudden, difficult, or complicated by other challenging life events. In other cases, a person's grief may be intensified by personal factors, such as physical health issues, mental health issues, (e.g., depression, addiction) or a personal, unrelated crisis. Social factors that may affect grieving are disenfranchised grief, difficult family dynamics, pre-existing challenges with the person who died, and lifestyle challenges resulting from illness and death. Examples of lifestyle challenges include the isolation entailed in long-term caregiving, a lack of financial resources, the need to relocate, having to quit one's job to provide care, and the changes in the bereaved person's ability to live independently. All these factors indicate that more specific grief support might be valuable.

As a nurse, you may see or hear from the grieving person, other family members, friends, or colleagues that the grieving person is struggling. While it is completely normal to lose one's appetite or not feel like getting dressed, it is a concern if the normal signs of grief seem exaggerated or occur over an extended time. You may notice that the person is not coping well if they show consistent and debilitating fatigue or an inability to take care of daily business, talk about self-harm, or express an ongoing sense of purposelessness.

You can make a big difference in a dying person's life by showing, through your words and actions, that you support them and care about them.

When circumstances of the death or social or personal factors have made grieving especially difficult, and when the grieving person appears to need extra support, it is important that you record this information and share it with the health care team.

The Bereavement Risk Assessment Tool (BRAT)

Use the Bereavement Risk Assessment Tool (BRAT) (see page 90 in Chapter 4, "Using Standardized Tools") to help identify whether a person is at risk of experiencing or is experiencing a difficult grief process and whether extra bereavement support may be needed (Victoria Hospice Society, 2014). Once these issues are identified, the person at risk can be referred to appropriate members of the health care team or appropriate community resources for specialized support.

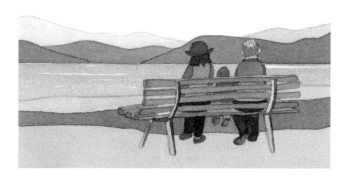

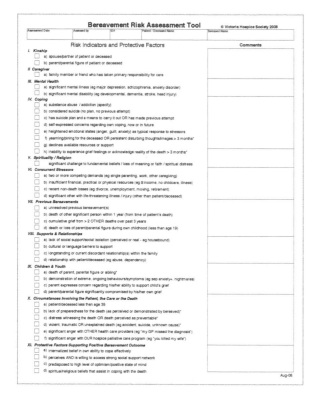

Bereavement Risk Assessment Tool (BRAT)

Leaving Room for Silence

It takes courage and confidence to witness deep grief and stay present, perhaps only offering a gentle touch or companioning in silence. Silence can be a sign that the person feels comfortable in your company. Sometimes the mere presence of another human can be comforting. Silence, however, can be awkward if the other person feels responsible for entertaining or engaging with you. It can be difficult to decide whether silence is welcome or not. It may be difficult for you to keep silent if you are accustomed to talking or feel it is your responsibility to keep the conversation going.

Many people associate silence with emptiness or just an absence of conversation. In fact, silence is full of presence; something is always going on in the spaces between words and actions. Embracing silence clears space for whatever needs to happen. When working with people who are profoundly ill, grieving, overwhelmed by change and loss, or anxious and fearful about what lies ahead, silence can be a gift that allows the person the time and space to collect their thoughts, to reflect on the immensity of death, or to consider questions like "Why me?" that have no answers. Being comfortable with silence requires being able to trust yourself and the person you are with, in order to give up control of the space that silence creates.

If conversation meets the needs of the person receiving care, then talking is appropriate. It's a good idea to check regularly to see if the person is tired of talking. A conversation can be a useful distraction from discomfort, but can also be exhausting. If you are not sure whether someone wants you to continue to talk, you might say, for example,

I don't want to tire you out with conversation. I can just sit here with you quietly if you would prefer.

Individualizing Care

Each grieving person has a unique grief experience and requires individualized care. You can be curious and focus on the person, and invite the person to describe what is helpful, what they appreciate people doing to help them. You know too that family members will grieve and will express their grief in different ways. Your compassionate response to each person will indicate that there are many normal ways to express grief and many ways to support a person in their grief.

You might say,

In every family or social group there will be people who express their grief in different ways.

What you are telling me is completely normal.

When Robert's wife died, people from the church and others that he barely knew in his neighborhood left many casseroles and baked goods on his doorstep. He had no appetite and felt guilty when the food went bad. Regina was the personal support worker caring for Robert. She wondered why Robert didn't eat the food and why he was not expressing gratitude for the meals. She resisted the urge to judge him and decided to be curious. One day she asked him, "Robert, of all the things that you have to deal with right now, what would you say is the most difficult for you?" He looked her in the eye and said, "I just miss her. I feel so awfully lonely I just want to lie down and die." Regina's heart felt like it was melting. She put her hand on his shoulder and sat down beside him. "What do you need the most right now?" She was very surprised when he said, "I want some company. I don't want the casseroles, I want someone to sit down and share a cup of tea with me." Regina and Robert then talked about how he could make that happen.

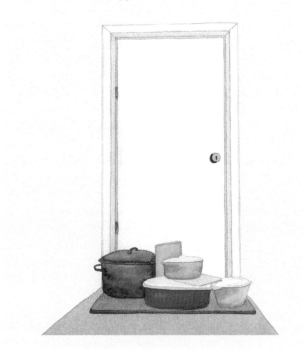

Making Room for Tears

Crying is a normal, healthy response to grief. Sometimes people try to stop people from crying by handing them tissues, patting them on the back and saying "Shhh," distracting them, or putting a positive spin on the person's grief. Silence and gently acknowledging that "It's so hard right now" may make space for tears. Sometimes other people's tears will trigger your own. This is normal and can be very comforting to the other person, because they can see that you understand. As long as the focus stays on the person you are with and does not move to you, it is okay to shed a few tears. (You may want to discuss your emotions later with a colleague or supervisor.)

Let us not underestimate how hard it is to be compassionate. Compassion is hard because it requires the inner disposition to go with others to the place where they are weak, vulnerable, lonely, and broken. But this is not our spontaneous response to suffering. What we desire most is to do away with suffering by fleeing from it or finding a quick cure for it.

(Nouwen, McNeill, and Morrison, 1981)

Remembering the Whole Picture— Emotional and Physical

The physical pains and discomfort discussed in Chapter 5, "Enhancing Physical Comfort," can often be decreased through the use of medications and comfort measures. However, when a person is dying, there are psychosocial pains that cannot be fixed. There is no "emotional morphine" that can ease deep suffering. The other reality is that it is not your job to fix deep suffering. It is your job to provide support. Chapter 3, "Preparing to Care," contains more information about this topic.

Facilitating Self-Determination and Autonomy with Advance Care Planning

In industrialized society, many people value self-determination and autonomy. Self-determination is the power or ability to make decisions for oneself without influence from outside. In hospice and palliative care, it is autonomy—the right of all competent people to choose to accept or refuse any or all medical therapy, even if refusal means they will die (Meisel, 1989)—that can significantly affect the dying person's and family's experience. Specifically, promoting autonomy with advance care planning as early as the time of diagnosis can benefit the dying person and their family by:

- Avoiding decision making when the person becomes more confused as disease progresses
- Providing space for difficult discussions before crises occur
- Preventing misunderstandings or misconceptions of the person's wishes by proxy decision makers
- Providing the opportunity for a longer survival time

(Zalonis and Slota, 2014)

Advance care planning (ACP) is a process in which the person identifies, records, and discusses their wishes for future health care and interventions that are based on their beliefs, values, hopes, fears, and priorities. Having conversations with their family and the physician/nurse practitioner and documenting their (the dying person's) preferences and wishes will inform the health care team if or when the person is no longer able to direct their own care. Both Canada and the United States have frameworks for advance care planning, available in digital and print formats on websites. ACP helps people to determine their own care through to death and following.

Tools for Advance Care Planning

In Canada: Speak Up Campaign
advancecareplanning.ca

In the United States: Five Wishes
agingwithdignity.org/five-wishes

Appointing a Substitute Decision Maker

In many states, provinces, and territories, a person may be able to legally appoint a substitute decision maker (SDM) (Canada) or durable power of attorney for health care (DPOA-HC) (United States) while mentally competent to do so. (To avoid repetition, the abbreviation SDM will represent both these roles in this text.) The SDM will make decisions and speak on the person's behalf if they become unable to speak for themselves. The theory is that the health care team consults the SDM when necessary, and together they can honor the wishes of the person through dying, death, and post-death care. An SDM is responsible for health care decisions for the person only if the person is no longer able to make their own decisions. An SDM is not able to, for example, contribute to financial decisions. The requirements to appoint an SDM vary in each jurisdiction. Providing the person and family with the specifics for your location will be helpful as they begin this process.

Selecting an appropriate SDM may be easier if the person considers people who:
- Know them well—their personality, likes, and dislikes
- Are actively involved in their care
- Are aware of current physical and psychosocial issues affecting them or that may affect them
- Are comfortable having ACP conversations with the person
- Understand that their role as SDM is to honor the person's wishes and make a decision they feel the person would make if they were able to speak for themselves in this particular situation
- Understand that they are not to make decisions based on what they themselves would want

In other words, an SDM should be someone who can respond to the question,

If your loved one was here today, given the current health concern and the available options, what do you think he or she would have wanted done?

In some families the SDM is assigned according to cultural tradition; for example, the eldest son is assigned to make decisions. In other families, the family may decide as a group what should be done even if one person is formally designated as the SDM.

Appointing an SDM that is appropriate for the dying person can substantially support their autonomy as disease progresses. If the person does not appoint an SDM, the health care organization will have a policy that identifies who is to be asked to make health care decisions. This may be a spouse, an adult child, or another relative. A problem would arise if the dying person does not have such people in their life to take on this role or is alienated from them, if those people do not want to make decisions on the dying person's behalf, or if there is considerable conflict within the family and an SDM is not appointed to make a decision.

Strategies to Assist with Creating an Advance Care Plan

ACP is a process that can be broken into individual steps. Informing the person and family about these steps can help them to more easily complete the advance care plan.

Think: What is right for you? What are your values, beliefs, and understanding about end-of-life care and specific medical procedures?

Learn! There are many medical procedures that can be offered at the end of life. Some may improve your quality of life, and others may only prolong life. Different people have different thoughts about these procedures.

Choose: Identify your SDM. Choose someone who would honor and follow your wishes, and is able to speak for you if you can't speak for yourself.

Talk: Share your wishes with your SDM, family members, and friends who are important to you. Tell your health care team. If you have a written plan, make sure they have a copy.

Record: It's a good idea to write down your wishes or make a recording or video about your wishes for end-of-life care. Find out what forms are available in your state, province, or territory.

Review: Update your plan regularly, especially when something in your life changes. Continue the conversation!

(CHPCA, 2016)

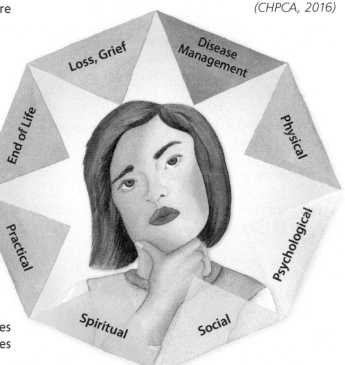

Case Study

Jimmy is a 64-year-old, Navaho Elder. Traditionally death is not talked about in his community. Recently an Elder was taken from the community when he was very sick, and he died in an intensive care unit at a big-city hospital. Jimmy does not want to leave his community, and he decided to talk with his family about what he wants if and when he is not able to speak for himself. Jimmy asked his granddaughter Alana, who is a nursing student, to talk with him.

Alana wrote a list of questions that she thought would help the family understand his wishes. She and Jimmy discussed the questions, and she summarized his answers on paper.

What makes my life meaningful?

Living in my community. Being with family. Traditional ways of healing and spiritual practices.

What three things do people need to know when they care for me?

I follow the traditional ways of healing.

I want to die in my community. I do not want to go to the big-city hospital.

I want to be heard.

What do I worry about when I think about death?

Being alone in a big hospital

Not being able to breathe

What do I want when I am nearing death?

My family around me

The burning of sweetgrass

A blessing from the priest

If I cannot speak for myself, who do I want to speak and make decisions for me?

I want my granddaughter Alana to make decisions about treatment for me.

I want my son to speak for me.

What treatments do I want or not want?

I do not want to live with machines keeping me alive.

I do not want dialysis.

I do not want to be taken to the big-city hospital for any reason.

What do I want my children to remember?

To follow the traditional ways

Who will I talk about this conversation with?

My children and the community nurse

Jimmy called his family together and shared with them what he wanted them to do when he is sick and when he is dying.

Ethics Touchstone
Respect can be difficult, and sometimes it can mean following through with the person's wishes even though others may not agree. How might you support this family to respect Jimmy's wishes if they disagree with them?

Goals-of-Care Conversations

Goals-of-care conversations are the extension or application of the ACP conversations in the decision-making process. These conversations occur when a physician or nurse meets with the person and/or the SDM and/or the family to review the person's current situation, progression of disease, and options for treatment or care. The person and their family are encouraged to identify current goals of care, and then, considering the goals, the health care team assists in identifying treatments, medications, and support that are most likely to help meet those goals. These conversations often result in a physician's order or a conversation with the physician (if the physician is not already present).

Goals-of-care conversations provide an opportunity for the person and family to share their observations, questions, and concerns. In addition to providing information and resources, as the nurse you can facilitate the process by raising the topics with the person and with the family, responding to concerns and challenges, and supporting the person and family to clarify or update the goals of care.

Goals-of-care conversations may be formalized and occur during a "family conference" initiated by the health care team or at the request of the person or the family. They may be planned, or they may occur spontaneously. They may be in a physician's office, or they may be at the person's bedside.

Facilitating Goals-of-Care Conversations

If you are leading the conversation, it may be helpful to identify the purpose of the meeting and then to provide a brief agenda. You might say, for example,

I wanted to talk with you today about your goals of care and together make a plan for next steps.

It is often helpful for people to share what they are experiencing and what they are seeing. You may ask,

Can you share with me a few snapshots of the last year? What did you notice a year ago? How much was your dad up and around? And six months ago? And four months ago? Two months ago? ... one week? ... the last few days?

It is helpful for the person and family to describe the changes over time, because in telling their story they may begin to absorb the reality of the person's impending death.

Alternatively, the person or family may be able to share their story of decline over the past months. You might ask,

Can you share with me what you are seeing? What you observe? How you are feeling? What things have changed in the past weeks, days ... ?

How do you feel the treatments are working? Are they meeting your goals?

Would it be helpful if I shared what I see, or if the physician visited and provided an update on the disease progression, and talked with you about treatment options?

Do you have a sense of the next steps? What are your goals and hopes for the next steps?

When the family asks what the purpose of the family meeting is, you may want to state that as the person's health declines, medical treatment decisions will need to be made, and that it is less stressful for the person and family to talk ahead of time, gain a good understanding of medically relevant and appropriate interventions, and have the support of the team to make decisions.

In the meeting you may also want to explore what the person understands of their disease, diagnosis, and prognosis, and what questions they want addressed in the meeting. Communicating this information to the team in advance will help the team be prepared to provide information, recommend treatment options that help the person meet their goals, and address any concerns or fears. Questions like these may help start the conversation:

Can you tell me about your illness?

As your illness progresses, what concerns or fears do you have?

What are your goals?

Developing Awareness of the Advance Care Planning Process

Nurses who develop their understanding of the ACP process will be better prepared to help others. Experiencing the process is one way to develop understanding. Use this exercise as a starting point.

Reflective Activity

1. Reflect on what is important to you as a person today, tomorrow, in a year, in 10 years.

What gives your life meaning? What gives you joy, strength, and support?

2. Talk with a friend or colleague and share your thoughts on what is important to you now and in the future.

3. Record on paper what values or ideas you want your SM to consider if you were to become unable to speak for yourself.

4. Who would you like to ask to be your SDM?

Understanding Physician Assisted Dying and Medical Assistance in Dying

Requesting and receiving medical assistance in dying/ physician assisted dying (see definitions in the next section) raise complex issues for the dying person, the family, and HCPs, and for hospice and palliative care communities. (For the purpose of this text, unless otherwise indicated the term "assisted dying" encompasses both medical assistance in dying and physician assisted dying.) This section of the book is not intended to be a discussion of whether assisted dying should be legalized. Laws in Canada and in certain jurisdictions in the United States have clearly established that assisted dying is a health care service that is or will be available to certain people at the end of life—people who meet specific criteria and who want to choose their time of death. The focus of this section is first to clarify terminology and identify hospice and palliative care principles that pertain to assisted dying, and second to provide stimulation that encourages you to consider your beliefs and identify challenges you may face when engaging with the dying person, the family, and your colleagues when assisted dying is being contemplated or pursued as an end-of-life care practice.

It is timely and appropriate to address assisted dying in this text because integrating a palliative approach includes relieving suffering, responding to difficult questions, and helping people explore care options. HCPs can apply their skills learned when responding to other difficult end-of-life questions to respond to requests for information about assisted dying. Nurses, as a community and as individuals, need to learn to engage in reflection, dialogue, and exploration to support the dying person and family in their process of considering assisted dying.

Terms Relating to Assisted Dying

In Canada and in the United States, laws are evolving in response to the requested death movement, a global social movement that is "concerned with the ultimate control of one's body at life's end" (McInerney, 2000). This movement seeks to empower people to choose the timing and manner of their own death. Terms relating to assisted dying vary by location and legislation, causing confusion for the dying person and the family, as well as for nurses and other members of the health care team.

In the United States, the term "physician assisted dying" refers to the legal practice of deliberately ending a dying person's life at their request; in Canada, the parallel term is "medical assistance in dying." As mentioned above, in this text the term "assisted dying" encompasses both medical assistance in dying and physician assisted dying.

Physician Assisted Dying

In the United States, "physician assisted dying" means:

A physician provides, at the patient's request, a lethal dose of medication that the patient can take by his own hand to end ... intolerable suffering.

(AAHPM, 2016)

In cases of physician assisted dying, the physician provides the prescription and the dying person receives it and self-administers the medication when and where and if they choose to do so; the presence of a physician or other HCP at the time of death is not required.

Oregon, Washington, Vermont, and California have legalized physician assisted dying, and legislative efforts are underway in at least 20 other states. In every jurisdiction in the United States, it is illegal for a physician or any other HCP to administer a medication or substance, regardless of route, with the explicit intention of ending the life of a dying person, even at that person's explicit request and for the purpose of alleviating their suffering.

Medical Assistance in Dying

In Canada, "medical assistance in dying" means:

The administering by a medical practitioner or nurse practitioner of a substance to a person, at their request, that causes their death; or

The prescribing or providing by a medical practitioner or nurse practitioner of a substance to a person, at their request, so that they may self-administer the substance and in doing so cause their own death.

(Government of Canada, 2016b)

Thus, medical assistance in dying is inclusive of physician assisted dying but is broader than the US practice in two ways: (1) medical assistance in dying provides the possibility of receiving a prescription for a lethal dose of medication for later self-administration, *or* receiving a lethal dose of medication that will be directly administered orally or intravenously by an HCP; (2) medical assistance in dying establishes the possibility for both physicians *and* nurse practitioners to provide assisted dying to their patients.

The term "medical assistance in dying" reflects the fact that not only physicians are involved in assisted death. In fact, Canadian federal law is explicit in conferring on both physicians and nurse practitioners the authority to prescribe, provide, and administer medical assistance in dying. The federal law also explicitly exempts any person from criminal prosecution for aiding a physician or nurse practitioner in providing medical assistance in dying.

Before the federal legislation was enacted, a law was passed in the Canadian province of Quebec that enabled physicians there to legally end the life of a dying person by injecting or providing intravenous medications, but it did not permit them to provide medications that the person would later self-administer orally with the explicit purpose of causing their own death. Thus, although the Canadian federal legislation now also applies in Quebec, existing policies in that province currently define assisted dying in a narrower sense than does the federal legislation. This is one example of regional and provincial differences in how the federal legislation is interpreted and applied, according to policies written by the provincial government, medical, nursing, and pharmacy regulatory authorities, and individual health care organizations, to name just a few. (See "Know and Be Clear about the Terms Used in Your Jurisdiction" on the next page.)

Eligibility Requirements for Assisted Dying

In the United States and in Canada, the person requesting assisted dying must meet specific eligibility requirements that are set out by law, and then follow the process outlined before receiving the life-ending medication.

Eligibility Requirements in Canada

In Canada, a person may receive medical assistance in dying only if they meet all of the following criteria:
- They are eligible to receive health services funded by a government in Canada.
- They are at least 18 years of age and capable of making decisions with respect to their health.
- They have a grievous and irremediable medical condition.
- They have voluntarily requested medical assistance in dying and did not do so as a result of pressure from other people.
- They give informed consent to receive medical assistance in dying after having been informed of the means available to relieve their suffering, including palliative care.

Eligibility Requirements in the United States

In the following named states, a person may receive physician assistance with dying only if they meet all of the following criteria:
- They are a resident of California, Oregon, Vermont, or Washington.
- They are 18 years of age or older.
- They are mentally competent, that is, capable of making and communicating their health care decisions.
- They are diagnosed with a terminal illness that will, within reasonable medical judgment, lead to death within six months.
- They are able to self-administer and ingest the prescribed medication.

All of these requirements must be met without exception.

A person cannot "qualify under aid-in-dying laws solely because of age or disability. Two physicians must determine whether all these criteria have been met"(Death with Dignity, 2016).

For further information on medical assistance in dying and related safeguards, and for clarification of terms, check the policy in your jurisdiction and facility.

The Process for Requesting Assisted Dying

The Joint Centre for Bioethics at the University of Toronto created a draft policy template to aid health institutions in responding to requests for medical assistance in dying. That document provides a detailed process for addressing and responding to requests for assisted dying. The process, detailed below, can be adapted to meet the laws and guidelines of your jurisdiction within Canada or the United States.

First, a dying person inquires about or explicitly requests assisted dying. This leads to a thoughtful and exploratory discussion between the person and their HCP or care team that probes the underlying factors motivating the person's interest in assisted dying. Questions that should be addressed at this stage include these:

- Have all care options that might be acceptable to the person been considered?
- Are the perspectives of all appropriate people (e.g., family members) known?
- Has there been meaningful involvement from palliative care and/or other specialist services (e.g., psychosocial services, including spiritual counseling) that might contribute toward alleviation of suffering?

The HCP must also consider whether she or he is comfortable discussing assisted dying as a care option with the person. If not, then a referral should be made to another HCP who can see the person through the process, although the original HCP can remain involved to the extent that she or he is comfortable.

A person who has discussed the issues described above with their HCP or care team, and who decides to choose assisted dying, must make a formal written request in front of two independent witnesses. A physician or nurse practitioner assesses the person's eligibility (see the "Eli-

gibility Requirements in Canada" section on page 211), and then a mandatory 10-day period of reflection ensues. During this period, the eligibility of the person to receive assisted dying must be confirmed by a second physician or nurse practitioner. The 10-day period may be shortened if the patient's death and/or loss of capacity for consent is imminent. (Mandatory reflection periods vary by jurisdiction. In Oregon, for example, two requests must be made, separated by a 15-day waiting period.)

The dying person pursuing assisted dying must understand that they have the right to withdraw their request at any time. At the time the dying person receives the prescription for the medication, the HCP or care team will advise the person and any other appropriate people (e.g., family members) about what to expect, and will provide specific instructions for self-administration of the medication (if applicable).

Know and Be Clear about the Terms Used in Your Jurisdiction

As a nurse, it is important to clearly understand the meaning of the terms used in your jurisdiction. These are some guiding questions for you to consider:

1. Is it legal for a physician or nurse practitioner to directly end a person's life, at the person's explicit request?
2. Is it legal for a physician or nurse practitioner to prescribe life-ending medications to a person, at their explicit request, to be taken later and in a different place?
3. If one or both of the above practices are legal, what criteria determine whether a person qualifies for assisted dying?
   a. Does the person need to be at the "end of life" and if so, how is this determined?
   b. Does the person need to be "suffering unbearably" and if so, how is this determined?
4. What does the relevant legislation say, if anything, about nurses' involvement in assisted dying?
5. What does the local state or provincial nursing regulatory authority say about nurses' involvement in assisted dying?

Reasons for Requesting Assisted Dying

The primary value underpinning the assisted dying movement is the autonomy of the person. As a guiding value for health policy, respect for autonomy establishes a person's right to decide what happens to their own body in situations of health and illness, including through dying and death. This means that the person's own preferences are what matters when deciding the appropriate course of action in health care decision making. The interests of other parties, including the government, HCPs, or even other members of the person's family, are important, but they cannot override what the person him- or herself chooses. The following quotations from people who want the option to choose assisted dying highlight their desire for autonomy:

> I want to be in control of my life as long as I can, I don't want doctors and nurses controlling me ... when I get to the [point] where I really can't cope anymore, where my quality of life is totally gone, I will tell my husband I want a really good day out with the kids, which is how he'll know that when I go to bed that night I won't wake up the next morning.
>
> (Chapple et al., 2006)

> I spent a month in the hospice ... So I have seen what happens at the end and, if I could avoid it happening to me, I would, simple as that ... if somebody was brave enough to help me, I'd be grateful to them. It's almost nonsense we can't decide what to do with our life at the end, isn't it? Why should a judge be able to say, no, I can't kill myself if I want to?
>
> (Chapple et al., 2006)

Another value that motivates the requested death movement is relief of suffering. Proponents of the requested death movement seek to provide people at the end of life with an option to avoid what could be intolerable suffering—to create end-of-life experiences that are consistent with values that are most important to them. For some people, values such as dignity, self-reliance, and bodily integrity are undermined by the physical and cognitive deteriorations associated with the dying process.

Although a desire for autonomy and relief of suffering do motivate some peoples' interest in assisted dying, it is important to understand what this interest is all about. A desire for *choice* to end one's own life in a situation of terminal illness is not the same thing as having *already decided* to die. Gloria Taylor, a public advocate in Canada for assisted dying, was the first Canadian to be allowed to end her life through assisted dying, before national laws changed. After her death, which was *not* by means of assisted dying, her family said that they were grateful that Gloria was given the solace of knowing that she had a choice about how and when she would die, enabling her "to live her final days free from the fear that she would become trapped in a body that had failed her" (BCCLA, 2012). Data from Oregon, where physician assisted dying has been legal for 20 years, substantiates the idea that while some people are comforted by having the option of assisted dying, they do not necessarily choose to die this way, even after being provided with the ability to do so (see "The Oregon Experience" below).

While some people will express interest in receiving information about assisted dying and want to have conversations with their family and HCPs about this option, that does not necessarily mean each person has decided that assisted dying is right for them.

The Oregon Experience

Data from Oregon collected since physician assisted dying was legalized in 1997 indicates that of those people who request and receive a prescription for life-ending medication, 60% of them use the medication, while 40% do not. In Oregon in 2015, 218 new prescriptions for life-ending medication were issued, and 132 deaths occurred due to ingesting life-ending medication. This means that the death rate attributed to physician assisted dying in Oregon was 38.6 per 10,000 total deaths, that is, only 0.386% of deaths are attributed to physician assisted dying.

(Oregon Public Health Division, 2016)

This is a textbook about hospice and palliative care; therefore, it is appropriate to examine the principles that guide hospice and palliative care and to reflect on assisted dying in that context.

Definitions of hospice and palliative care, for example, the World Health Organization's definition, are clear that hospice and palliative care neither hastens nor delays death, and that death is a natural phenomenon. Because assisted dying deliberately hastens death, some people in the hospice and palliative care community feel that assisted dying contradicts the principles of hospice and palliative care.

Currently, the public lacks understanding about hospice and palliative care services, often believing that hospice and palliative care is only for people who are dying imminently and that involvement with such care will hasten death. Therefore, many people in the hospice and palliative care community are concerned that if hospice and palliative care programs were to provide assisted dying, the mistaken perceptions and beliefs about hospice and palliative care services would increase.

The definition of hospice and palliative care suggests that the person and the family are the focus of care, that care should be individualized, and that the goal of care is to reduce suffering. If, for any reason, hospice and palliative care is not available to the dying person, or if symptom management has not been effective, assisted dying may seem the best way to address the person's unique needs and reduce their suffering.

The previous reflections are from hospice and palliative care professionals as they consider how to respond to the legalization of and requests for assisted dying. Some hospice and palliative care programs have policies that clearly indicate that they do not support or provide assisted dying, while other programs have developed specialized teams to respond to requests for it. Other programs have policies that are somewhere in between.

On an individual level, nurses have beliefs, values, and ethical assumptions about assisted dying that affect their desire and willingness to participate in discussion about, referral to providers of, and the actual providing of assisted dying. One nurse may believe that life is sacred and that assisted dying is terminating a life and therefore is not ethical, while another nurse may believe that the person requesting assisted dying must be a competent adult and has the right to decide how and when they want to die.

It is not surprising that it is stressful for HCPs to struggle as they wrestle with new legislation, develop policies, and determine next steps.

Responding to a Person's Request for Assisted Dying

As a nurse, it is important to listen carefully to the dying person and their family. Support them, by helping to clarify their values, hopes, expectations, and fears, to arrive at a decision that they feel is best. These skills are the same as for dialoguing more generally with people at the end of life, as they come to terms with the realities of their illness and contemplate the implications of different choices available to them.

A dying person interested in assisted dying may say to you,

I want to know about assisted dying.

I want to die.

I have had enough! Can someone just give me a pill?

I want assisted dying.

While these statements reflect a range of emotions and can mean many different things, it is most important first to respond with compassion and empathy, and second to clarify meaning. As suggested in earlier chapters, you can offer compassion and empathy by sitting in silence and providing appropriate touch. The essence of compassion, and of hospice and palliative care, is to be with a person in their suffering, to walk with them on difficult pathways, and to convey along the journey empathy, warmth, acceptance, and love in professional practice. This is a time for nonjudgmental presence, no matter what your personal beliefs are about assisted dying.

Best practice includes providing compassion, warmth, empathy, and respect for the person requesting assisted dying.

When a person asks for assisted dying, pause to consider what the person is requesting:
- Is the person expressing a thoughtful and deliberate interest in assisted dying?
- Is the person expressing an emotional response to the difficulties of the dying process?
- Is the person requesting factual information about their legal options with respect to assisted dying?
- Does the person need accompaniment and support as they grieve their losses?

When asking questions is appropriate, you might clarify the person's meaning by asking questions such as these, or adaptations of them:

Can you tell me more about what is happening, what you are wanting [thinking] about?

Do you want to talk for a bit?

Can I clarify what it is that you are asking for?

Asking open-ended questions will help clarify the person's needs and interests in assisted dying. Whether the person is seeking more information about assisted dying or wanting to access it, the next steps include documenting the request and collaborating with the health care team. Policies and guidelines relating to assisted dying will identify the parameters of these steps and will depend on the legal policies of your professional college or organization and the resources available in your work setting.

The role of the health care team is to address the needs of the dying person and help the person make decisions based on his or her own values, goals, and circumstances.

When a person wants to explore the option of assisted dying, remember that psychosocial factors (e.g., perceptions of dignity), more than physical factors (e.g., pain), often lead a person to consider medical assistance in dying. The team will want to reflect on some critically important questions such as these:
- What suffering is this person experiencing that they feel is intolerable?
- Are there palliative care options that might help minimize suffering? Specifically:
  - Is this person receiving optimal pain and symptom management?
  - Is this person receiving the necessary psychological, social, and spiritual support from an appropriately trained interprofessional care team?
  - Has the health care team done everything possible to provide dignity-conserving care?

The Nurse's Role in Assisted Dying

As a nurse, you share a special proximity to the dying person and their family. This means that in your care of people who contemplate or pursue assisted dying, there will be important personal and professional implications for you. As a nurse you may experience strong emotions in engaging with someone who expresses a desire to die. You may find the intensity of the experience daunting. You may be concerned about the well-being of the family members of the dying person. You may find that the interprofessional dynamics of your setting are such that you need to advocate for the dying person's wishes for assisted dying so that the rest of the care team understands those wishes and takes them seriously. Conversely, you may have personal moral objections to some or all dimensions of caring for people who request assisted dying.

One thing is certain: the therapeutic relationship that you will develop with the dying person is unique and can be a source of important insights that need to be a part of collaborative interprofessional decision making (Wright and Brajtman, 2011).

The exercise that follows is provided to help you reflect on your beliefs, assumptions, and values. Self-reflection will help you feel more comfortable in responding in an ethical way when you care for someone who wants to talk about or who requests a hastened death.

Reflective Exercise

This exercise is designed to help you clarify your beliefs and feelings about participating in assisted dying.

The care process relating to assisted dying is complex. This is a list of necessary activities that nurses may participate in as part of the assisted dying process. Consider how comfortable you would be doing each activity. Identify where on the continuum you would place yourself for each activity.

1. Responding to a request from a person you are caring for about the possibility of assisted death as a care option

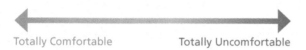

Totally Comfortable   Totally Uncomfortable

2. Responding to a request from the family of a person you are caring for about the possibility of assisted dying as a care option
3. Discussing a person's request for assisting dying with interprofessional colleagues, including physicians
4. Assessing the underlying meanings of a person's request for assisted dying
5. Teaching a dying person and family members how to administer a lethal prescription
6. Preparing medications to be used for the explicit purpose of ending life
7. Inserting an IV catheter so that a person can receive a life-ending infusion of medication
8. Directly administering medications to end the life of a dying person
9. Supporting family members after a person dies by means of an assisted death

After completing the exercise, consider activities that make you feel *uncomfortable*. Explore, through journaling or in dialogue with a friend or colleague, whether your discomfort comes from a *professional* or a *moral* stance. Consider the following:

- **If you are uncomfortable having an open dialogue** with a dying person about the possibility of assisted dying, is this because you lack confidence in your knowledge and skills to have these conversations, or because you have an ethical objection to the idea of assisted dying as a care option?
- **If you believe assisted dying is not ethical** and if you do not want to participate in providing assisted dying, investigate organizational policies and find out whether they include a policy for people who have a moral objection to assisted dying. Find out whether staff can choose not to be involved in providing referrals, information, or counseling related to assisted dying, and/or to the administration of medication for assisted dying. Consider other ways you can contribute to your team.
- **If you are unsure of what you believe**, and you are not comfortable in supporting or participating in assisted dying for any reason, consider your needs for education, support, and skill development, and seek continuing education in the areas you identify.

- **If you support assisted dying**, you may also want to identify areas where you want further education and/or skill development. Consider ways you can contribute to the well-being of the health care team, and how you might offer empathy and support to those who do and those who do not participate in offering assisted dying. You may want to volunteer to respond to requests for assisted dying, and provide information and counseling supports.

The results of the reflective exercise above may help you to clarify your current level of comfort with respect to engaging in the care of people who might request assisted dying, and to identify directions for your professional development.

It is important to involve yourself in dialogues with other team members about what the dying people you care for experience and what should be done to support them. If you practice in a jurisdiction where assisted dying is legal, ensure that your organization has a policy that delineates clearly the nurse's role in responding to requests for assisted dying, and in participating or not participating in the care of dying people who request assisted dying.

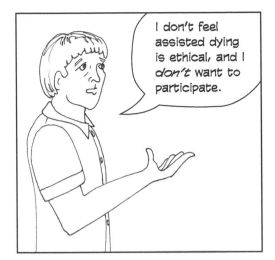

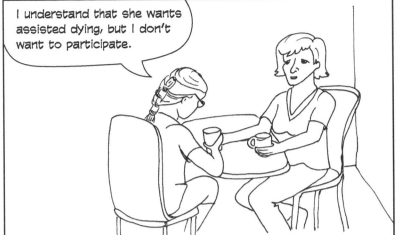

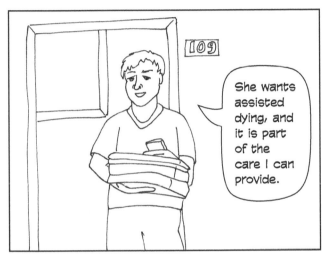

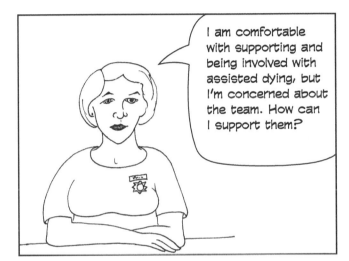

Spirituality and the Search for Meaning, Purpose, and Connection

The majority of patients with advanced illness view religion and/or spirituality as personally important and experience spiritual needs.

(Balboni et al., 2010)

People who received spiritual support from the health care team reported better quality of life near death, chose less aggressive treatments as death neared, and were more likely to accept hospice care (Zalonis and Slota, 2014; Balboni et al., 2010). This is a significant finding if quality of life is one of the goals of care! These findings also align with the principles of hospice and palliative care. It follows, then, that a nursing responsibility, or role as part of the health care team, is to participate in providing spiritual care.

What Is Spirituality?

When asked, nurses reported feeling less competent in providing spiritual care than in any other self-assessed competencies (iPANEL, 2014). They are not alone in this feeling. Many people struggle to define spirituality and provide spiritual care. The United States Consensus Project developed this definition:

Spirituality is the aspect of humanity that refers to the way individuals seek and express meaning and purpose and the way they experience their connectedness to the moment, to self, to others, to nature, and to the significant or sacred.

(Puchalski et al., 2009)

The European Task Force on Spiritual Care worked with that definition and began building a definition of spirituality that would best suit European populations, acknowledging that the multidimensional aspect of spirituality makes it more difficult to develop a meaningful definition that meets the needs of diverse populations. Because spirituality is included as a component of the WHO definition of palliative care, it is important for an appropriate definition to emerge that resonates with people who work with the dying.

For the purpose of this text, spirituality is as defined by Dr. Christina Puchalski:

> *Spirituality is a dynamic and intrinsic aspect of humanity through which persons seek ultimate meaning, purpose and transcendence, and experience relationship to self, family, others, community, society, nature, and the significant or sacred. Spirituality is expressed through beliefs, values, traditions and practices.*

(Puchalski, 2008)

Puchalski's definition suggests that spirituality includes the search for meaning and purpose of life, transcendence and connection with others, community, nature, and the sacred. A person's beliefs, values, traditions, and practices are expressions of spirituality. Ideally, spirituality helps a person find strength, peace, and comfort (Puchalski, 2008).

Relating to Spiritual Needs

The person and family you care for might find meaning and address these needs through formal cultural or religious beliefs and language. They may identify as atheists, agnostics, or Humanists. They may find strength in connecting to nature, the arts or sciences, or human goodness. And they may not have considered concepts of meaning making, purpose, and connection.

A person's spiritual needs guide their search for meaning, purpose, transcendence, and connection. Spiritual care, then, would refer to care that supports the person in their search for meaning, purpose, transcendence, connection, and experiencing the sacred.

Individualizing Care: Spirituality

The concept of spirituality may not resonate with everyone. If the concept does not not resonate with you, consider instead the search for meaning, purpose, transcendence, and connection as different ways of approaching the same concept.

What beliefs and ideologies provide you with strength, hope, connection, and purpose?

As you read this section of the text, substitute your own concept for what other people term "spirituality." How might you relate to and care for someone whose concept of spirituality is different from yours?

Ethics Touchstone
How can you support a person's spiritual requests if their beliefs are different from your own?

Is it possible that nurses provide spiritual care without realizing it? Nurses who integrate best practice as identified by Davies and Steele (Davies et al., 2016), provide compassionate care (Nouwen, McNeill, and Morrison, 1981), and integrate love in professional practice (Butot, 2005) are, in fact, providing spiritual care. The purpose of this section is to help illustrate what spiritual care might look like, and to help you as a nurse discover ways that you might integrate spiritual care into your practice.

Strategies for Providing Individualized Spiritual Care

Many nurses report discomfort when discussing meaning making, existential issues, and cultural and religious traditions, and consequently they might avoid these topics consciously or unconsciously, being neglectful in terms of spirituality in their care. At the other end of the spectrum are nurses who breach professional boundaries by inappropriately sharing their personal beliefs and ideologies in a prescriptive manner with people when providing care to them. The Reverend Dr. Carla Cheatham refers to the practice of sharing one's personal ideology (especially with the goal to convert) in professional practice as "spiritual abuse," and she refers to both spiritual neglect and spiritual abuse as "spiritual malpractice" (Cheatham, 2016). Cheatham suggests that the place in between neglect and abuse is the "sweet spot" where a nurse can connect and provide ethical and competent spiritual care.

Spiritual care, just like any comfort measure or support strategy, needs to be individualized. Best practice HCPs approach spiritual care by being open and curious about the person's definition of and needs for spiritual care, then by connecting and providing compassionate care.

Guidelines for Providing Spiritual Care

These guidelines are organized into lists of "dos" and "don'ts" to help nurses avoid being spiritually neglectful or abusive. Using these guidelines may help nurses increase their competence and comfort with providing spiritual care. This will ultimately benefit the person, who will receive enhanced spiritual care, individualized to their needs and provided by a nurse who is comfortable with spiritual care.

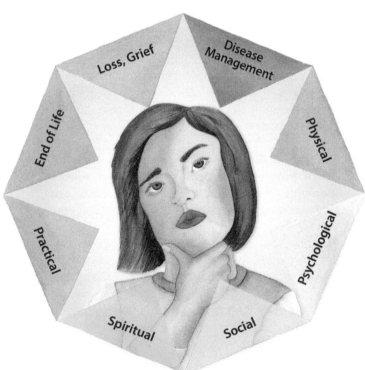

Dos

1. Reflect on your own spirituality before engaging with the person, to avoid imposing your beliefs and practices onto their spirituality. Consider how you make meaning, what you value and believe, what you hold sacred, and who you turn to for support in times of need.
2. Acknowledge that the process of being diagnosed with a serious illness, disease progression, and facing death can stimulate the person to ask some of the deeper questions of life, including "Why me?" and "Why now?"
3. Be curious and help the person explore their questions, values, beliefs, and ways of making meaning, finding strength, and connecting with others. Understand that these may change over time.
4. Individualize your approach and language to meet the needs of the person.
5. Integrate love in professional practice as you provide best practice care and compassion.
6. Collaborate with and support the person's spiritual care providers as appropriate.
7. Be willing to explore unknown territory and know that you do not need to have "all the answers."
8. Be confident that the process of exploration is an important part of the journey.
9. Understand that when you are invited, your role is to be fully present.
10. Offer to participate in spiritual practices to the extent you are comfortable doing so and as appropriate.

Don'ts

1. Do not use words that the person does not use in describing spiritual understanding or practices. For example, if the person talks about the "creator," do not automatically use the word "God."
2. Do not feel responsible for answering the big questions of life, for example, about meaning, purpose, and suffering.
3. Do not use this opportunity to proselytize, prescribe, or promote your personal beliefs or values.

Spiritual care: it is less about what you do and more about how you do it.

Exploring Beliefs and Traditions as Part of Spiritual Care

One of the simplest ways to open the door to exploring spirituality is attributed to Dame Cicely Saunders. When she completed a physical assessment, she would ask the question "How are you within?" It was an invitation for the dying person to talk about their experience beyond the physical aspects of their dying. This simple question indicated to the person and their family members that Saunders wanted to learn about their emotional or inner experiences as well.

Puchalski and Romer developed the FICA Spiritual Assessment Tool (see page 91 in Chapter 4, "Using Standardized Tools"), which contains questions to assist HCPs to learn about a person's faith and beliefs (Puchalski and Romer, 2000). "FICA" stands for Faith, Importance, Community, and Address in Care.

On the George Washington Institute for Spirituality and Health website at smhs.gwu.edu/gwish /clinical/fica/spiritual-history-tool, Dr. Puchalski offers suggestions for asking the FICA questions.

FICA

"FICA" can be a useful device to help providers and patients discuss the role of religion and spirituality as relevant to health and illness. FICA is a device that can assist the health care provider in taking a patient's spiritual history and facilitate discussion of the role of spirituality and religion in a patient's physical well being. By using FICA and addressing spiritual issues, an environment of intimacy and trust may be established, leading to patient comfort in revealing fundamental information about his/her worldviews and sources of personal meaning.

Faith or beliefs: *What is your faith or belief? Do you consider yourself spiritual or religious? What things do you believe give meaning to your life?*

Importance and Influence: *What influence does it have on how you take care of yourself? How have your beliefs influenced your behavior during this illness? What role do your beliefs play in regaining your health?*

Community: *Are you part of a spiritual or religious community? Is this of support to you and how? Is there a person or group of people you really love or who are really important to you?*

Address: *How would you like me, your healthcare provider, to address these issues in your healthcare?*

FICA Spiritual Assessment Tool

Dr. Carla Cheatham offers the following questions to be used as part of the FICA assessment:

Faith: "Is there any particular faith tradition in which you were raised?"

Asking this question allows room for the possibility that the person is not of a particular faith tradition, decreases the chance that the person will feel judged by asking about faith, and will provide them space to share their story of their spiritual journey from childhood to the present day. Their response may provide insight into what has been helpful and what has been hurtful for them in their journey.

Importance: "Which of your current beliefs/ ideologies are most helpful for you right now as you cope with your circumstance and make decisions for your future?"

The purpose of asking this question is to identify spiritual beliefs and strengths that are supporting the dying person and family and that may influence their health care decisions.

Community: "If there is a crisis at 2 a.m., whom do you want me to call to come and be with you and your family?"

One person might identify their community as a group of friends that they hiked with for years. Another person might identify their spiritual leader. For one woman it was her accountant, who came from a different community and a different religion, but was trusted to be exactly the person needed during a crisis.

Address in Care: "What do we need to know about how your particular culture and beliefs/ ideologies will influence your decisions, and how we may be most respectful of you and your views?

The more you understand about their beliefs and values, the better you can fine-tune the care plan to meet the unique needs of the dying person and their family.

In addition to offering support for the family, it might be helpful to include spiritual leaders who are important to the person in the discussions about goals of care.

Hello, I understand that you are Mr. Singh's clergy. He has given me permission to talk with you about how he is doing and what he is choosing for care and treatment.

As you know, this is his fifth admission to hospital this year. He has undergone a number of tests and treatments. Each time he hopes that he will gain strength and improved appetite and start to feel better. He is disappointed that he is not improving.

What is your sense of how he is doing? How do you feel that we might best support him? Do you have any questions for me?

Offering and Responding to Requests for Prayer

Of all the supportive comfort measures offered, offering to pray with or for someone, or responding to a request for prayer, requires the most delicate and sensitive communication. Key ingredients to discussing prayer include:

1. **Acknowledging and respecting** the person's and family's views and boundaries.

2. **Offering prayer as one of many options.** You may identify the variety of comfort measures you can provide:

   Some people want to talk, others want me to sing or read with them, some just want to sit quietly, some want me to pray, and others just want to play a game. Whatever it is you would like, I'm happy to do.

   Then, before leaving them, I ask if there's anything else I can do for them. I trust them to take the lead by asking for what they need and want.

3. **Knowing and working within your comfort zone.** Determine your comfort zone and, if you are not comfortable praying or praying out loud and someone requests that you pray, you might acknowledge the request, apologize if you feel unable to offer a prayer, and identify what you feel comfortable doing:

   Praying out loud isn't something I'm comfortable with [or good at or experienced with] but I'd be happy to sit with you and hold your hand while we both pray silently, or while you pray aloud. And I'll definitely be holding you in my heart.

There is no reason for the dying person or the HCP, to feel obligated or offended.

4. **Finding and using their words.** Strive to find and use the words and a format that honors the person's and family members' beliefs. You may want to ask,

   How do you typically begin and end your prayers?

5. **Asking what the person would like you to pray for.** If you are asked to pray, for example, for healing, ask the person what healing looks like to them. Then, equipped with words from their heart, you can offer those words back, out loud, as a prayer that respects their needs.

6. **Asking for assistance.** If you do not feel comfortable offering a prayer, ask if you can request the support of a chaplain or other spiritual care person to visit and to pray.

7. **Following up.** It is good practice to connect with the spiritual care counselor with whom you work. Coordinate care with the professional responsible for overseeing the spiritual aspect of a person's care plan. This will help to build the team and resources available to the person, and will also respect interprofessional boundaries.

(Cheatham, 2016)

His wife and daughter brought him to the city to see a specialist. The specialist told him that he was dying. He chose to remain in the city instead of returning to his remote community, and together they requested registration with the hospice program.

I arrived at the home early in my night shift. In that initial assessment visit, they shared a brief story of their life, they shared some of what gave their life meaning, and they shared their grief about their disconnection and falling away from their church community. If I remember correctly, they left the church because of a disagreement with the minister. They never felt comfortable enough to return, and it appeared that they had never found another church or community that addressed their desire for community and spiritual connection.

At about one in the morning, I was called back to the home. The man had died suddenly, peacefully, in his sleep. The family described their last hours with him.

They shared their surprise at his sudden death and found meaning in the fact that he did not linger. I pronounced the death, and together we cared for his body.

While caring, I thought of their grief at losing their connection with their church community. I thought of them in this city, removed from their home. I wondered how I might create a sacred moment, a ritual that might meet their needs. "Would you like to have a moment of silence, a song, or a prayer before I leave?" I asked. The wife jumped at the invitation and asked if I would pray.

We gathered around the bed, and, using the language that reflected the language they had used earlier and the language of their faith tradition, I offered a prayer. Warm silence, tears, and hugs followed. I hoped that in some way, I was able to provide them with a ritual that met their needs in that tender moment. A week later I arrived at work to find a thank-you note from this family. "Thank you, nurse, for the prayer."

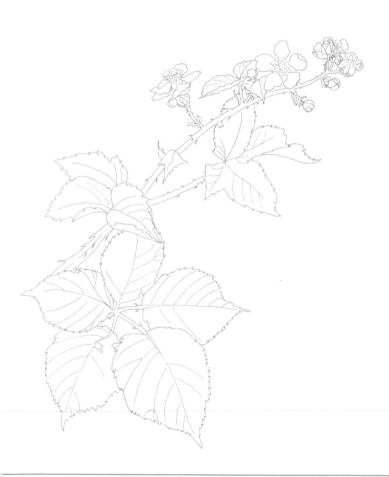

Supporting Intimacy and Sexuality

He was coming home after a lengthy stay in hospital. It appeared to the health care team that he would die in the coming weeks, but he was not yet ready to discontinue the treatments. My first task was to transfer him, and all the tubes that were coming and going from his body, from his wheelchair to his bed. I reached under his buttocks to loosen the tubing that was caught beneath him. I said, "Excuse me." He responded, "No worry, it feels great."

When I finished all the tasks that were required to support him and his spouse for the next 24 hours, I reflected back on that statement and asked him, "Can I give you a massage?"

"Oh yes!" he replied.

"Can I ask your wife if she would be comfortable learning how to give you a massage?"

"Sure" he said. "Maybe she hasn't touched me because I was in a busy hospital room, and maybe she was afraid to touch me with all these tubes in me."

With his wife standing near me, I started with his back (as much as I could do with him lying on his side), his lower back, his buttocks, and then down to his legs. Somewhere in there, he said, "It has been a long time since I was really touched! This feels sooo good." Reaching down to give him a kiss, his wife said, "I've been so afraid of hurting you, but it's good to see how relaxed you are, now I can give it a try."

A person's interest and desire for physical intimacy and emotional closeness may change with the diagnosis and progression of a life-limiting illness. The needs may vary from the desire to hold and be held, to the desire to hold hands and kiss, to the desire for sexual intercourse (Rando, 1984). It is important to remember that intimacy and sexuality can continue to be a part of a person's life through to death, and that a loss of intimacy and sexuality can negatively affect the dying person's well-being and quality of life (Bevan and Thompson, 2003). Despite the value of intimacy and sexuality for many people when they are ill, sexual health is rarely assessed or investigated by clinicians (Matzo, 2015). When HCPs do not ask or talk about sexuality, that suggests to the person that the topic is not open for discussion (Katz, 2016). For example, Rawlings explored issues related to being lesbian, gay, bisexual, and transgender (LGBT) at the end of life. He reported that people in the LGBT community experienced barriers to sexual health that were secondary only to the negative social attitudes of society. People in this community experienced two types of loss: first, negative social attitudes toward their lifestyle and second, a lack of acknowledgment of their sexual health when undergoing treatment or dying (Rawlings, 2012).

Intimacy and sexuality may be disrupted by life-limiting illness due to lack of privacy (in hospice or residential care), changes to the body, the effects of symptoms and treatments (e.g., fatigue, dyspnea, pain, nausea, anxiety),

changes in elimination, and changes in mobility (Lemieux et al., 2004). Family may be concerned that sexual activity will hurt the person or that being both the caregiver and the partner will be too challenging.

A first step in addressing sexuality is to acknowledge the person's concerns and fears. When HCPs offered people in their care an opportunity to address their intimacy concerns, the people were not offended by these discussions (Lemieux et al., 2004). The second step is to remember that sexuality is holistic and therefore encompasses more than just the body.

People within the same family and within a relationship will have different levels of comfort in talking about the need for intimacy, and will have different needs for intimacy. Therefore, it is very important to approach these conversations gently, with respect for individual preferences, without making assumptions or judgments about how people "should" feel or act. Be sensitive to timing issues and the need for privacy. Use language that is acceptable to the person, and be prepared for some people to initially feel reluctant to discuss a topic they may never have before.

Consider opening up a conversation about intimacy when you are alone with the dying person. You might ask the person one or more of the following questions to open the door to this conversation:

In our experience, sometimes people have questions or concerns about how to have their needs for intimacy or touch met. I wonder if you want to talk about that?

Sometimes it is nice to have a loved one close by. Is there someone you would like to have lie on the bed with you? Or would you like someone to sit on the bed next to you?

Massage can be a lovely way to feel connected with those we love. Do you enjoy receiving massage? Would you like someone to give you a massage? We can teach them how to give a massage if that would be helpful. Would you like that?

Would you like some privacy when a loved one is visiting?

In our experience, it is not uncommon for people to have questions or concerns about intimacy and sexuality when they are ill. Do you have any questions or concerns that you would like to talk about with me or another member of the health care team? Would you like me or one of the team to talk with your partner?

Considering the Family

Observe how family members visit, where they sit, their physical distance from the person, and the positioning of the furniture. Are family members comfortable, or do they strain to reach out to hold a hand or give a hug? Do they sit near the bed, or are they far away? Do they sit on hard chairs or on a commode or the seat of a walker? Is it possible to help them be more comfortable? Is it appropriate to talk with them about their needs for closeness?

Seven days before my mother died she started to develop fevers early in the morning. The first time this happened, she went to the room where my brother was sleeping and climbed into bed with him to get warm. The second day I came upstairs and found her on the couch, under a blanket, chilled and shaking. I lay next to her, put my arms around her, and held her. She relaxed in my arms. I held her until her fever settled. She was comforted by being held. I was comforted by holding her. Holding her was foreign to me, but it was perfect in the moment. After those two snuggles, we all had times when we lay next to her. It was one of the most relaxing ways of being with her in those last days. I think it was healing for all of us.

Discussing concerns about intimacy and sexuality may be empowering for both the person who is ill and their partner. Consider using the following four steps of the P–LI–SS–IT model to guide your assessment and consideration of interventions when difficulties arise in intimacy and sexuality (Taylor and Davis, 2007). Match the level of intervention to the intensity of the problem. These are the four steps:

Permission: Invite the person to discuss their concerns and provide an atmosphere of safety in which to do so. You might say,

Do you have any questions or concerns about intimacy or sexuality?

Limited **I**nformation: Provide basic information that the dying person and their partner need about sexual functioning and the impact their illness has on it. Information in pamphlet form may be available to address disease-specific concerns.

Specific **S**uggestions: Provide specific suggestions that relate to the person's problems.

Intensive **T**herapy: When limited information and specific suggestions are not sufficient, with the person's permission you may want to engage a mental health professional or counselor with the appropriate training, or a specifically trained sex therapist.

The experience of dying can be lonely and isolating. Addressing the desire for intimacy and sexuality is a component of holistic care and can help maintain and strengthen relationships.

Strengthening the "Social" in "Psychosocial"

While death is a personal experience, it is also a family and a social experience. The person does most of their living and dying in their community, among people they have interacted with throughout their lives. Their community may include the people in the grocery store, their bankers and hair stylists, waiters, a car mechanic, a furnace technician, teachers, and many more people.

In the past, family and community members cared for the dying and the deceased. However, today's community members may not be involved in caring for the dying. They may feel that dying, death, loss, and caregiving are foreign and difficult and may want to avoid them. It is not uncommon for hospice nurses and professionals to hear, "You must be special, I could never do that … you are an angel."

Community has cared for the dying and their caregivers for millennia. It is essential that community is not neglected at a time when the dying person and their family are in need, and as society faces such an increase in the number of people dying. The reality is that death will come to everyone. Dying and death are one part of being in a community. Responding to the needs of a dying person and their family is part of supporting community.

A growing movement considers palliative care to be a public health issue, as discussed in Dr. Allan Kellehear's book *Compassionate Cities: Health and End-of-Life Care*. He suggests that because public health activities in palliative care are participatory and conceived, partnered, and nurtured by community members, they could be instrumental in:

- Helping to prevent social difficulties related to dying, death, loss, and caregiving
- Minimizing difficulties that cannot be prevented
- Intervening early along the journey of dying, death, loss, and caregiving
- Altering or changing a setting or environment for the better in terms of responses to dying, death, loss, or care
  (Kellehear, 2005)

My favorite example of a public health palliative care idea is a beer coaster, which on one side reads "Dying for a beer" and the other side reads "Ten ways to support a grieving friend." One of my favorite teaching memories was hearing stories from a bartender who participated in one of the Life and Death Matters online courses. She told stories of listening to people in the bar, hearing their struggles, and sharing information about educational re-

sources and community support groups with them. I *loved* her stories and thought, "We missed the boat. We need to be sharing education with the bartenders and the hair stylists; they provide community counseling daily!"

Nurses can integrate a public health approach into palliative care in conversations with the person and the family by:
- Asking about friends, neighbors, book clubs, social groups, and so on
- Exploring ways their community might provide support and ways they might respond when people offer to help, for example, what to say when people ask, "Is there anything I can do?"
- Exploring their concerns about the discomfort of dealing with social stigma related to dying, death, diagnosis, and so on when in social situations or meeting with friends
- Discussing concerns, misunderstandings, or myths that friends express about the person's illness, dying, being a caregiver, and so on

More information about helping to involve community, family, and friends in caregiving is available on the websites of Lotsa Helping Hands (lotsahelpinghands.com) and Caring Bridge (caringbridge.org) and in books, such as "Share the Care: How to organize a group to care for someone who is seriously ill" (Capossela and Warnock, 2004).

You may be inspired by the words of Dr. Julian Abel, a palliative care consultant: "End-of-life care does not begin with palliative care, it begins with community" and "Don't leave death to the experts" (Abel and Kellehear, 2016).

The idea of health promotion in palliative care—that we can decrease the negatives by including community—is one that resonates with me and makes sense. We *cannot* afford to forget that the community has cared for the dying for millennia and that HCPs are *new* to the scene.

Ethics Touchstone
When nurses care for the dying person, it can be easy to forget that other people are available and willing to provide care. How can nurses involve the team and community in providing care that nurses are not able to address?

Supporting Children Whose Loved One Is Dying

Many people find it challenging to support a child when a person close to the child is dying or has died. The separation of dying and death from ordinary life has raised more issues than it has solved. When the dying process happens behind closed doors, adults may separate children from their dying loved one, often with the unintended effect of interfering with children's ability to say good-bye to the person. In addition, the separation denies children the opportunity to learn about death, one of life's greatest teachers. Current research-based principles on supporting children whose loved one is dying suggest that children should be included and communication with them should be open and honest.

Applying the principles discussed below can help nurses and families feel more confident when supporting children whose loved one is dying, as well as help children in their grieving process.

Principles for Supporting Children Whose Loved One Is Dying

Include Children

People often ask questions such as "Should my daughter visit her grandfather who is dying?" Children benefit by having the choice to visit family members or friends who are dying. Children of all ages can be asked whether they want to visit and should be allowed to participate to the extent that they are comfortable doing so. Children must also have the option not to visit. If they choose not to visit, they can be asked if they would like to draw a picture or write a story as ways to participate. What is most important regarding children is that they are asked and given choice.

Prepare Children

Some parents are hesitant to let a child visit a dying person due to concerns that the person's appearance or the equipment in the person's room may frighten the child. Andrea Warnick, a social worker and child and youth counselor, states that preparing a child to visit their dying loved one will help make the experience a positive one (Warnick, 2015a). Before the visit, set the stage for the child:

- Describe how the person's room will look—the equipment in the room, the lights on the equipment, and the sounds that may be present in the room.
- Describe how their loved one looks now compared with when the child last saw the person, including any dramatic changes such as weight loss, hair loss, or pallor (a child could be shocked by seeing a person who customarily wears dentures without them).
- Explain:
  - Where the child is allowed to go and what the child may touch when visiting someone in a hospital or hospice setting
  - What the child is allowed to do in the presence of, say to, or talk about with the dying person
  - What will happen during the visit (e.g., both laughter and tears may occur).

Be Honest

Adults may try to protect children from the news that a family member is dying. However, most children sense when something is wrong in the family, and if they are not told the truth, they invent a story to explain what is wrong. Quite often their imaginations create scenarios that are worse than reality. This means that withholding the news that a family member is dying tends to be more frightening than the truth and denies children access to accurate information and appropriate emotional support. When children sense they have not been told the truth or they learn the truth after the fact, their sense of security and ability to trust the adults around them may be damaged.

Invite Participation in Caregiving

Children may want to participate in caregiving but probably will not know what to do or how to help. They can be included in caregiving by inviting them to:

- Assist with personal care, such as mouth care and applying nail polish or skin moisturizer
- Help create a comfortable atmosphere by means of music, decorations, storytelling, or reminiscing
- Share daily events, do homework, or do other quiet activities at the bedside
- Sit quietly at the bedside and hold hands with their loved one

Invite Questions

Children often have many questions about what is happening to their dying family member and the care that the person is receiving. It is important to invite children to ask questions with statements such as "You are welcome to ask me any questions."

When a child asks questions, be prepared to repeat your answers, as the child may ask the same questions repeatedly. If you do not have an answer, be honest and tell the child that you do not know the answer. If someone else on the care team or in the family might know the answer to the question, ask that person to respond to the child.

Whatever questions children ask, thank them for asking and let them know that their questions are good ones. Also encourage children to share their questions about dying and death with other caregivers.

Ethics Touchstone

Sometimes people will exclude children from visiting or supporting a dying person. How can you help support a child asking questions about dying when the family is clear that they do not want to talk about it with the child? How can you support the family to see the child's point of view?

Use Correct Language

In an effort to protect children, adults often avoid using the name of the disease by instead saying that the person is sick or has an illness. This can confuse children. When an adult says, "Your grandma is sick and will die," the child may start to think that anyone who is sick will die. Andrea Warnick suggests that using correct language that names the illness (e.g., "Your grandma has leukemia") will help prevent such confusion (Warnick, 2015b).

It is also common for adults to avoid using certain words around children, specifically "dying," "death," and "died," and substitute other words, such as "passing" or "passed away." Substituting words can confuse children. Use the correct language and avoid using unclear terms such as those below to describe dying and death:

- "Passing" or "passed away." These terms do not indicate what has happened to the person and will be difficult for children to understand.

- "Mommy went to a better place." Children may interpret this to mean that Mommy chose to leave the family and go somewhere else.
  - "We lost Grandpa." Children frequently lose things and find them later. Saying that someone is lost may lead children to believe the person will be found later, or children may think that they themselves could get lost and not be found.
  - "Dad will never get better." This phrase doesn't accurately indicate that Dad is dying. Children may think that Dad will live forever in his current state of functioning.
  - "It's like a big sleep." This phrase may make children believe that falling asleep is dying and therefore cause them to fear falling asleep.

Instead of using unspecific phrases, such as those listed above, explain that "Death is when a body stops working and will never work again."

Understanding Children's Concerns: The Three C's

Children whose loved one is dying often have three concerns, which Andrea Warnick terms the "Three C's" (Warnick, 2010).

1. Did I *cause* it?
Children often feel more responsible for what is happening around them than adults realize. If, for example, the child had been angry with the person who is dying, the child may believe they caused the dying to happen or that it is a punishment for their misbehavior. Even if a child shows no signs of feeling responsible for the illness, it is important to let the child know that nothing they did or thought caused or can cause illness or death.

2. Can I *catch* it?
Children often think that all illnesses are like the common cold or the flu and can be spread from one person to another. It helps to explain to children that some diseases, such as amyotrophic lateral sclerosis and cancer, are not contagious and one person cannot catch such diseases from another person.

3. Who will take *care* of me?
If a child's parent or guardian is dying, it is important that the child be told who will take care of them following the person's death.

Recognizing Children's Grief

Children, like adults, have a range of responses to death and dying. Adults are often surprised to see children who are very upset one moment about a family member's dying and then are playing happily the next. It is important to allow children, like all people, to express their sorrow in their own way and in their own time. Children will naturally regulate the amount of time they spend experiencing intense emotions by taking breaks from the feelings through play and continuing to enjoy life (Goldman, 2012). It is also important to realize that because children get up from crying and go out to play, they are not over their grief but rather are dealing with it bit by bit, as they are able.

Children's grief may include the following:
- Sleep disturbances
- Stomach aches and headaches
- Difficulty concentrating in school
- Angry outbursts
- Fears about seemingly unrelated things

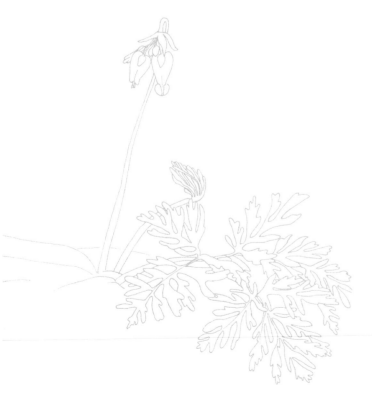

Grieving Together

Adults who hide their emotions from children in an effort to protect them may inadvertently teach them that grief should be hidden. It is important for kids to know that all of the feelings they are experiencing are normal, and that adults experience them too (Warnick, 2015b).

Grief can be described to children as "all of the feelings people experience when someone is dying or has died. This includes being sad, mad, worried, and lonely, as well as being happy and continuing to enjoy life."

Children learn how to grieve by watching the adults around them (Goldman, 2012). Nurses can let families know that it is okay for them to cry together, be mad together, and be sad together, and that moments of happiness and laughter are all part of the process. Sometimes children will ask questions or make comments that are surprising or disturbing to other people. These questions or comments may be developmentally appropriate to the age of the child.

Supporting children through the death of someone they care about can be a heartbreaking experience during what is already a difficult time. However, death is an inevitable part of life and ultimately not something from which children can be protected. Adults can help prepare children for a loved one's death by including children at the bedside and providing them with ongoing emotional support. Preparing kids for dying and death can help prepare them for life and living. By doing this, HCPs, parents and guardians, and other family members can play a powerful role in shaping children's experience of the death while at the same time equipping them to deal with future adversity.

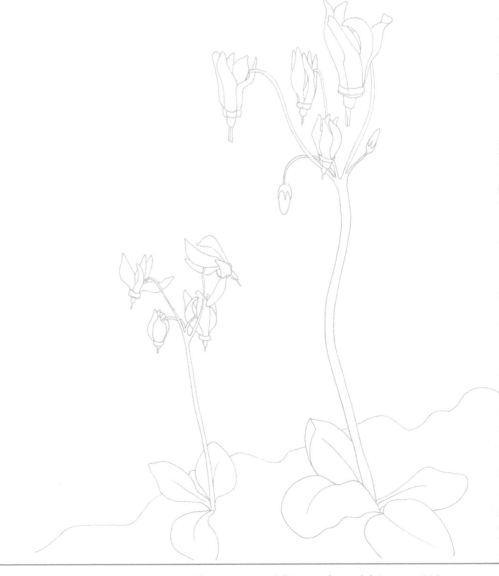

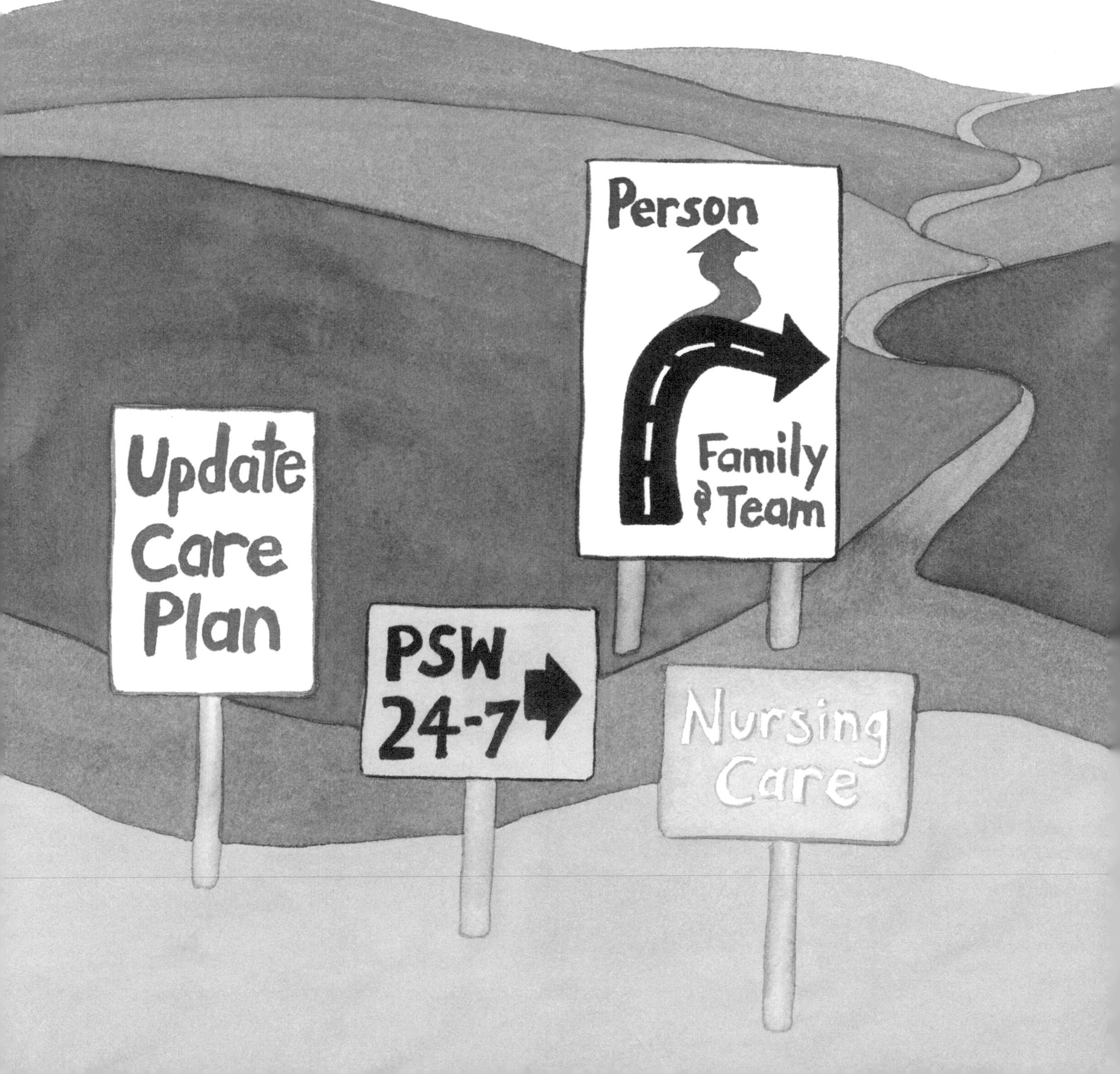
Person
Family & Team
Update Care Plan
PSW 24-7
Nursing Care

Caring in the Last Days and Hours

Preparing the Person and the Family for the Last Days and Hours

Some people will want to know what dying will look like and how to care for the dying person before death is imminent, and others will not want to know until the person is actively dying. The authors of *Transitions in Dying and Bereavement: A Psychosocial Guide for Hospice and Palliative Care* suggest that the family is often ready to discuss the changes that may occur in the last days and hours when the dying person's score on the Palliative Performance Scale (PPS) has decreased to 30% to 20% (Victoria Hospice Society, Wainwright, W., and Thompson, M., 2016). The person's condition will change in the last days and hours, and in some cases changes are rapid. Health care providers (HCPs) will need to anticipate changes in medications and needs for support, develop a plan for the time of death, and identify rites and rituals that are relevant to the dying person and their family.

Assessing, sharing information, and responding to questions and concerns are part of preparing the person and family for the last days and hours. In some cases, HCPs may need to consider how to offer support if the family or the person is *not* interested in talking about death.

Assessing and Sharing Information

Assessing what the family knows about the dying process, the last days and hours in particular, what they want to know, and what they may need to know if they are providing care will facilitate excellent care for the person and family.

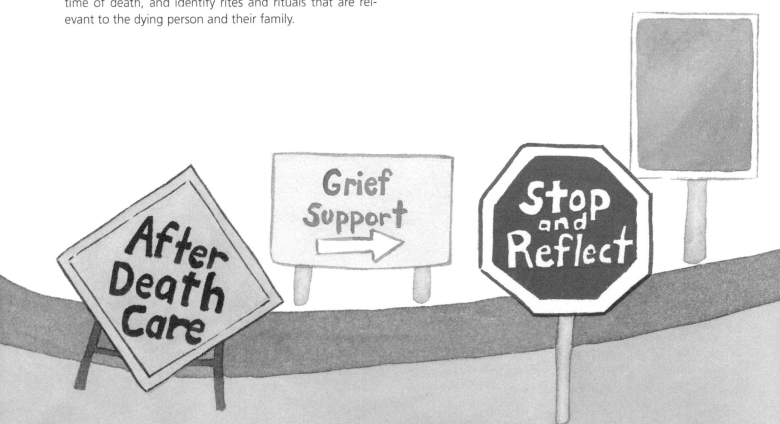

In her research, Davidson found that family members want information (Davidson, 2011). They want to understand what to expect. As death draws near, the person and the family may have questions, and they may be concerned but not know what questions to ask. Forbes Hospice developed a Question Prompt Sheet (QPS) (Table 1), based on actual questions caregivers asked to help the family identify and ask questions (Hebert et al., 2008).

Table 1. Question Prompt Sheet

Medical	<ul><li>How long does my loved one have?</li><li>Will my loved one recover?</li><li>What should I expect to happen over the course of the illness?</li><li>What caused the illness?</li><li>What are the common side effects of my loved one's medications?</li><li>What can I expect when my loved one is dying?</li><li>What does dying look like?</li><li>Will my loved one be in pain?</li><li>Is my loved one in pain?</li><li>Can the pain medicine cause my loved one's heart or breathing to stop?</li><li>What if my loved one stops eating—will they starve?</li><li>Will my loved one need a feeding tube?</li><li>Will my loved one need IV fluids?</li><li>What are the risks of the treatment my loved one is receiving?</li><li>Will the pain medicines stop working if used too often?</li><li>Will the pain medicines cause addiction?</li><li>Can my loved one hear me?</li><li>What do I do if my loved one seems depressed?</li></ul>
Practical	<ul><li>Who can I talk to about insurance? Financial concerns?</li><li>How do I get information about home health services, assisted living or nursing homes?</li><li>Who can I call if I have questions or need help?</li><li>How can I get in touch with the doctor?</li><li>How do I get information about hospice?</li><li>How do I get information about living wills?</li><li>How and when should I make funeral arrangements?</li></ul>
Psychosocial	<ul><li>What do I do if family members disagree about treatment or disagree about what should be done for my loved one?</li><li>Should I discuss death and dying with the my family? With our loved one?</li><li>How can I help the children understand what is happening?</li></ul>
Religious or spiritual	<ul><li>Who can I speak to about religious and spiritual concerns?</li><li>Why is this happening? Why is God allowing this?</li></ul>

(Adapted from Hebert et al., 2008)

When you provide the family member with the QPS, you are communicating that it is normal to have questions and that questions are welcomed. The QPS can be adapted to address the unique needs of any community. Sharing information about what to expect in the last days and hours can validate what family members are seeing, help them anticipate what might come next, and help them participate in providing care.

Ethics Touchstone
Do any of these questions surprise you? How would you answer these questions if your loved one was dying?

Responding to the Family's Questions

Families often ask questions that HCPs may not know how to answer. Knowing how to respond to these questions in a supportive way will help build the dying person's and their family's trust and decrease their anxiety.

Consider this example:

How much longer will my loved one will live?

To meet the family's needs, it is helpful to consider what prompted the question and to explore what the family understands about the timing of death. An HCP might respond to that question by acknowledging and validating it:

That's an important question. It is not an easy question to ask, and it is not an easy question to answer. But let's talk about it.

After acknowledging and validating the question, the HCP should try to find out what brought the family to ask the question. Knowing this will help the HCP understand what type of response would be most helpful. For example, the family may want to arrange for people to visit from out of town, or might need to decide whether to return to work, or might need to figure out how to balance work and being with the person, or might just be trying to decide whether there is time to go home and shower. You might say,

If I can better understand your needs, then I will be more able to help you. Is there a specific reason you are asking this question now?

Often the family will ask health care workers (e.g., personal support workers, nursing assistants, hospice aides) how much time their loved one has before dying. You can suggest to them that although it is not their job to prognosticate, it is their job to respond to the question. They might say, for example,

That is a really good question. I don't have the answer to that question, but I can ask the nurse to talk with you about this. Can you please tell me more about your needs and why you are asking the question? Then I can share that with the nurse, who can help you.

In this response, the health care worker acknowledges and validates the question, finds out the needs of the family, and gathers information to report to you, the nurse.

Exploring what the family perceives is happening will help you provide the information in a way that best suits the family's understanding. You might ask the family,

What changes have you noticed? How long do you think your loved one has to live?

It is often helpful to ask the family for insights about the person and their personality that might affect the time of death. The family may be able to provide information that will help you and the family decide what care is the most appropriate for this person at this time. For example, the family may respond,

I think she is waiting for her grandchild to be born.

She always does everything very carefully and never rushes at anything, so I think she might linger for a while.

On the other hand, the family may have no idea when their loved one will die and may need the help of the health care team to prepare for an imminent death.

Acknowledging and validating the questions are the first steps. Next is exploring the reason for the questions, as necessary, which may help in formulating answers that meet the needs of the family. Third, exploring the family's understanding of the situation may help the health care team know how to help the family prepare for their loved one's death.

Note that in the responses above to the question about an estimated time until death, no definitive prognosis was given, but the nurse did respond! Answering all questions with an "all knowing" answer is impossible much of the time, but responding to difficult questions, trying to understand the needs, and preparing to respond and address the needs are important.

> *I asked an adolescent daughter if she had a sense of how long her mom might live.*
>
> *She replied, "I used to think that she had a long time, but now I don't think she has very long … maybe six months."*
>
> *I was concerned when I heard this, as I figured that the mom had only days to live. I gently suggested that I thought that she would not have months and that it might be much shorter than that. We talked for a while, and then I arranged for her to meet later that day with the counselor and the physician.*
>
> *Over the next few days, we continued to educate the daughter on what was happening, the changes we saw, and what dying looks like, and helped her come to understand that her mom was dying imminently. I was glad that I had not told her my estimate of a few days.*

Talking about Death When People Do Not Feel Ready

It can be difficult to help the person or family prepare for the last days and hours when either are not ready to talk about the possibility that death is nearing.

Assessing the needs of individual family members and the person who is dying will help identify who is reluctant to talk about and prepare for death, and why they might be feeling this way. People may be reluctant to talk about death because they are focused on life, hopeful for more time, find talking about death awkward, don't know what to ask or how to ask, or perhaps want to protect family members from painful information or engaging in difficult conversations.

Again it is helpful to ask, "What do I need to understand?" and "What do I need to ask?"

The dying person might say,

> *I don't want to talk about death and dying. I don't want to hear any more bad news.*

The following responses are intended to help you develop ways to open the door to discussions about decline and death:

> *I understand that there are certain topics that you do not want to discuss at this time, and I respect that. However, I would like to check out a couple of things with you to be sure that I understand your preferences, so that we don't fail to have a conversation that you might actually want to have.*
>
> *First of all, can you tell me why you don't want to talk about death and dying?*
>
> *Are there any circumstances in which you would want to talk about death or dying, for example, if you are declining and actively dying? Would you want to talk about death then?*
>
> *If we, your health care team, think that you are dying in the coming few days, would you want to be informed?*
>
> *If you knew that you were dying, would you do anything differently than you are doing now?*
>
> *Sometimes people don't know the questions that they want to ask. Would it be helpful if I showed you some of the questions that people find helpful to ask?*

When people are reluctant to talk about death or to even use the "D" word, you may find it helpful to speak gently. For example, using the words "declining" or "changes in your physical condition" may make it easier for the person to engage in conversations. Adopting the phrases and terms that the person and family uses may help to increase their comfort. If the family use the phrase "pass away," it may be best to use the same phrase.

There are times, however, when you need to be bold, such as when a person is dying imminently and the family is not registering or understanding that this is the reality. You may need to say, "If you want to be with your dad when he dies, you may need to stay close by, as he is dying imminently."

I remember a woman who did not understand that her mother was dying. The nurses asked her if she was okay. She did not register until *after* the mother's death that the nurses were asking her because they knew the mom was dying.

Another woman told me of how she sat at her mother's bedside and was thinking that death was a number of hours or days away. When the health care worker said, "If you need to go to the bathroom, let me know and I can come and sit with her," the woman realized that death would be soon.

Preparing to Meet the Person's Needs in the Last Days and Hours

When a person is dying, their needs for personal care, medications, and support will change. When a person's score on the PPS declines from 30% to 20% to 10%, you can anticipate the changes in care needs and help prepare the team to respond. When preparing to respond, knowing the preferences of the person and the family is helpful.

Developing a Plan

When I was pregnant with my first child, I was keen to develop a birth care plan. I wanted to be sure that the care team knew what I wanted and would respond to the needs that arose during the birthing process as discussed in our prior conversations and noted in my care plan.

And so it is with dying. When the time comes, I want my caregivers to know what is important to me. I want my caregivers to know my hopes and preferences for my dying and the care of my body after I die. And I expect that, just as my birthing plan was adjusted to meet my and my baby's needs during the birthing process, my family and care team will honor my preferences when I am dying and will adjust to meet needs as they arise. Whether I die at home or in a hospital, hospice, or residential care setting, the essence of who I am, what I am, and what I hope for can be honored.

As death approaches, the more hypothetical discussions that may have occurred in the preceding years and months, and the care plans that were developed weeks or days ago, will need to be adapted and fine-tuned to best meet the current needs of the person. The Psychosocial Assessment Form (see pages 83 to 88 in Chapter 4, "Using Standardized Tools") provides guidance for discussing practical, financial, and spiritual topics with the person and family to help you prepare for the last days and hours, when death occurs, and after death. Keep this tool with the person's chart, and update the plan as necessary.

Psychosocial Assessment Form

Consulting with the Physician/Nurse Practitioner for New Orders

When the person's score on the PPS declines to 20%, it is important to consult with the physician/nurse practitioner to obtain orders for medication changes, and for pronouncement and notification of death. Questions to discuss include:

- What medications should/can be discontinued now or when the person becomes unable to swallow?
- What medications will be continued or required through to death but require a route change?
- Would a urinary catheter be a useful comfort measure for this person?
- Are there other comfort measures that require a physician/nurse practitioner's order?
- Who will pronounce or certify the death?
- Does the physician/nurse practitioner want or need to be notified at the time of death?

Preparing in advance for changing needs will help to prevent crisis calls and inappropriate or unnecessary admissions to the emergency department.

CPR Does Not Prevent Death in the Chronically Ill

Cardiopulmonary resuscitation (CPR) was originally developed to assist people who had suffered a sudden heart attack but were relatively healthy otherwise. Sudden death is the least common trajectory of decline and characterizes less than 5% of deaths; however, CPR has become the default treatment for all people experiencing cardiac failure, regardless of their trajectory.

Unfortunately, CPR is not an effective strategy for preventing death and disability in people who have a terminal illness, progressive organ failure, or chronic frailty (see table below). Less than 15% survive CPR.

Death Rates after CPR for People with Chronic Illness

Death Rate after CPR	Illness
80%–85%	People with a terminal illness, progressive organ failure, or chronic frailty
90%	People without a shockable heart rhythm (i.e., patients with rhythms other than ventricular fibrillation or pulseless ventricular tachycardia, such as asystole or pulseless electrical activity)
95%–99%	People who are very ill and in the intensive care unit

For people at the end of life who survive CPR, 30% to 70% live with diminished function and decreased quality of life, and are discharged to a hospice, residential care facility, or another hospital.

During advance care planning, nurses can help the person and family to understand the risks and benefits of CPR for people at the end of life, and support the person and family to make decisions that align with the person's goals of care.

(Heyland, 2016)

Inactivating Implantable Cardioverter Defibrillators Decreases Pain and Anxiety

Implantable cardioverter defibrillators (ICDs) are used to prevent sudden cardiac death in people with congestive heart failure. However, when a person's heart ceases functioning for other reasons, the ICD may continue to deliver shocks at inappropriate times, causing the person significant pain and anxiety. Goldstein reported that among people in hospices who had an ICD, an average of only 42% of the ICDs were inactivated prior to death (Goldstein et al., 2010). Unfortunately, discussions about inactivating ICDs are rare, and, be-

cause of this, the person and the health care team are not clear about the reasons for deactivating the ICD before death is imminent.

Inappropriate shocks from an ICD can be prevented with advance care planning and discussions about when to turn the ICD off (Sherazi et al., 2013). An excellent article for the person and family—"End of Life and Heart Rhythm Devices" (Heart Rhythm Society, 2014)—is available from the Heart Rhythm Society (hrsonline.org).

Arranging 24/7 Access to Support

The family may hear about the physical changes that often occur in a dying person's last days and hours, but that does not mean the family will feel comfortable with those changes, feel a sense of "normalcy" when witnessing the changes, or feel capable of providing care through to death. While the physical changes may be normal in the context of the dying process, they will be new, different, and probably very strange for the family.

When a person wants to remain in their home in the community, ensure that the person or family has ways to contact the health care team for support and advice 24/7. If the person lives in a small community, you may want to arrange for the family to be able to call a friend, the local hospital, or a home care service in a neighboring community if there are not enough personnel in their own community.

Make sure that the family knows the answers to these questions:
- Whom do I call if I have questions or concerns?
- Who is available at night and on weekends to respond to my needs and questions?
- How do I get help if my loved one is uncomfortable in the night?
- What other resources are available to us for providing care in the home?

Arranging Ongoing Support

"It takes a village to raise a child," my mother, Yetta, repeated frequently in her last weeks, and then she would add, "And it takes a community to care for the dying." This is particularly true for people dying at home. Providing care for someone right through to death in the home setting can be especially difficult when only one or two family members are providing the care.

In the United States, hospice programs may include funding for health care workers to provide personal care in the home and in residential care. In Canada, the dying person may be registered with hospice or with a palliative care benefits program while living in the community, but may require further assessment to access government-funded health care worker services.

For the dying person and their family, having a health care worker they do not know come into the privacy of their home to provide care can be helpful, but it can also be difficult for them.

In addition to arranging for the family to have access to the resources hospice or palliative care programs provide,

HOSPICE CONSULT TEAM

If you have questions, call
555-6786
day or night

it may be appropriate to talk with family members about people in their social network who might want to and be able to assist in caregiving, in supporting the caregivers themselves, or in helping with any chores and errands that need to be done. Websites of organizations such as Caring Bridge (caringbridge.org) and Lotsa Helping Hands (lotsahelpinghands.com) help the family identify and communicate their needs for support, and provide ways for people to offer their help and sign up online for different tasks. The book *Share the Care: How to Organize a Group to Care for Someone Who Is Seriously Ill* provides insights into ways to help the family access support from their community (Capossela and Warnock, 2004).

Referring to Hospice or a Palliative Care Consultant/Team

As the dying person reaches their last days and hours, consider whether the person is comfortable and whether their goals of care are being met with the services you and your team can offer. Consider whether the person would benefit from a referral to a hospice or palliative care team or consultant. If a person living in the community or in residential care is not comfortable or is in distress, it may be necessary for them to be admitted to the hospital for assessment and symptom management, and then either to receive care through to death there or be discharged to their home.

Identifying Rituals and Care Preferences

In preparation for the time of death, it is helpful to ask the person and family whether they have certain traditions, rituals, and care preferences for the time of death and after it occurs. The following comments and questions can be adapted to help you open conversations with the person and family to discuss their preferences relating to death.

Some people have specific preferences or hopes for the last hours, time of death, and following death. Do you have any thoughts about what you want or do not want to happen? Would you like to discuss this with me?

As a nurse, it is helpful for me to know if you have any fears or concerns about dying. For example, if you are afraid of having a certain symptom as you are dying, then I can record and report that to the team, and we will work extra hard to make sure that symptom is controlled.

These are suggestions for helping the person or family consider what they want at the time of death and following death:

The time following death can be a special and a sacred time. Is there anything special you want to do or have happen when death occurs or following death?

Are there any traditions important in your family, culture, or religious community that you would like to observe? Is there someone in your extended family that you want to talk with in case there are traditions of which you are not aware?

Do you have any cultural requirements or preferences that relate to not touching the body following death?

Is there someone you want to have here with you when death occurs or following death?

Some people like to have the person's body removed soon after death. Others want the body to remain in the home for a time. Have you thought about this?

What might be helpful to you as a person or as a family after death has occurred?

Whom do you want to be present at the time of death or following death? Whom do you want to be notified that death has occurred?

Is there anyone you would like me to notify?

If you or members of the family are concerned that integrating preferred rites or rituals during or following death might be difficult, consult with the leadership in the organization to explore possibilities. It is helpful to address concerns in advance and prevent unpleasant surprises and disappointments in the moment. I have been impressed with the capacity of health care teams to be creative and facilitate a variety of rituals that are important to the person and family.

The Home Funeral Movement

The home funeral movement is growing. An increasing number of families are choosing to provide care for the person while they are dying and to provide care for the body following death, through to burial or cremation. The family may want to make a coffin, sew a shroud to wrap the body in, wash and dress the body, keep the body in the home for several days, register the death, transport the body to the church, crematorium, or burial ground, and help to bury the body.

This growing interest in "do-it-yourself" death care is giving rise to new types of caregivers: death doulas and death midwives. Like hospice and palliative care teams, death doulas and death midwives provide holistic, family- and person-oriented care for the dying and deceased. Funeral celebrants lead services and rituals that are personalized to the beliefs and style of the deceased and their families. Resources for home funerals are available online at the website of the (U.S.) National Home Funeral Alliance (homefuneralalliance.org) and at the Canadian Virtual Hospice website (virtualhospice.ca under the menu for Decisions).

Palliative Sedation Therapy

The explicit use of medications to decrease or obliterate awareness for the purpose of relieving refractory symptoms is termed "palliative sedation therapy." Refractory symptoms are those that have not responded to any treatment (Fraser Health Authority, 2011; Olsen, Swetz, and Mueller, 2010).

Palliative sedation will decrease the person's awareness of living and may shorten life. This therapy is usually only considered when death is days or short weeks away. Palliative sedation is different than physician assisted dying, where medication is administered to cause death. In addition to excellent assessment, information sharing, and supporting the person to choose treatments that are in line with their goals of care, it is essential to ensure that the person meets the criteria identified by the health care organization, and then to follow guidelines for administering sedation.

Caring with Compassion: It's Hard to Be Family

The need to provide care compassionately is discussed in Chapter 3, "Preparing to Care." However, people who are involved in caring for the dying have been heard to say, "Caring for the dying person is easy. It is caring for the family that is difficult."

The point to remember is that people respond to the dying of a family member in all kinds of different ways, and this is to be expected. It is also true that the ways in which people respond when a loved one is dying are strongly related to their history as a family, including the nature of their relationships with one another and the physical and emotional distance that separates them, as well as their existing obligations to work and so on. Remember that family members need your understanding, your compassion, and your warmth. They do not need you to take sides, judge, or share your personal opinions. Be kind. Empathize. Support. Acknowledge. Inform. Encourage.

It may be helpful to remember the following:
- The dying person and the family are the unit of care. While you work to create a safe place for the person to die, try to create a safe place for the family too.
- Stress and grief may be a family's constant companions. Accept the wide range of emotional responses that various family members experience and express.
- Respond to questions and concerns, even if it is simply to reply, "That is a good question. Let's talk about that."
- Provide accurate information in a timely way to allow family members to anticipate changes, validate what they see, and participate in caregiving. Information may also reduce fears and prevent unnecessary crises.
- Provide messages that are consistent with those of the health care team. Receiving conflicting messages from various members of the team is difficult for the person and the family. If a family is struggling with conflicting messages, talk with the team.

Providing Care in the Last Days and Hours

Physical changes often occur during the last days and hours when a person is actively dying. Not all dying people experience every change, nor do they experience the changes in any specific order. Share information about such changes with the family so that they can anticipate them and participate in providing care.

The following sections about the common changes that may occur during the last days and hours suggest ways that, together with those discussed in Chapter 5, "Enhancing Physical Comfort," you can support the person and the family.

Decreased Physical Strength and Increased Drowsiness

As death nears, the dying person's strength decreases and the time spent sleeping increases, until eventually the person is sleeping most of the day. This is a natural change in the dying process.

Supporting the Dying Person

Adapt the care plan to meet the needs and changing priorities of the person. For example, sleeping may be more important than a daily bed bath, and visiting with the family may be more important than visiting with friends. Keep the care team informed of the changing needs and priorities.

Supporting the Family

The dying person's increased need for sleep can be difficult for their family members, who may feel they are missing time with their loved one. You may hear them say,

I knew she was dying in a few weeks, but I did not realize she would be sleeping most of that time.

You can acknowledge that it is common for people to sleep more as death nears. You might say,

It is normal for a dying person to sleep more and more as time passes.

If the family expresses concerns that medication may be causing their loved one's drowsiness, review the goals of care and the rationale for medications, explore the consequences of decreasing medications, and, if necessary, talk with the physician/nurse practitioner about adjusting medications for a trial period.

Share information about the dying person's patterns of wakefulness. Let the family know what times might be best for visiting. Explain that even enjoyable visits can be exhausting for the person, and discuss ways to limit visitors or the length of visits. These are some other ways to support the family when the person is drowsy and needs rest:

- Help the family find ways of being with their loved one whose energy is low. Depending on the interests of the person, this could include playing their favorite music, reading a special book, or reminiscing about good times.
- Encourage family members to continue talking with the dying person and one another, because hearing familiar voices may comfort the person. The person's hearing might be the last sense to go.
- Explore the person's preference for touch. Even if a person is too weak to respond, they may find it reassuring to have physical contact.

Reduced Intake and Difficult Swallowing

In the last days and hours, a person's intake naturally decreases and changes from solids to fluids, from a mouthful to sips of fluids, and from sips to nothing by mouth. The person may begin having difficulty swallowing, followed by forgetting to swallow and then becoming unable to swallow.

Supporting the Dying Person

You can help the dying person in these ways:
- If the person has difficulty swallowing clear fluids, try offering thickened fluids.
- If the person forgets to swallow, remind them to do so.
- If the person is unable to swallow and/or chokes on fluids or coughs after swallowing, do not give anything by mouth.
- Provide excellent and regular mouth care to help keep the person's mucous membranes moist.

Supporting the Family

The dying person's transition from eating and drinking to no longer doing either can be particularly difficult and emotional for the family. You can help in these ways:

- Inform the family of changes in the person's intake and ability to swallow. Use family-friendly language. You might say,

    She is only taking sips of water.

    She is no longer able to swallow but seems comforted when I freshen her mouth.

- Acknowledge that decreased intake and eventually no intake at all are normal when a person is dying.

- Support family members who may find it very difficult to witness their love one not eating or drinking.
- When family members have concerns about the effects on their loved one of decreased intake and what the experience may be like for that person, encourage them to talk to or ask questions of the dietitian and other members of the health care team.
- Explain to family members the benefits of good mouth care, and demonstrate how to provide mouth care if they want to participate in providing comfort measures.
- Explore other ways that the family might nurture. You might ask,

    Were there any activities that your mom liked that you might do now, like playing music, singing, sharing stories, giving her a gentle massage?

When Family Expresses Concerns That the Person Is Dehydrated

When the family is concerned that their loved one is dehydrated, they may want to consider artificial hydration—the provision of fluids through intravenous or subcutaneous routes. Deciding whether to provide artificial hydration can be ethically challenging when the benefits may be questionable, especially when the person is thought to be in their last days of life. A study by Bruera and colleagues suggests that artificial hydration does not improve symptoms associated with dehydration for people with advanced cancer who are experiencing mild to moderate dehydration and are within days or weeks of death (Bruera et al., 2013).

Because of their cultural beliefs and values, some families may consider artificial hydration to be a basic need. They may also believe that artificial hydration promotes comfort and quality of life. In other words, some families may not consider the decision to provide artificial hydration to be a medical one, but instead to be an ethical decision based on their values and beliefs. These perspectives must be considered when making decisions about the use of artificial hydration (Danis, 2015).

It might be helpful to ask if the dying person appears uncomfortable, has a dry sore mouth, is very thirsty, or shows signs of confusion and delirium. If the person does not have any of these signs of dehydration, you might discuss the possible advantages of dehydration in the last days. You might say, for example,

When people have less fluid in their system in the last days, they will have decreased urinary output and may be less likely to experience respiratory congestion.

When the prognosis is unclear, when there is a question of a reversible cause, when the person appears to be uncomfortable because of dehydration, or when the person and family need time to transition to the idea that death may be imminent, artificial hydration may be appropriate. The physician/nurse practitioner may order a trial period of artificial hydration using a small amount of fluids delivered via hypodermoclysis. The following day, before the provision of fluids is continued, the person should be assessed to determine whether the fluids increased their comfort.

> *Christine, a student nurse on the medical unit, reported that Mrs. Boyd's daughter, Jennifer, was upset that her mother had stopped eating and drinking. She knew her mother was in her dying phase, but Jennifer was worried that her mother was now getting dehydrated. When I reviewed Mrs. Boyd's condition with Christine, it was clear that Mrs. Boyd was in her final days of life and that the goals of care were to have comfort measures only. She had stopped eating and drinking; her difficulty with swallowing made taking anything by mouth impossible.*
>
> *We sat with Jennifer, acknowledging how difficult it was for her to watch her mom as she was dying. We reflected on her mom's wish to be peaceful and not prolong her dying time. We reviewed the events of the last few days with Jennifer, how her mother's body was slowly closing down, step by step. Jennifer nodded and added her own observations about her mother's decline. We pointed out that as part of her whole body declining, Mrs. Boyd's digestion was slowing too, as well as her circulation, and how we did not want to add any extra work to her mom's body that was trying to slow down as part of the dying phase. Adding fluid to a body at this point may not help, and may actually cause more burden. The swelling in her arms and legs showed the changes in her circulation that were already occurring.*
>
> *Holding Jennifer as she sobbed, Christine said, "It is hard work, watching your mom die.*

Delirium and Confusion

It is common for dying people to have periods of delirium in the last few days of life. The delirium may include confusion, misperceptions, and difficulties with focusing and separating events of the past, present, or future. If the person is very sleepy, the delirium may be less noticeable. If the person is awake, restless, and agitated, medications may help settle the person. If appropriate, artificial hydration may help to decrease the delirium.

Supporting the Dying Person

These are some comfort measures to support the person who has delirium:
- Promptly report early signs of delirium to the health care team and the physician/nurse practitioner.
- Reorient and provide reassurance if the person is afraid or paranoid. You may say,

   Can you tell me what is happening? I don't see what you are seeing, but I know that you do. You are safe. I am here with you and I have contacted the nurse.

- Allow the person to be in their delirium without reorientation if they appear to be comfortable.
- Offer soothing comfort measures such as warm blankets, massage, or healing touch.

Dying people may see deceased loved ones or other entities during delirium or in the last days and hours. In hospice and palliative care, this is referred to as "nearing death awareness," as defined by Maggie Callanan and Patricia Kelley in their classic book *Final Gifts: Understanding the Special Awareness, Needs, and Communications of the Dying* (Callanan and Kelley, 1993).

It may be appropriate for you to explore with the person what they are seeing. You might say,

   Tell me, what do you see?

   Tell me more about what you are experiencing.

Supporting the Family

Family members need compassion, information, acknowledgment, and encouragement. Witnessing a loved one who is confused, agitated, or paranoid can be extremely upsetting. Caring for someone with delirium can be exhausting for family members. You can help in these ways:
- Acknowledge how stressful it is to witness a loved one experiencing delirium.
- Share information on ways to be with a person with delirium:
  - Walk with them if they want to walk.
  - Listen to them if they want to talk.
  - Orient them to reality if they are afraid.
- Encourage family members to care for themselves, whether by having time away, time to rest, or time to be with the person without having to be the main caregiver.

Final Gifts

Maggie Callanan and Patricia Kelley, two hospice nurses, wrote about "nearing death awareness" in their book *Final Gifts: Understanding the Special Awareness, Needs, and Communications of the Dying* (Callanan and Kelley, 1993). They found that many dying people have visions of people who have already died. The authors relate how common it is for dying people to use metaphorical language and to experience restlessness and agitation as they talk about what they need in order to have a peaceful death. Callanan and Kelley suggest that rather than trying to point out reality to the dying person, people involved in their care instead help the family connect with the person and consider whether the symbolism has meaning for that person.

Although in their book Callanan and Kelley present many case studies in which dying people used symbolic language and saw visions, the authors leave the interpretation of such language and visions up to the families of the dying person.

Carol had suffered a series of small strokes followed by a massive stroke that left her blind, mute, and partially paralyzed. Her large family had gathered around her in the hospital to say their last farewells. Carol's death was marking the passing of a generation in their family: her brother, Charles, had died only the year before, leaving his wife, Victoria, a widow but consoled by their many grandchildren.

As the physical changes of the last days and hours of death began to occur, Carol's eyes started to track across the room, almost as if she could see something despite her blindness. A smile broke across her face and she lifted her arms and acted as if she were embracing the air above her. Her family stood bewildered, watching this. Carol gestured for a pen and paper, making urgent writing motions as she continued to radiate a joyful smile. When the paper and pen were placed in her hand, she scrawled for a few moments, then relaxed back against the cushions, still smiling as she closed her eyes.

Her family began to weep at she took her last breaths. One of them took up the paper Carol had written on. Barely legible were the words, "Tell Victoria Charles says hi."

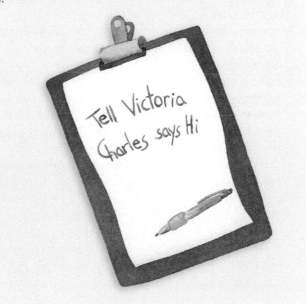

Agitation and Restlessness

As death approaches, the dying person may want to be on the move, without knowing what they want to do or where they want to go.

Supporting the Dying Person

Consider the causes of agitation, such as pain, a full bladder, constipation, and emotional or spiritual issues. Record and report agitation and restlessness. Address restlessness promptly. Not addressing restlessness during the day can lead to a sleepless night for the person and the family. If the person is not confused, guided imagery and other visualization and relaxation techniques may be helpful.

Supporting the Family

It can be distressing and exhausting for the family when their loved one is unable to settle. It may be helpful to:
- Acknowledge the fatigue and stress the family is experiencing, and how difficult it is to care for someone who is restless and moving all the time
- Encourage the family to continue to discuss their concerns and questions with the health care team
- Share information:
  - Explain that restlessness is common in the last days and hours.
  - Provide and model comfort measures to help the person settle, but acknowledge that medications may be needed.
  - Offer family members opportunities to rest and take breaks. You might say,

    While I am here would you like to have a nap?

    If we have someone sit with your mom, would you like to get some fresh air or go home and have a shower?

Unresponsiveness

It is normal for people nearing death to respond less to stimulation. Initially they may seem to be sleeping lightly and can be woken. At other times they may appear to be in a deep sleep and unable to respond to verbal or physical stimuli.

Supporting the Dying Person

Reposition the person regularly to protect their skin and increase their comfort. Continue to talk with the person as though they are able to hear you. Introduce yourself when you arrive at their bedside, let them know what you are going to do, and talk as you provide care. Consult with the team to adjust routines as necessary.

Supporting the Family

The family may have adapted to their loved one not being able to talk and visit, but may reach yet another emotional landmark when the person is no longer able to respond at all. You can help by acknowledging the family's sense of loss when their loved one does not respond and is no longer able to talk with them. Family members should be encouraged to continue to talk to the person if they are comfortable doing so. You might say,

It is our experience that people can still hear even when they cannot respond, so feel free to continue to talk as though she is able to hear you. You do not need to speak any louder than normal.

It is also important to share information. You can help family members explore ways to connect with their loved one by using touch or music, by simply being a quiet presence, or by reminiscing and recalling family stories in the presence of the dying person.

You might suggest the possibility of the dying person talking with other friends or relatives by telephone if they cannot be present. Putting the phone to the person's ear will enable them to have a private, perhaps final conversation, even if the dying person can only listen.

Another way you can be supportive is by teaching family members to position the person, using large and small pillows to support joints and weakened muscles and maintain good body alignment. Massage, touch, and energy work may be relaxing and nurturing to both the giver and the receiver.

Irregular Breathing

When a person is dying, their breathing will usually become irregular, with periods of not breathing (known as apnea). The gaps in breathing can be very long, and family members may find themselves holding their breath and wondering if this is their loved one's last breath. Irregular breathing is not the same as gasping for air. Irregular breathing does not appear to cause discomfort for the dying person.

Supporting the Dying Person

You can help by positioning the person in a way that supports their breathing and by providing verbal assurance. Some people appear to find comfort in following the voice of a caregiver.

That's good, you're doing fine … just breathe easily.

Modeling this coaching strategy for the family may be helpful.

Supporting the Family

The family may feel concerned when their loved one's breathing pattern changes. It is important to acknowledge that irregular breathing is normal for people in the last days and hours. You might say,

Breathing can become very irregular in the last days, with long periods of apnea followed by short or long periods of irregular breathing.

Irregular breathing is normal and in our experience does not appear to be uncomfortable for the dying person.

Please ask if you have questions or concerns.

In addition, you can support the family in these ways:
- Provide contact information to enable the family to access a member of the health care team 24 hours a day.
- Explain the difference between what distressed breathing as opposed to what irregular breathing might look like. For example, if the person is frowning, looking tense or anxious, or becomes agitated, that may indicate discomfort, and the nurse should be contacted.
- If the family is interested in helping with care, demonstrate how to freshen and moisten a dry mouth if the person is breathing through their mouth. Show the family how to use an atomizer and apply lip balm.

Congested Breathing

Respiratory congestion is common in a person's last days and hours. Moisture from the mouth, throat, or lungs collects in the airways, and the person is unable to clear the secretions by swallowing or coughing. The person can have a little congestion or can become very congested. Most likely, the person will be unresponsive, unaware of, and not distressed by the congestion. Occasionally a dying person will be responsive and uncomfortable or distressed. If medication is given at the first sign of congestion, it often helps decrease secretions, thereby preventing or decreasing distress.

Supporting the Dying Person

When you first notice moist respirations, review agency policies and guidelines, and consult with the physician/nurse practitioner. Report the congestion and observations of the person's breathing and behavior; for example, note whether the person is relaxed and breathing regularly, agitated, sitting up, lying down, struggling to breathe, gasping for air, attempting to cough, conscious, alert, aware, responsive, or distressed. You can help in these ways:
- Provide a calm and reassuring presence.
- Give frequent mouth care.
- Reposition the person to facilitate easier breathing and prevent pooling of secretions in the back of the throat:
  - Elevate or lower the head of the bed. Help the person into a semi-supine position if they are very congested.
  - Place pillows under the person's arms to provide support if that makes them more comfortable when they are sitting up.
  - Lay the person flat, turn onto the side on which they are most comfortable, and put a facecloth or small towel under the mouth to absorb any fluids. Gently clean the mouth. (If the fluids are in the oral cavity rather than being deeper in the lungs, suctioning may be helpful. Most people find deep suctioning very uncomfortable.)
- Record and report to the health care team the positions in which the person appears to be most comfortable.

Supporting the Family

The family may be uncomfortable with the sound of the moist respirations of their loved one. Acknowledge that people may find the sound upsetting to hear. Provide a number to call if the congestion increases, the person starts to look uncomfortable, or the family just needs someone to be with them.

Changes in Skin Color and Temperature

When a person is near death, various changes may occur in the color and temperature of their skin. Sometimes the skin warms up and cools down again. Cooling of the skin usually begins at the tips of the fingers and toes and gradually works back toward the core of the body. The feet and legs may become bluish, mottled, and cool to the touch. The area where the person's body rests on the mattress may also become bluish.

Supporting the Dying Person

If the person is sweating, you can provide clean clothing and bedding. If the person is cold, you can offer another blanket; however, be aware that the person's skin temperature might change again and should be checked regularly.

Supporting the Family

You can help the family in the following ways:
- Acknowledge their concerns about the comfort of their loved one. For example, if the person seems to be cold, it may be helpful to say to the family,

  When a person is dying, they do not appear to feel cold. If we put too many blankets on the bed, the person may begin to sweat.

- Consider the person's physical need to be washed and their personal preferences for bathing and touch. More frequent washing may be necessary if the person is sweating or is incontinent. Full baths may not be necessary if the person remains clean and dry.
- Share information:
  ○ Changes in body temperature (e.g., a fever) may indicate an infection or that the circulatory system is not working well and is shutting down.
  ○ Skin color may change and body temperature may cool as death nears.

Other Changes as Death Nears

Muscle Twitching

Sudden twitching of the muscles in the arms or legs when a person appears to be resting is referred to as "myoclonic" twitching. Metabolic changes may cause this twitching just prior to death. Myoclonic twitching that occurs infrequently or occasionally does not distress the dying person. If such twitching occurs more frequently, it may disturb the person's sleep and may be difficult for the family to witness. If this symptom is disturbing to the person or to the family, medication may be required to decrease the twitching.

Dry Eyes

The person's eyes may be open, partially open, or shut during the last days. Seeing a person with only the whites of their eyes showing can be distressing for the family. Remember that families often carry mental images of their loved one's death for a long time after the death. If the person's eyes are open for long periods of time, you can provide comfort by moistening the eyes with artificial tears. In some cultures, the caregivers place a facecloth over the eyes to keep them closed.

Bowel and bladder Incontinence or Lack of Urinary Output

Urinary output decreases as kidney function declines in a person's last days. This results in dark, concentrated urine. Urinary incontinence is common among people who are dying. Some prefer that a urinary catheter be inserted, while others prefer the use of incontinence pads. It is important to remember that people's preferences may change. Talk with the person if possible, or speak with the family to decide which option is most consistent with the person's preferences given the current needs.

People sometimes lose control of their bowels as they are dying. Having an incontinence pad in place is practical and may provide a sense of comfort for the person and family.

Last Breaths

Last breaths occur in a variety of patterns. Some dying people stop breathing suddenly. Others progress from irregular breathing to deeper breaths that alternate with shallow breaths. Eventually, the person's breathing becomes even shallower, followed by mouth breathing and then none. The person may open their mouth as if to take a last breath.

Sometimes the person's face wrinkles or grimaces at the time of death. This occurs even in people who do not seem to be experiencing any pain. I have been told that adherents of Eastern religions believe that the spirit exits through the head. I wonder if this little grimace is the final little tug of the spirit separating from the body.

When Death Occurs

What You Will See

At the time of death, the person does not have a pulse and does not breathe. Their pupils are enlarged, their eyes are fixed in one position, either open or closed, and their mouth and jaw relax.

If the person dies in their home in the community, a specific care plan may be in place for what to do at the time of death. If the person dies in a facility, it will have a protocol about what to do following a death. In addition to following the protocol, it is important to consider and, if possible, adapt to the needs of the family.

Following a loved one's death, the family may respond in a variety of ways. Each person is unique, and the family's responses reflect cultural traditions and family and personal styles and ways of being. Watching people express deep emotion can be difficult, and you may be tempted to "shush" the person, pat their back, and tell them to breathe or to be quiet. Instead of doing that, you might consider that crying and sobbing may be how the person needs to express their grief. I have never heard of a person who did not eventually stop crying. Breathe deeply yourself so you can relax and be fully present.

Some people respond to death by becoming silent and withdrawn, or get busy with phone calls and organizing the funeral, or reminisce and laugh or cry about old memories. Some people express anger or frustration at the unfairness of the loss, or their perception of a difficult death or a health care system that did not meet their needs.

All of these responses are normal. You do not need to guide, control, or judge people's responses. It is important for you to be present in a calm and supportive way for all involved.

What You Can Do

At the time of death, *if there is a signed do-not-resuscitate (DNR) form*:

- Note and record the time of death—when the person's breathing and pulse stopped.
- Breathe. This is not an emergency. Nothing has to happen right away.
- Do not call 911, the ambulance, the police, or the fire department.
- Notify the attending physician/nurse practitioner.
- Notify the family if the family is not present when death occurs.
- Ensure that the appropriate HCP pronounces and certifies the death.
  - The HCP confirms that the person's heart is not beating, the person is not breathing, and the person's pupils are fixed and dilated.
- Confirm (if this has not already been done) with the family whether any rituals or special preferences regarding care of the body need to be observed. If appropriate, create a space in which the rituals can take place.
- Offer the family nourishment, space, and privacy.
- Position the person's body on their back, place a small pillow under the head, and place the hands either at the person's sides or across the abdomen.
- Declutter and simplify the space around the person to help create space for the family to be with the person.
- Check that the care plan has been followed.

If death occurs in the community and *there is no signed DNR form* in the home or on the chart, and the family is not present to refuse cardiopulmonary resuscitation, then be sure to follow agency policies about responding to death. In this situation, you may need to call 911.

When an "Expected Death" Form Has Been Signed

In some communities in Canada, if the physician has previously signed an "Expected Death" form, the death does not need to be pronounced by an official. The form directs the family to contact the funeral home following the death.

Caring for the Body after Death

Over the past century, the responsibility for washing and preparing the body slowly transitioned from family members to HCPs and funeral professionals. Interestingly, families are currently re-involving themselves in washing and preparing the body. Regardless of who takes on this responsibility, it is important to consider agency and facility policies for care of the body. These are the steps to follow in caring for the body:

- Position the person lying flat with a pillow under their head.
- Close their eyelids if their eyes are open. If the eyes do not stay closed, you might place a facecloth over the eyelids to hold them closed.
- Wash the face and hands, and the body if the person was incontinent or diaphoretic (sweating).
- Put in the person's dentures if this is important to the family.
- Place an incontinence pad under the buttocks in case of further incontinence.
- Dress the person in a fresh gown or clothing, as appropriate.
- Change soiled linens and arrange the bedding and pillows.
- Follow facility procedures and the family's wishes with respect to the removal of personal effects, such as jewelry.
- Prepare the body as respectfully as you would if the family were present.

About three or four hours after a person dies, chemical changes cause stiffening of the body, known as rigor mortis. For this reason, caring for the body in the first few hours after death is easier than waiting until the body cools and become less flexible. The work of digestion continues after death, which means that gases may escape the body when it is being washed or moved. Sounds emitted while this is occurring are normal.

Creating Space for Special Moments and Rituals

As a person is dying and following their death, there may be opportunities to create a special or sacred space and a moment in time dedicated to the person who has died and to their life. The family may want the opportunity to observe or create rituals or traditions, or to be in the moment in a way that brings meaning and understanding.

Rituals can help create a sacred or special place. They can honor and show respect for the person who has died, and respect for traditions, beliefs, and heritage. When faced with a person's dying and death, rituals can help people find meaning in what has occurred, enabling them to transition to a new place in grief. Rituals can provide anchors for creating memories. Angeles Arrien, a cultural anthropologist, author, and teacher, suggests that rituals can support, strengthen, balance, and comfort:

> *Ritual provides the bridge between inner and outer worlds, and creates a context of connecting to our souls. The result of all ritual is increased balance, strength, energy, and comfort.*

(Arrien, 2001)

Although people may think of rituals as formalized ceremonies and services that are repeated, rituals can also be behaviors that occur only once, in relation to a specific person. When such a behavior is repeated as part of the human family over generations, it becomes a ritual for that family. In this way, rituals also include those activities that are used to create special moments.

Religious or spiritual rituals include praying, chanting, smudging, communion, blessings, lighting candles, ringing bells, singing, opening windows, covering mirrors, touching or not touching the body, reminiscing, and sharing stories. Rituals that involve caring for the body may include bathing the person, rubbing the skin with special oils, dressing the body in particular clothing, washing the feet, and placing flowers in the hair or a memento in the hands or on the chest. Rituals can be as simple as thoughtfully covering the person's face when the body is placed in the casket. Rituals can last for moments or extend over days. Rituals may be performed by spiritual leaders or offered by family members. Rituals may be passed down through the centuries or created in the moment.

Follow the Family's Lead Regarding Rituals

Ideally the person and family have had advance care planning conversations and their preferences for rituals at the time of death have been identified. If the family has not yet explored the idea of rituals or traditions, you might want to ask a few questions and open the door to exploring the idea. Be mindful to ask in a neutral manner that allows the family to decline. You might ask,

Are there any important traditions in your family, culture, or religious community that you would like to honor or observe?

It can also be useful to gather information about the needs or restrictions regarding rituals, by asking questions such as these:

Are there restrictions on touching the body or who is supposed to bathe the body?

Is there anything that I can do that would help you carry out a ritual that is important to you at this time?

If the family identifies traditions or rituals that are important to them, it may be helpful to:
- Create a comfortable, private area
- Remove medical equipment, linens, and health care supplies
- Tidy the room and empty the garbage
- Put fresh linen on the bed and/or tidy the bed

If death occurs in an acute or residential care setting (as in the following story), you can still explore the family's preferences for rituals and then work with the health care team to create a special space in which the family can be with the deceased.

Rituals can develop spontaneously. As a nurse, you can step back and watch as the family finds ways to create ritual that has meaning to them and brings them together.

Sometimes, by being attentive to nature people discover ways to give meaning to events that occur at the time of death or during the dying process. By listening to and watching the natural world, they find meaning in an event that others may not have noticed. And in making the meaning, they create a sacred, special, or healing space, and open the door to larger possibilities. In some ways, the act of listening and attending could be considered a ritual, or it could be considered an alternative to ritual. People have shared examples about finding meaning in events in nature at the time of a death, such as a ray of sunshine falling across the bed of the dying person, a bird singing loud and clear nearby, a gust of wind blowing through the window, and eagles soaring overhead as a First Nations (Native) Elder died.

Supporting people in their culture, being curious, and learning from these experiences can open the doors of possibility in the experience. It is possible to create a space that allows the family to observe or create rituals or to be in the moment in a way that brings meaning or understanding to the death. Lindsay Borrows, who writes about the cultural rituals in her Anishinaabe community, shares the story below.

When someone is dying, many of the older people know how to listen to the dying person's breath, and they can tell when the person only has a few days left on the earth. There are signs in nature as well, which indicate when someone is close to dying. When my great-grandpa passed away, his friend saw four ducks circling in a pond. Then he looked up and, as if in reflection of the ducks, four birds circled overhead. He felt this was not a coincidence but was a message with important symbolism of the circle, the number four, and the birds. The circle represents the continuity of life, that endings bring new beginnings. The number four speaks to each of the four directions, and when someone passes they head home to the north—giiwedin. Birds are the messengers of death. He immediately went home and his wife informed him that my great-grandpa had died. He was not surprised, knowing that nature can provide comfort and closure.

Lindsay Borrows, Anishinaabe community member

Supporting at Time of Death

Supporting the Family

The family of a person who has died may feel exhausted, hungry, thirsty, tired, emotional, and tearful. They may not remember what they are supposed to do following the death and may need to be reminded. HCPs can help in these ways:

- Offer nourishment, such as a hot drink and a snack. Companioning someone through to death can be tiring. Physical nourishment provides the family with a break before taking care of the body. It can also provide space for spiritual support.
- Invite individual people or the family to sit with their loved one. You might say things like the following:

> *Some people like to have some quiet time with their loved one following death. Would you like to have some time together as a group or some time alone with your dad?*

Some people don't really know what they want to do or say when they sit with their loved one after the person has died. Some people talk as though the person is still alive and able to hear them. Others prefer to sit quietly in prayer or meditation. You might say,

> *I can sit with you if that would help you feel more comfortable.*

It is also important to consider the needs of people who are not present at the time of death and those coming from out of town. You might say to the family,

> *Sometimes people who were not present at the time of death want an opportunity to see or have time with the loved one's body. You can keep the body at home for a few more hours, or you can arrange for a visitation at the funeral home. What would you like to do?*

In the minutes and hours following death, the physical presence of the deceased can help to make the death "real." For those who may have watched their loved one struggle in the last days and hours, it may be a time to see the body "at peace." Sitting with the deceased person can help people understand in a new way, perhaps a deeper way, that the death really has occurred. Caring for the body, as described previously, can help to create ritual and meaning in the experience.

Advocating for the family for more time with the deceased

Some facilities require that the room be ready as soon as possible for the next person to be admitted. This happens in acute care, emergency care, and residential care facilities. If the family members feel very strongly about being with the deceased, you may need to advocate on their behalf. If hospital policy is not flexible enough to accommodate the needs of the family, the family may want to arrange time for visitation at the funeral home.

In some facilities, finding an appropriate space for rituals can be difficult. Fortunately, the cultural competency of health care personnel has improved over the past decades. Sometimes a little creativity can help the health care team come up with options that work for the family and allow them to observe the rituals important to them.

Supporting Other Residents

In residential care homes and hospices, the residents often come to know each other. These people also need support when a person who lived among them dies. In residential care facilities, the residents closest to the deceased are sometimes invited into the room to say their farewells before the body is removed.

Supporting and Debriefing Residential Care Staff

Just as the residents need time to say good-bye and to honor and remember the person who has died, the staff may also appreciate the opportunity to say good-bye. In a residential care facility, sharing information about a death and supporting staff can be relatively easy given that people work day to day at the same location. Rituals can help the staff acknowledge their own grief about the death of yet another resident, may help them develop a sense of satisfaction in having provided good care, and may support them as they continue to provide compassionate care to the dying.

The following stories are from Jackie McDonald, a participant and leader in the Quality Palliative Care in Long Term Care research project. In the first story, she shares what the staff at that the care home where she works do after the death of a resident. In the second story, she shares the experience of leading a staff debriefing after the death of a resident.

Immediately after a person dies, we open a window. We believe this freshens the room; some believe it is a pathway out for the spirit. A staff member puts a butterfly on the frame of the door to let everyone know that the resident has died. We tidy up the resident if needed, tidy the bed, put all bed rails down, and give the family privacy to say their good-byes.

Staff come to say good-bye to the family, because we are losing them when we lose the resident.

When the family leaves, we say good-bye to our resident.

When the funeral home staff come, we place a dignity quilt over the body bag, and a member of our staff walks the resident's body out to the funeral van and returns with the quilt.

We place a decorated memory box on the bed of the resident. On the lid of the box is a beautiful poem and information on grief counseling from one of our community partners, which also donates the boxes to our home.

We put a sympathy card on our table in the staff room for staff to sign and write stories about our resident. Within a week, it is mailed to the family. It is a beautiful moment when you look down at this card and see the many stories and signatures of the many people who have worked hard to make sure this resident left this world with dignity and love.

(McDonald, 2013a)

A few years ago, almost half of our residents died in one year. We called it the "pancake effect," with one death on top of another. There was no way to grieve or say good-bye. Staff could not always go to the funeral, as they were working. We decided to have a peer-to-peer debriefing to care for ourselves after a person died. Management has supported this initiative from the start. As a health care worker, I was trained to lead these debriefings.

We try to have a debriefing within hours of a death. Staff gathers for 15 to 20 minutes. Attendance is always voluntary—people attend because they want or need to. Sometimes there are a few people while at other times there is a full room with someone from all departments. There is no hierarchy, just co-workers remembering our special resident. The debriefing is led by a personal support worker, which helps people feel equal in the debriefing. There is no expectation that you have to talk.

We use the acronym INNPUT to give structure to the meeting.

I—*Information about resident: name, how long in home, and any other pertinent details.*

N—*Need to do. What we can do to help staff finish the shift, get through the day or the week. Staff members may need a hug, reassurance, or recognition that the person was very special to them.*

N—*Need to say. Exchange stories about what made this person special to you. What was important to you about the resident and/or their family?*

P—*Plan for self-care. What will you do to help yourself? Go for a long walk, go to the funeral, sign the card for the family?*

U—*Understanding. We need to understand that everyone grieves in a different way. Understand that it is all right to feel sad, to be angry, and/or to feel as if something is missing. These are all parts of the grieving process. We need to understand that these feelings will pass. To understand that it's all right to seek help through one another, to access the employee assistance program or your own counselor/spiritual person.*

T—*Thank you. We acknowledge and thank everyone for their contributions to the well-being of our resident, family, one another, and themselves.*

(McDonald, 2013b)

Supporting and Debriefing Community Care Staff

In community care situations, sharing information about a death and supporting staff can be more complicated, because people work daily in different locations in the community. In your role as a nurse, it may be helpful for you to advocate for a debriefing to include the health care workers who have provided care. You may want to encourage the agency to do the following:

* Notify the staff members (regardless of role) who were involved in the person's care to let them know when a person has died.
* Identify when you need to debrief after a death.
* Develop a buddy system that provides you with an opportunity to debrief with a colleague while maintaining confidentiality.
* Develop a personal ritual to remember and honor the person who has died, to say good-bye, and to let the person go.

Death affects everyone. Take care of yourself.

Preparing to Transfer the Body

Each agency or facility has policies on how to care for the body and prepare it for transport. Nurses need to be familiar with these policies and follow them.

The following list exemplifies what occurs in some hospitals or residential care homes:

* The health care worker or nurse dresses the body in a gown and covers it with a sheet, leaving the face exposed.
* In hospitals, some means of identification (e.g., an armband), including the person's name and birthdate, is secured around the person's wrist.
* The nurse often calls the funeral home when the body is ready to be removed, but the family can complete this task if they want to.
* The funeral home staff put the body in a body bag, close the zipper, place the body on a stretcher, and transport the body to the funeral home.
* The family may want to accompany the body to the funeral van.
* In a home setting, the family may request that the zipper be left partially open and that the person's face be exposed. This provides an opportunity for the family to kiss the person, put a flower on the chest, or observe some other ritual in saying good-bye.

It may be helpful to inform the family that the removal of the body can often feel as final as the death itself. The family may want to be present when the body is removed, or may prefer to go to another room or leave the unit before the body is taken away.

When Death Is Sudden and Unexpected

It is hoped that preparing for death will prevent a sense of crisis when death does occur. If people have not prepared for the death or the death is sudden and unexpected, then there is a need to respond quickly. If you discover a person has died suddenly and unexpectedly in a residential or acute care setting, follow policy and protocol.

When a sudden and unexpected death occurs in a person's home:
* Call 911
* Notify the physician and follow agency/organization policies
* Leave the person and the room as you found it
* Remain with the body until the paramedics arrive

The Role of the Coroner When Death Is Sudden

The coroner may be involved when a person's death is sudden, unexpected, or occurs within 24 hours of admission to a hospital. The role of the coroner is to confirm the identity of the person who died and the probable cause and time of death. The coroner classifies the death as natural, accidental, suicide, homicide, or undetermined.

If the coroner determines that the death is due to natural causes, usually no further investigation takes place. If there are concerns about the identity of the person or the cause of death, then the coroner will investigate. If you are the person who discovered the dead person and the coroner is involved, you may be interviewed and asked to describe what you saw. The coroner's role is to protect the public and help identify factors that contribute to preventable causes of death. The coroner also helps the family by providing links to resources and support.

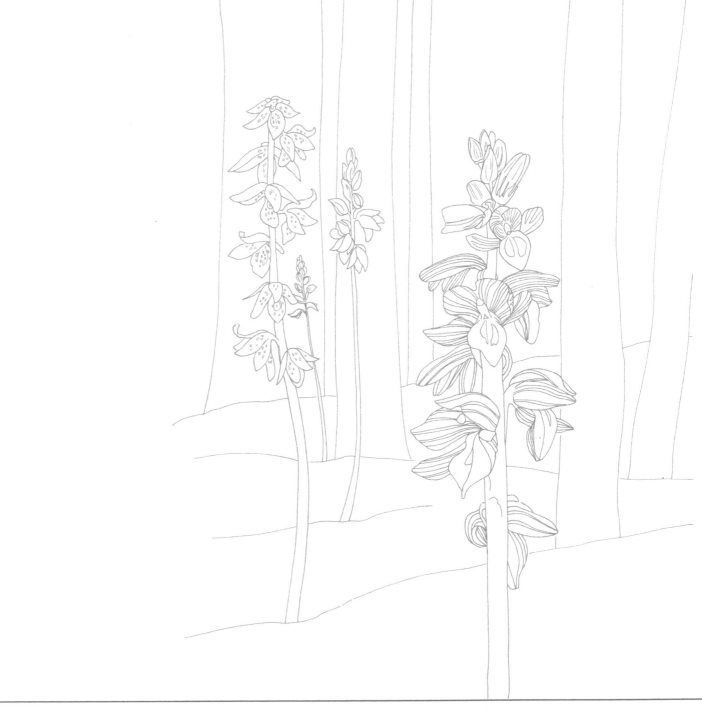

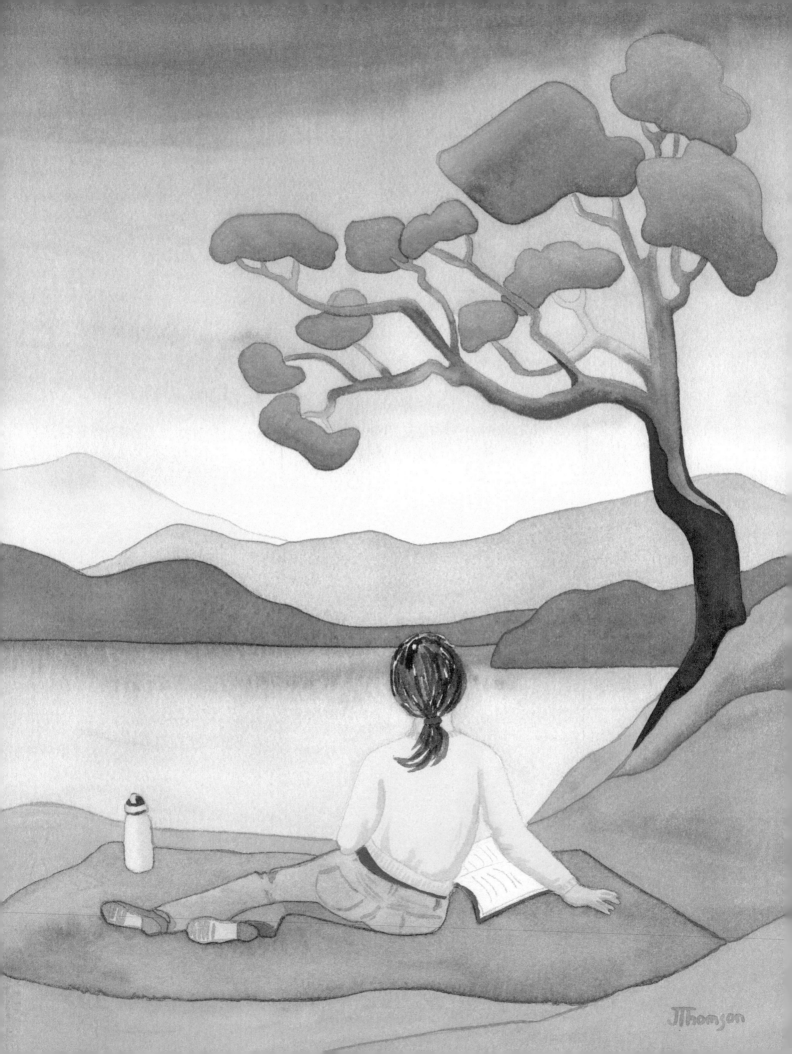

Caring for *You!*

Providing Care for the Dying Will Change You

Caring for the dying will touch you and change you. In her book *Kitchen Table Wisdom: Stories That Heal*, Rachel Naomi Remen says,

The expectation that we can be immersed in suffering and loss daily and not be touched by it is as unrealistic as expecting to be able to walk through water without getting wet.

(Remen, 1997)

There are both positive and negative consequences to providing hospice and palliative care. On the positive side, being with people during their dying process may enhance your enjoyment of living, increase your appreciation of simple things, strengthen your ability to empathize, and increase your awareness of the challenges that people experience. These benefits may increase your capacity to care and may inspire you to face your own challenges with renewed strength and determination.

On the negative side, there may be times when your work and the sorrow you witness leave you grieving, sad, and feeling exhausted. You may find yourself grieving the dying person's losses as though they were your own. You may feel guilty that you are mobile while the person you care for is immobile, and that you are living while they are dying.

The purpose of this chapter is to stress the importance of caring for *you*! You do invaluable work, and you need to care for yourself as well as you care for others. Activities that may nurture and strengthen you include developing strong social support networks; learning and growing through education; and seeking out supervision, counseling, and coaching. In addition, activities that may help you to refuel include stepping back, reflecting, shaking things up, and practicing mindfulness strategies. If your compassion is in alignment with your intentions and the work that you do, then your work can energize you rather than deplete your energy.

Considering Compassion Fatigue

Françoise Mathieu, a mental health counselor and compassion fatigue specialist, and author of *The Compassion Fatigue Workbook* (Mathieu, 2012), encourages health care providers (HCPs) to care for themselves as well as they care for others. She works with organizations to help them develop ways to better support their staff. I am honored by Mathieu's significant contribution to this chapter and thank her for it.

Nurses require self-care in order to prevent burnout and compassion fatigue. The term "compassion fatigue" encompasses the emotional and physical exhaustion that can occur when a nurse (or any other HCP) is unable to refuel and regenerate quickly enough to meet the emotional and physical demands of her or his work. Nurses doing this work—providing care for the dying person and their family, and witnessing suffering day after day and year after year—are at high risk of developing compassion fatigue. In addition to the demands of the work itself, challenges such as high workloads, insufficient staffing, and policies and procedures contribute to compassion fatigue. Self-care can help you withstand the negative effects and benefit from the positive effects of caring for the dying. Without the buffer provided by self-care, you may lose your capacity to provide excellent care for the dying. For example, nurses with compassion fatigue may be impatient, cynical, and irritable, be less sensitive to or less able to empathize with people, and be neglectful or dismissive of the suffering of the dying person and family.

Checking In: Signs of Compassion Fatigue

People who care for the dying differ greatly in the type and amount of self-care they need. Your needs for self-care may also change as you develop skills and learn from your experiences as an HCP.

Françoise Mathieu developed a chart (Figure 1) of thoughts and feelings that HCPs can use to assess their self-care needs in relation to compassion fatigue and to assess which zone on the chart they are in (Mathieu, 2012).

Figure 1. Assessing self-care needs

Green Zone	Yellow Zone
Feeling	**Feeling**
You are at your absolute best: well rested, organized, and feeling on top of the world. You are enthusiastic about your work and excited to go to work each day. You love it.	You are not coping as well. Things are not as smooth as they were. Perhaps you are more tired, more irritable. You are starting to feel overworked, and perhaps overwhelmed by the demands placed on you. You once loved the work you did, but now you are bored when people tell you their problems. You ignore problems that you cannot fix and ask only those questions that will result in a discussion that is easy and positive.
Thinking	**Thinking**
Life is good. Work is good. Let's go!	*I loved my work, for years I loved it. Then with all the cutbacks, fewer staff, fewer resources, no flexibility to switch shifts or take time off, no vacation relief … the recent policy changes, I am starting to hate work. And not only am I mad with management, I don't even feel the same joy in caring for the people I am assigned to care for. I hate it. And I hate myself for not working with the joy that I always worked with.*
Reflection	**Reflection**
Are you in the Green Zone? If you are not in the Green Zone now, can you remember being there? What does being in the Green Zone feel like for you? Take a minute to feel it and enjoy the feeling of energy and inspiration. In your life, how do you care for yourself so that you can stay in the Green Zone?	Have you been in the Yellow Zone? What does the Yellow Zone feel like for you? Sometimes people live in this place feeling overloaded and are barely aware of it. What brought you to this place of increasing fatigue? Do you have any physical symptoms of fatigue? Chronic pain? Headaches? Back pain? What about emotional symptoms? Irritability? Tearfulness? Some people find it more difficult to take care of themselves in the Yellow Zone: they eat more junk food, exercise less, and get less sleep. What are your health behaviours when you are in the Yellow Zone? Can you imagine anything that might push you further toward the Red Zone? What can you do to move back to the Green Zone?

Mathieu uses the colors of a traffic light to indicate when you are safe to go ahead (green), when you should proceed cautiously (yellow), and when to stop (red). Although the colors indicate zones, it is useful to think of the zones as a continuum from healthy to unhealthy and suffering from severe immobilizing fatigue. The goal is to encourage nurses and other HCPs to become aware of their overall health and to use strategies that help you remain healthy and in the green zone.

I invite you to use the chart below to assess where you are on the continuum.

Red Zone

Feeling

You feel unable to cope. If you can even fall asleep, you wake up wondering how you can get out of bed, care for the kids, go to work, and care for those people you are assigned to for one more day.

You are not interested in hearing about any problems, or advocating for anyone who needs any changes, and you hope that no one asks anything extra of you.

Your co-workers, if they are not aware, should be aware to leave you alone and not ask for your help.

Or:

You are frequently tearful at the drop of a hat. You feel angry if someone even looks at you.

Someone suggested you take a stress leave, but you can't imagine how much work it might take to make that happen.

You wonder if it would be easier to quit your job.

You have never been depressed before, but wonder if this is what depression looks and feels like.

Thinking

I didn't realize I had a problem. I knew I was tired. I knew I was frustrated … But one day I woke up and I could not get out of bed. I could not care for my kids, or go to work. I was totally and completely immobilized. My partner took me to the doctor. She signed me off work for a month. I could not believe it. A month … surely I would feel better in a few days. Nevertheless, a month went, and the numbness was just wearing off and the pain was just beginning. It took me nine months before I was back at work.

Reflection

Have you been in the Red Zone? Are you in the Red Zone now?

What does the Red Zone feel like for you?

If you are in the Red Zone now, speak to your doctor or counsellor.

Get support from an employee assistance program.

Is there anything that you can do today to nourish yourself?

Can you connect with a friend or a supervisor to talk about how you are doing?

Can you ask friends/family for support to help you get professional support and develop some strategies to get out of the Red Zone?

Preventing Compassion Fatigue

The following strategies may help you refuel, refocus, care for yourself, and keep you in the Green Zone. If you are emotionally exhausted, you may need to seek professional help, as well as integrate self-care strategies into your daily routine.

Developing Self-Awareness

Personal reflective practices, as discussed in Chapter 3, "Preparing to Care, can be valuable strategies for exploring personal issues and understanding your needs. Writing in a journal or talking with a friend or counselor are other useful reflective strategies.

Self-care means checking on your energy levels and emotions.

Maintaining therapeutic boundaries is part of effective self-care.

Considering the following may help develop your reflective skills:

- Mentally scan your body and "listen" to what it tells you about how you feel. How is your energy level? How does your body communicate to you when you are feeling tense, stressed, hurt, angry, resentful, or other emotions? For example, do you get rashes, an upset stomach, pain, headaches, or other physical discomfort? Reflect on how you process your emotions.
- What do you do when you feel angry? Do you talk about it, exercise, explode, or swallow your anger?
- What do you do when you are sad?
- What you do when you feel overwhelmed?
- Listen to your conversations. What do you talk about? How do you describe your work, your colleagues, the people you care for?
- When you start to feel stressed, examine your decision making. Do you:
  - Agree to do things you don't have time for?
  - Take on more responsibilities?
  - Drink alcohol or eat excessively?
  - Cancel self-care appointments, doctor's appointments, haircuts, and other appointments relating to you?

Remembering Your Boundaries

Establishing and maintaining therapeutic boundaries when caring for the dying can be difficult for many reasons. The dying person or their family may ask you to do tasks or answer questions that are outside of your scope of practice. If you work in the community (especially a small community), the person and family may begin to think of you as part of the extended family rather than as an HCP who has been hired to provide care. Your employer's expectations about your work may be different from those of the person or the family.

Your stress level will increase if you do not have clear boundaries. Setting boundaries may become even more difficult when you are stressed and fatigued.

Blurred boundaries lead to emotional exhaustion and can be a sign of work overload. If you are near the Red Zone, boundaries become more and more muddled. Some people become very rigid when their energy is depleted; others may become excessively flexible and work outside the limits of their job description, perhaps because they feel guilty about being healthy or feel sorry for the person they are caring for.

Strategies for Maintaining Boundaries

Listen to what you say about your work at work and at home; for example, expressions of anger or resentment:

I am not hired to bring the family tea, and I don't do it. I am not staying after work one more day. They cannot expect us to stay!

Consider these strategies:
- Talk with a trusted colleague, mentor, or supervisor when you want to provide care outside of work hours:

The client's wife needs help just as much as he does. I have reported this to the team, but so far the wife has not received any help. I took time from another visit and I helped her get washed and dressed. Last week on my day off, I did errands for them. I would like to talk to you about this and about setting boundaries.

- Review your job description and employee policies to remind yourself what is expected of you.
- Write about boundaries in your journal.

If you live and work in a very small community, coaching or counseling may be available via phone to help you get some perspective on local issues without breaking confidentiality.

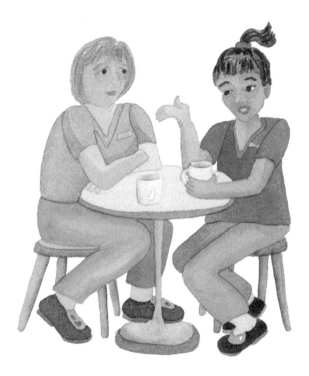

Strategies for Developing a Strong Support Network

Explore ways to meet with colleagues:
- Develop relationships with people away from work.
- Seek out like-minded colleagues for conversation and inspiration.
- Develop a buddy system (with two or three people) or study group and meet to explore relevant topics. Together you could try a few of the suggestions below or come up with your own topics that reflect your needs in your workplace.

Develop strategies for exploring self-care:
- Debrief and learn from stories of caregiving (while honoring confidentiality).
- Study a chapter of *The Compassion Fatigue Workbook*.
- If you cannot connect with other people in person, consider meeting on the phone or joining an online support group.

- Talk with a partner, friend, or roommate about the work you do, the fatigue you experience, and what is helpful when you are feeling very depleted.
- Have fun! Make time for fun with friends! Take a kid on a date!

Strategies for Developing Support When Working Alone in the Community

It can be difficult to meet and interact with other HCPs when you work alone or in home and community care settings. In these situations, it is even more important to create a support network for yourself. These strategies may be helpful:
- Find a few colleagues with whom you can connect regularly for a snack, phone call, or power walk, or to share some common interest.
- Meet with your employer to discuss these topics:
  - Your desire to do an excellent job, continue to learn and grow, maintain your health, and prevent compassion fatigue
  - Your desire to connect with colleagues
  - Guidelines on confidentiality
  - Ways that your agency supports debriefing, ongoing education, peer support, and workload management
  - Your offer to help organize a room in your workplace where the nurses can gather to talk, eat, and have education sessions. You might suggest to your employer that strong social networks help balance mind, body, and spirit, and that having a room for this purpose would be a good investment.

Supporting Yourself in an Uncomfortable or Toxic Work Environment

A negative or toxic work environment can lead to workplace burnout. Feeling overwhelmed with your workload and frustrated that the organization does not respond to your need for support can create feelings of distancing and job dissatisfaction. Whole teams can be affected by this. Instead of working together and supporting one another, staff may turn against one another, gossip, backbite, bully others, and develop an "us versus them" attitude. Here are some things you can do to try to prevent this happening in your work environment:
- Commit to avoid starting or spreading gossip.
- Develop relationships with colleagues who are positive and are interested in being constructive and proactive at work.
- Express gratitude openly and anonymously (e.g., write a note, put a flower on someone's desk).

Consider Coaching or Counseling Resources

As a society, we bring who we are and what we know to work, and then we use the experiences that happen at work to further our learning. Coaching, counseling, and feedback from supervisors can help you learn from your work experiences and may help you cope with a toxic work environment. You may have your own counseling support, or you may want to obtain support through an employee assistance program. Many companies provide this type of service to employees, yet often it is not used. If you have not accessed counseling through such a program, consider doing so.

Coaching is an emerging field that uses a positive, strengths-based approach to help people achieve personal and professional growth. I was first introduced to coaching when a friend needed a guinea pig for part of her coaching training program. I was thrilled to assist. You may be able to access coaches through a coaching school; you could offer to help the coaching students learn. Coaching is frequently provided by telephone, so you do not need to live in the same geographic area as the coach. Distance coaching can be especially useful if you live in an isolated community.

Learning

Education is one of my very favorite self-care strategies. I am inspired by new ideas and use the creative process to apply what I learned to my practice. I am also thrilled when I learn skills that enable me to do my job better. Being prepared to do your work and having the necessary education can help you continue to be balanced in your work. Expand your knowledge to keep up with the expanding scope of practice, new developments, and changes in policy and practice. No basic program can prepare you to do everything that you will do.

Strategies for Learning

These are some strategies to help you increase your knowledge:
- Reflect on what type of education and learning makes you excited.
- Try to identify what topics you need to learn more about.
- Watch for and take advantage of educational opportunities, such as workshops, conferences, and lunchtime lectures in your area.
- Request feedback from supervisors or a trusted mentor.

- Meet with colleagues and supervisors to develop educational opportunities.
- Search for educational opportunities online (you can do this at home, in your pajamas, with the cat on your lap!).
- Offer to help with research projects and champion skill development in areas that you are passionate about. Believe in your ability to influence care.

Refueling

Refuel yourself using the many self-care strategies that nourish you and your spirit. Choose strategies that are meaningful to you and will energize you. You need to schedule them into your life regularly enough to keep yourself fueled up. The important part of refueling is to make the effort even though sometimes you do not feel you have the time or energy to do so. It is then that these strategies are most important to your well-being. Sometimes the most helpful thing you can do is call on your social support network to work together on refueling.

Some ways to refuel are listed below. The list is not comprehensive and does not provide instruction. If an idea interests you, then explore it further using books, websites, and courses to guide you.

Eat Food That Nourishes You

Keeping your body in good working condition assists with developing emotional resilience.

During a busy shift it is easy to fall into the pattern of grabbing a quick bite on the fly. Try to prepare healthy, easy-to-eat, nutritious snacks in advance, take them to work, and enjoy them throughout the day. Avoid turning to sugar and carbohydrates for a quick fix. (I say this as I dream of my favorite dark chocolate ice cream!)

Drink Water

Drinking water is a bit like having a shower: it cleanses your insides just as a shower cleanses your outside. Water increases energy, relieves fatigue, helps cleanse your body of waste, and boosts the immune system. Keep a water bottle with you at work, and try to develop a habit of drinking water between clients and at breaks.

Exercise Regularly and Stretch Often

Exercise for at least 30 minutes a day! (The first 30 minutes of exercise provides the most benefit.) If you work in isolation, you may find it helpful to exercise with another person. If you work in a group, you may prefer to exercise on your own. If the physical care you provide requires a lot of strength and exertion, consider attending a fitness class to strengthen the muscles you use regularly at work, or get a group together and consult with a personal trainer to develop an exercise routine that will increase your strength and so help prevent injuries.

Stretching is another good practice. It can increase your flexibility, range of motion, circulation, and energy level, as well as reduce stress, muscle tension, and lower back pain.

> *I do yoga as a way to relax. At work, when I feel my muscles tighten I find a quiet space. I breathe deeply and stretch the area that is tight. By doing this I am able to prevent my back muscles from going into spasm.*

Sleep Well

Sleep well and sleep long enough. Integrate "sleep hygiene" habits in the hour or so before you go to bed: go for a walk, have a warm bath, pray or meditate, read a soothing book, listen to calming music, and avoid using devices with backlit screens (e.g., tablets and smartphones) at least for the hour before you go to bed. If you work night shifts or have difficulty sleeping, research additional strategies to help you get the best sleep possible.

Be in Nature

Being in nature and even seeing nature (including trees and green space) help to reduce stress and improve health.

> *The pack is on my back ... I breathe the fresh air ... walk the first steps of the trail and already life is better.*

> *I sit by the ocean, the waves lapping at the shore ... I sense ... I am energized.*

Laugh

One of my favorite songs is from the movie *Mary Poppins*: "I love to laugh, long and loud and clear, I love to laugh ... it's getting worse every year!" What a fabulous song! I do love to laugh! The relatively new field of "laughter yoga" helps people obtain the benefits of laughter through laughter exercises. What might start as fake laughter soon becomes real laughter. Years ago I read that "laughter is internal jogging," and I am sure that this is one form of exercise that I can get hooked on!

Develop an Attitude of Gratitude

Feeling and expressing gratitude not only feels good, but can also benefit your body and your social network. Thank-you notes, flowers, sticky notes with positive comments ... all help create a positive environment.

Keep a daily gratitude journal. At the end of each day, write three things that you are grateful for. Make it your goal to find something to be grateful for at work each day.

Enjoy "grateful" music. One of my other favorite songs is "What a Wonderful World." I joke that when my husband, Ted, and I die, one of our tombstones will read "What a wonderful world" and the other one, to the right, will read "But the best is yet to come!"

Create a Transition Ritual Between Work and Home

Create a ritual that is a clear divider between work and home. Play a certain type of music when you are going home, change clothes once you arrive home, or routinely go for a walk after work. The important part is sending your mind a clear message that "work is over, leave the concerns behind." Regular use of this type of ritual will help you shift from a work mindset to a home mindset. If your home is busy and full, try to create a few minutes of peace before entering the door.

> *I placed a bird feeder in my backyard. When I get home I sit and relax for 5 to 10 minutes by the feeder before seeing the family.*

> *I listen to relaxing music on the way home to transition gently into the next phase of my day.*

Build Capacity with Compassion

The Stanford University Center for Research in Compassion and Altruism found that "the practice of compassion is seen to be as important to health as a balanced diet and physical activity."

Darcy Harris, thanatologist, counselor, and author, provided a webinar titled "The Sustaining Capacity of Compassion in the Midst of Loss and Grief" that stated, "Compassion fatigue is really more akin to empathic overload or empathic disruption ... compassion, when sustained by the various components that comprise it, is truly self-sustaining" (Harris, 2016).

If you refer back to the GRACE Model mentioned in Chapter 3, "Preparing to Care," you will find the core domains of compassion as they pertain to practice. The core domains are:

G: Gathering Attention—getting grounded within yourself

R: Recalling Intention—recalling what brought you to this work in the first place

A: Attuning to Self and Other—checking in with yourself and tuning in to the other person, to family, or to team members

C: Considering What Will Serve—asking "What will best serve here?"

E: Engaging and Ending—releasing, letting go, and recognizing both internally and externally that this particular encounter is now over

Harris (2016, handout) identifies "edge states" as markers of empathic overload. Edge states occur when one or more of the core domains of compassion are blocked or not supported. When core domains of compassion are blocked, then true compassion is not expressed, which leads to exhaustion in caregiving. Empathic overload happens when HCPs are attuned with dying people and their families but are out of balance with their own ability to ground themselves and align with their intentions. For example, perhaps you identify yourself as being in the Yellow Zone of the compassion fatigue table presented earlier in this chapter. To move to the Green Zone, look at the core domains of compassion, identify whatever is blocked for you, and find ways to address and release that blockage.

The Center for Contemplative Mind in Society developed the "Tree of Contemplative Practices" (Figure 2) as a way to help people practice and create the habit of being mindful and intentional in their professional and personal lives. You may find that you are more naturally drawn to some of the suggestions than others, and that is fine. It is not necessary for you to attempt to do all of the practices; use just the ones that appeal to you.

Understanding the Tree

On the Tree of Contemplative Practices, the roots symbolize the two intentions that are the foundation of all contemplative practices. The roots of the tree encompass and transcend differences in the religious traditions in which many of the practices originated, and allow room for the inclusion of new practices that are being created in secular contexts.

The branches represent different groupings of practices. For example, stillness practices focus on quieting the mind in order to develop calmness and focus. Generative practices may take many different forms but share the common intent of generating thoughts and feelings, such as thoughts of devotion and compassion, rather than calming and quieting the mind. (Note that such classifications are not discrete, as many practices can be included in more than one category.)

It is not possible to include all contemplative practices on the tree. Fortunately the Center for Contemplative Mind in Society offers free downloads of a blank tree for you to customize with your own practices. This blank tree is available at the organization's website (contemplativemind.org/practices/tree).

Activities not included on the tree (including those that may seem mundane, such as gardening or eating) may be understood to be contemplative practices when done with the intent of cultivating awareness and wisdom.

Figure 2. The Tree of Contemplative Practices

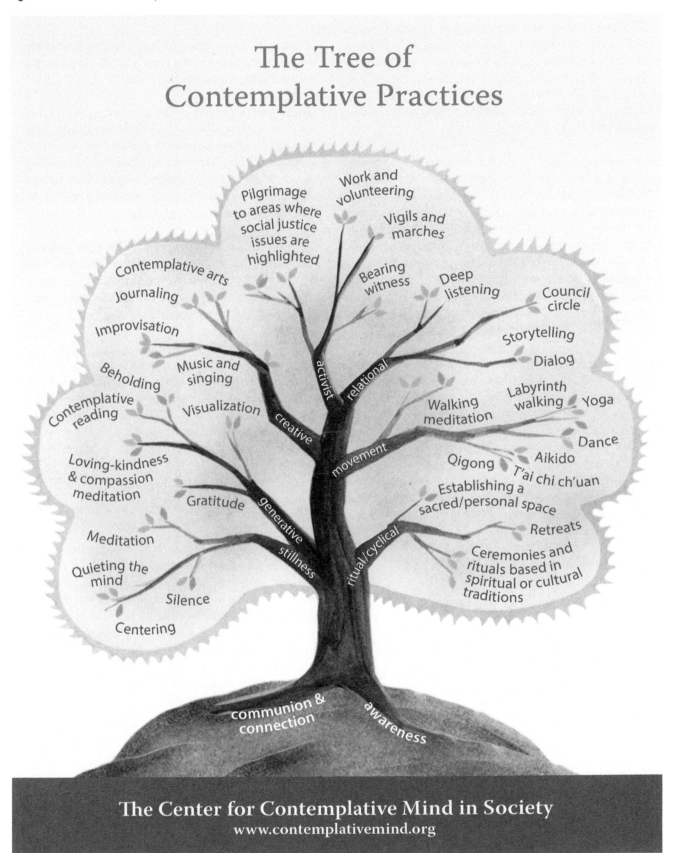

Practice Mindfulness

Mindfulness is one of the most effective strategies for reducing compassion fatigue. Consistent, regular training in mindfulness develops your awareness of your thoughts, feelings, and sensations as they naturally arise, so that when you are in a stressful situation, you can recognize your judgments and reactions without being automatically controlled by them.

There are many ways to practice mindfulness. One very popular and well-researched approach is Mindfulness-Based Stress Reduction (MBSR), developed over 30 years ago by Jon Kabat-Zinn, professor of medicine and founder of the Stress Reduction Clinic at the University of Massachusetts Medical School. Kabat-Zinn defines mindfulness as "paying attention in a particular way; on purpose, in the present moment, and nonjudgmentally" (Kabat-Zinn, 1994). MBSR training typically consists of an eight-week program to introduce mindfulness practices as tools for stress reduction and self-discovery.

Mindfulness can be practiced anywhere. You can apply mindfulness to your daily tasks; for example, when you are washing dishes, pay attention to the feeling of warm water on your hands, the shine and texture of the soap bubbles, the sound of scrubbing a pot. When you notice that your mind has wandered from your task, gently refocus your attention on it. This may sound simple, yet it can be surprisingly difficult to achieve at first! Focusing on breathing is a method often used to teach mindfulness. Here are some directions for a basic meditation on mindfulness of breathing.

An Exercise in Mindfulness

Choose a quiet space where you are not likely to be disturbed for the next 5 to 10 minutes. Sit comfortably, or lie on the floor.

Focus on the feeling of the air coming in and out of your nostrils. There is no need to breathe in a special way; just notice the natural sensations of your breathing, without interpreting or judging them. If closing your eyes helps you to relax and focus, feel free to close your eyes; it's also fine to keep them open or partly open.

Unless you are very tired (in which case you will probably fall asleep), you might find yourself distracted by a million thoughts. Don't worry—that's normal. Just gently bring your mind back to noticing the air coming in and out of your nostrils.

You may need to bring yourself back to the present a thousand times during the 10 minutes. That's all right; simply bring yourself back as often as you need. If you do this regularly, over time it will become easier to maintain your attention and restore your focus.

(Kabat-Zinn, 1994)

Shake It Up

As you reflect and review your life and your work, you may feel a need for a change. It may be as simple as asking for a new assignment or a transfer to a new unit, or you may need to work for a different company or employer. You may want to decrease the number of hours you work in a week or the number of hours you work as an HCP, or maybe you want to take a few months away from your professional caregiving altogether. You may be energized by doing totally different work, for example, in a flower shop or a grocery store.

Closing Thoughts

Self-care is essential to maintaining your ability to continue caring for others and to maintaining your own health. Compassion fatigue can be a consequence of working with people experiencing life-threatening diseases. One strategy is to notice where you are in terms of compassion fatigue and get help and support before you are suffering from total emotional exhaustion. Another strategy is to learn more about compassion and how to focus your intentions, be open to all possibilities, and bring about endings to each encounter so that fatigue does not occur.

Care for yourself as well as you care for others. Access social and counseling support, enjoy opportunities for further education, and refuel regularly. When you are fatigued, step back, reflect, shake things up a bit, and get some extra support. Let your work as an HCP strengthen and enrich your life. That is possible if you pay attention to the intentions that brought you to this work in the first place.

In closing, I share a favorite poem by Deanna Edwards, a singer-songwriter who made it her profession to help other people through music.

Teach Me to Die
Teach me to die
Hold on to my hand
I have so many questions
Things I don't understand
Teach me to die
Give all you can give
If you teach me of dying
I'll teach you to live

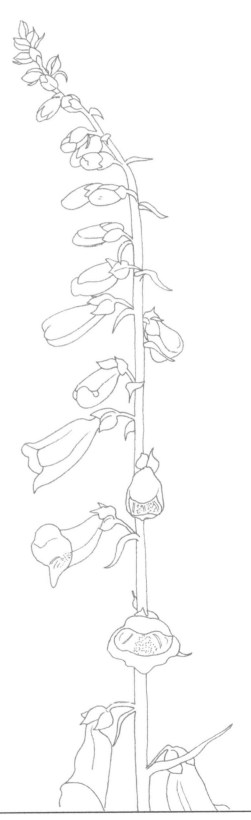

Appendices

Appendix 1
International Council of Nurses Code of Ethics

This is the preamble from the International Council of Nurses Code of Ethics which provides the cornerstones for ethical nursing practice throughout the globe. The detailed code of ethics from the ICN can be found at their website, http://www.icn.ch/images/stories/documents/about/icncode_english.pdf .

(International Council of Nurses, 2012)

"Nurses have four fundamental responsibilities: to promote health, to prevent illness, to restore health and to alleviate suffering. The need for nursing is universal.

"Inherent in nursing is a respect for human rights, including cultural rights, the right to life and choice, to dignity and to be treated with respect. Nursing care is respectful of and unrestricted by considerations of age, colour, creed, culture, disability or illness, gender, sexual orientation, nationality, politics, race or social status. Nurses render health services to the individual, the family and the community and coordinate their services with those of related groups"

Appendix 2
Canadian Nurses Association's Code of Ethics for Registered Nurses

There are two parts to the Canadian Nurses Association code of ethics for registered nurses (Canadian Nurses Association, 2008).

Part I—Nursing Values and Ethical Responsibilities:
Identifies core responsibilities central to ethical nursing practice and is grounded in nurses' professional relationships with people, families, groups, populations and communities as well as with students, colleagues and other health-care professionals. The core responsibilities are described in the following seven primary values, and are expanded on in the accompanying responsibility statements (available on the website).

A. Providing safe, compassionate, competent and ethical care
B. Promoting health and well-being
C. Promoting and respecting informed decision-making
D. Preserving dignity
E. Maintaining privacy and confidentiality
F. Promoting justice
G. Being accountable

PART II—Ethical nursing practice involves endeavoring to address broad aspects of social justice that are associated with health and well-being.

(The Canadian Nurses Association's Code of Ethics (2008) is being revised. The new code is expected to be released in 2017.)

Appendix 3
Code of Ethics for Licensed/Registered Practical Nurses (LPN/RPN) in Canada

(CCPNR, 2013)

The Canadian Council for Practical Nurse Regulators (CCPNR) is a federation of provincial and territorial members who are identified in legislation, and responsible for the safety of the public through the regulation of Licensed Practical Nurses (LPNs). The College of Licensed Practical Nurses of Alberta (CLPNA) contributed to and adopted this code as their code of ethics.

These five principles provide a framework for the ethical responsibilities of licensed and registered practical nurses in Canada. The Canadian Council for Practical Nurse Regulators is the author of the Licensed Practical Nurses Code of Ethics.

The document can be retrieved at: http://www.ccpnr.ca /wp-content/uploads/2013/09/IJLPN-SP-Final.pdf

PRINCIPLE 1: Responsibility to the Public
Licensed Practical Nurses, as self-regulating professionals, commit to provide safe, effective, compassionate and ethical care to members of the public.

PRINCIPLE 2: Responsibility to Clients
Licensed Practical Nurses provide safe and competent care for their clients.

PRINCIPLE 3: Responsibility to the Profession
Licensed Practical Nurses have a commitment to their profession and foster the respect and trust of their clients, health care colleagues and the public.

PRINCIPLE 4: Responsibility to Colleagues
Licensed Practical Nurses develop and maintain positive, collaborative relationships with nursing colleagues and other health professionals.

PRINCIPLE 5: Responsibility to Self
Licensed Practical Nurses recognize and function within their personal and professional competence and value systems.

Appendix 4
American Nurses Association Code of Ethics

These provisions are the foundation of the American Nurses Association Code of Ethics. More detailed information is available at the website of the American Nurses Association, at http://www.nursingworld.org/Main MenuCategories/EthicsStandards/CodeofEthicsforNurses /Code-of-Ethics-For-Nurses.html .

(ANA, 2015a)

Provision 1

The nurse practices with compassion and respect for the inherent dignity, worth, and unique attributes of every person.

Provision 2

The nurse's primary commitment is to the patient, whether an individual, family, group, community, or population.

Provision 3

The nurse promotes, advocates for, and protects the rights, health, and safety of the patients.

Provision 4

The nurse has authority, accountability, and responsibility for nursing practice; makes decisions; and takes action consistent with the obligation to promote health and to provide optimal care.

Provision 5

The nurse owes the same duties to self as to others, including the responsibility to promote health and safety, preserve wholeness of character and integrity, maintain competence, and continue personal and professional growth.

Provision 6

The nurse, through individual and collective effort, establishes, maintains, and improves the ethical environment of the work setting and conditions of employment that are conducive to safe, quality health care.

Provision 7

The nurse, in all roles and settings, advances the profession through research and scholarly inquiry, professional standards development and the generation of both nursing and health policy.

Provision 8

The nurse collaborates with other health professionals and the public to protect human rights, promotes health diplomacy, and reduce health disparities.

Provision 9

The profession of nursing, collectively through its professional organizations, must articulate nursing values, maintain the integrity of the profession, and integrate principles of social justice into nursing and health policy.

Appendix 5
Canadian Hospice Palliative Care Association: Domains of Care

(CHPCA, 2013)

DISEASE MANAGEMENT

Primary diagnosis, prognosis, evidence

Secondary diagnoses (e.g., dementia, psychiatric diagnoses, substance use, trauma)

Co-morbidities (e.g., delirium, seizures, organ failure)

Adverse events (e.g., side effects, toxicity)

Allergies

PHYSICAL

Pain and other symptoms*

Level of consciousness, cognition

Function, safety, aids:
- Motor (e.g., mobility, swallowing, excretion)
- Senses (e.g., hearing, sight, smell, taste, touch)
- Physiologic (e.g., breathing, circulation)
- Sexual

Fluids, nutrition

Wounds

Habits (e.g., alcohol, smoking)

PSYCHOLOGICAL

Personality, strengths, behaviour, motivation

Depression, anxiety

Emotions (e.g., anger, distress, hopelessness, loneliness)

Fears (e.g., abandonment, burden, death)

Control, dignity, independence

Conflict, guilt, stress, coping responses

Self-image, self-esteem

LOSS/GRIEF

Loss

Grief (e.g., acute, chronic, anticipatory)

Bereavement planning

Mourning

PATIENT AND FAMILY

Characteristics

Demographics (e.g., age, gender, race, contact information)

Culture (e.g., ethnicity, language, cuisine)

Personal values, beliefs, practices, strengths

Developmental state, education, literacy

Disabilities

SOCIAL

Cultural values, beliefs, practices

Relationships, roles with family, friends, community

Isolation, abandonment, reconciliation

Safe, comforting environment

Privacy, intimacy

Routines, rituals, recreation, vocation

Financial resources, expenses

Legal (e.g., powers of attorney for business, for healthcare, advance directives, last will/ testament, beneficiaries)

Family caregiver protection

Guardianship, custody issues

END OF LIFE CARE/ DEATH MANAGEMENT

Life closure (e.g., completing business, closing relationships, saying goodbye)

Gift giving (e.g., things, money, organs, thoughts)

Legacy creation

Preparation for expected death

Anticipation and management of physiological changes in the last hours of life

Rites, rituals

Pronouncement, certification

Perideath care of family, handling of the body

Funerals, memorial services, celebrations

PRACTICAL

Activities of daily living (e.g., personal care, household activities)

Dependents, pets

Telephone access, transportation

SPIRITUAL

Meaning, value

Existential, transcendental

Values, beliefs, practices, affiliations

Spiritual advisors, rites, rituals

Symbols, icons

* Other common symptoms include, but are not limited to:

Cardio-respiratory: breathlessness, cough, edema, hiccups, apnea, agonal breathing patterns

Gastrointestinal: nausea, vomiting, constipation, obstipation, bowel obstruction, diarrhea, bloating, dysphagia, dyspepsia

Oral conditions: dry mouth, mucositis

Skin conditions: dry skin, nodules, pruritus, rashes

General: agitation, anorexia, cachexia, fatigue, weakness, bleeding, drowsiness, effusions (pleural, peritoneal), fever/chills, incontinence, insomnia, lymphoedema, myoclonus, odor, prolapse, sweats, syncope, vertigo

Appendix 6
CHPCA: Six Steps for Providing Excellent Hospice and Palliative Care

(CHPCA, 2013)

ASSESSMENT
- History of active and potential issues, opportunities for growth, associated expectations, needs, hopes, fears
- Examine with assessment scales, physical examination, laboratory, radiology, procedures

1

CONFIRMATION
- Understanding
- Satisfaction
- Complexity
- Stress
- Concerns, other issues, questions
- Ability to participate in the plan of care

6

INFORMATION SHARING
- Confidentiality limits
- Desire and readiness for information
- Process for sharing information
- Translation
- Reactions to information
- Understanding
- Desire for additional information

2

SIX STEPS

CARE DELIVERY
- Careteam
  - Composition
  - Leadership, coordination, facilitation
  - Education, training
  - Support
- Consultation
- Setting of care
- Essential services
- Patient, family, extended network support
- Therapy delivery
  - Process
  - Storage, handling, disposal
  - Infection control
- Errors

5

DECISION-MAKING
- Capacity
- Goals for care
- Issue prioritization
- Therapeutic options with potential for benefit, risk, burden
- Treatment choices, consent
- Requests for:
  - withholding, withdrawing therapy
  - therapy with no potential for benefit
  - hastened death
- Surrogate decision-making
- Advance directives
- Conflict resolution

3

CARE PLANNING
- Setting of care
- Process to negotiate and develop plan of care that:
  - Addresses issues and opportunities, delivers chosen therapies
  - Includes plan for:
    - Dependents
    - Backup coverage
    - Respite care
    - Emergencies
    - Discharge planning
    - Bereavement care

4

Appendix 7
The CHPCA Process of Providing Care

(CHPCA, 2013)

		Process of Providing Care					
		Assessment	Information Sharing	Decision-Making	Care Planning	Care Delivery	Confirmation
Common Issues	Disease Management						
	Physical						
	Psychological			Patient and Family Care			
	Social						
	Spiritual						
	Practical						
	End of life/ Death Management						
	Loss, Grief						

Appendix 8
Domains and Recommendations from the National Consensus Project (NCP) Guidelines in the United States

(Ferrell et al., 2007)

NCP Domain	Recommendations
Domain 1: Structure and Processes of Care	• Comprehensive interdisciplinary assessment of patient and family. • Addresses identified and expressed needs of patient and family • Interdisciplinary team consistent with plan of care • Education and training • Emotional impact of work • Team has relationship with hospices • Physical environment meets needs of patient and family
Domain 2: Physical Aspects of Care	• Pain, other symptoms, and treatment side effects are managed using best practices • Team documents and communicates treatment alternatives permitting patient/family to make informed choices • Family is educated and supported to provide safe/appropriate comfort measures to patient
Domain 3: Psychological and Psychiatric Aspects of Care	• Psychological and psychiatric issues are assessed and managed • Team employs pharmacologic, non-pharmacologic, and complementary therapies as appropriate • Grief and bereavement program is available to patients and families
Domain 4: Social Aspects of Care	• Interdisciplinary social assessment • Care plan developed • Referral to appropriate services
Domain 5: Spiritual, Religious, and Existential Aspects of Care	• Assesses and addresses spiritual concerns • Recognizes and respects religious beliefs and provides religious support • Makes connections with community and spiritual/religious groups or individuals as desired by patient/family
Domain 6: Cultural Aspects of Care	• Assesses and aims to meet the culture-specific needs of patients and families • Respects and accommodates range of language, dietary, habitual, and ritual practices of patients and families • Team has access to/uses translation resources • Recruitment and hiring practices reflect cultural diversity of community
Domain 7: Care of the Imminently Dying Patient	• Signs and symptoms of impending death are recognized and communicated • As patients decline, team introduces or reintroduces hospice • Signs/symptoms of approaching death are developmentally, age, and culturally appropriate
Domain 8: Ethical and Legal Aspects of Care	• Patient's goals, preferences, and choices are respected and form basis for plan of care • Team is aware of and addresses complex ethical issues • Team is knowledgeable about relevant federal and state statutes and regulations

Bibliography

AAHPM (American Association of Hospice and Palliative Medicine). (2016). *Statement on physician assisted dying*. Retrieved July 6, 2016 from http://aahpm.org/positions/pad

Abel, J., & Kellehear, A. (2016). "Palliative care reimagined: A needed shift." *British Medical Journal: Supportive Palliative Care*. doi:10.1136/bmjspcare-2015-001009

American Geriatrics Society. (2002). "The management of persistent pain in older persons. AGS Panel on Persistent Pain in Older Persons." *Journal of the American Geratrics Society*, 50(6), 205–224.

American Geriatrics Society Ethics Committee. (2015). "American Geriatrics Society care of lesbian, gay, bisexual, and transgender older adults position statement." *Journal of the American Geriatrics Society*, 63, 423–426.

ANA (American Nurses Association) (2015a). Code of Ethics for Nurses. MD: Nursesbooks.org.

ANA. (2015b). "Demystifying delirium." *The American Nurse*. Retreived from http://www.theamericannurse.org/index.php/2015/08/31/demystifying-delirium/

American Psychiatric Association. (2000). "Diagnostic and statistical manual of mental disorders" (4th ed). Washington, DC. Retrieved from http://www.wai.wisc.edu/pdf/phystoolkit/diagnosis/DSM-IV_Criteria_Delirium.pdf

Arensmeyer, K. (2012). "Nursing management of patients with cancer-related anorexia." Retrieved from https://www.oncolink.org/healthcare-professionals/o-pro-portal/articles-about-cancer-treatment-and-medications/nursing-management-of-patients-with-cancer-related-anorexia

Arrien, A. (2001). "Using extraordinary experiences to cope with loss and change." In Louis LaGrand (Ed.), *Gifts from the Unknown*. San Jose: Author's Choice Press.

Austerlic, S. (2009). "Cultural humility and compassionate presence at the end of life." Santa Clara University: Markkuola Centre for Applied Ethics. Retrieved from https://www.scu.edu/ethics/focus-areas/bioethics/resources/culturally-competent-care/from-chronic-to-critical/cultural-humilitycompassionate-presence/

Balboni, T.A., Paulk, M.E., Balboni, M.J., Phelps, A.J., & Trice, E. (2010). "Provision of spiritual care to patients with advanced cancer: Associations with medical care and quality of life near death." *Journal of Clinical Oncology*, 28, 445–452. doi:10.1200/JCO.2009.24.8005

Barnard, A., Hollingum, C., & Hartfiel, B. (2006). "Going on a palliative journey: Understanding palliative care nursing." *International Journal of Palliative Nursing*, 12(1), 6–12. doi:10.12968/ijpn.2006.12.1.20389

BCCLA (British Columbia Civil Liberties Association). (2012). "In Memory of Gloria." Retrieved from https://bccla.org/2012/10/in-memory-of-gloria/

Beernaught, K., Deliens, L., De Vleminck, A., Devroey, D., Pardon, K., Van den Block, L., & Cohen, J. (2014). "Early identification of palliative care needs by family physicians: A qualitative study of barriers and facilitators from the perspective of family physicians, community nurses and patients." *Palliative Medicine*, 28(6), 480–490.

Bevan, D., & Thompson, N. (2003). "The social basis of loss and grief: Age, disability and sexuality." *Journal of Social Work*, 3(2), 179–194.

Brady, A.J. (2016) "Helping families cope with cancer-related anorexia and cachexia." *Oncology Nurse Advisor*. Retrieved from http://www.oncologynurseadvisor.com/general-oncology/helping-families-cope-with-cancer-related-anorexia-and-cachexia/article/483636/3/

Brignell, A. (2009). "Facial Grimace Scale." In A. Brignell & I. Tigchelaar (Eds.), *Guidelines for developing a pain management program (5th ed.). A resource guide for long term care facilities*. Ontario: Beach House Press.

Bruera, E., Hui, D., Dalal, S., Torres-Vigil, I., Trumble, J., Roosth, J. ... Tarleton, K. (2013). "Parenteral hydration in patients with advanced cancer: A multicenter, double-blind, placebo-controlled randomized trial." *Journal of Clinical Oncology*, 31(1), 111–118.

Bruera, E., Kuehn, N., Miller, M.J., Selmser, P., & Macmillan, K. (1991). "The Edmonton Symptom Assessment System (ESAS): A simple method for the assessment of palliative care patients." *Journal of Palliative Care*, 7, 6–9.

Buchanan, G.F., & Richerson, G.B. (2009). "Role of chemoreceptors in mediating dyspnea." *Respiratory Physiology & Neurobiology*, 167(1), 9–19.

Burki, N.K., & Lee, L.-Y. (2010). "Mechanisms of dyspnea." *Chest*, 138(5), 1196–1201.

Bush, S.H., Leonard, M.M., Agar, M., Spiller, J.A., Hosie, A., Wright, D. ... Lawlor, P.G. (2014). "End-of-life delirium: Issues regarding recognition, optimal management and the role of sedation in the dying phase." *Journal of Pain and Symptom Management*, 48(2), 215–30.

Butot, M. (2005). "Reframing spirituality, reconceptualizing change: Possibilities for critical social work." *Critical Social Work* (University of Windsor), 6(2). http://www1.uwindsor.ca/criticalsocialwork/

California Health Advocates. (2007). "Are you practicing cultural humility?—The key to success in cultural competence." Retrieved from http://www.cahealthadvocates.org/news/disparities/2007/are-you.html

Callanan, M., & Kelley, P. (1993). *Final Gifts: Understanding the special awareness, needs, and communications of the dying.* Toronto: Bantam Books.

Canadian Coalition for Seniors' Mental Health. (2006). "National guidelines for seniors' mental health—The assessment and treatment of delirium." Retrieved from http://seniorspolicylens.ca/Root/Materials/Adobe%20Acrobat%20Materials/Delirium_Guidelines.pdf

Canadian Nurses Association (2008) "Canadian Nurses Association's Code of Ethics for Registered Nurses. Centennial Edition" https://www.cna-aiic.ca/~/media/cna/page-content/pdf-fr/code-of-ethics-for-registered-nurses.pdf?la=en

Canadian Thoracic Society. (2011). "Managing Dyspnea in Patients with Advanced Chronic Obstructive Pulmonary Disease." Retrieved from http://www.respiratoryguidelines.ca/sites/all/files/CTS%20COPD%20Dyspnea%20Slide-Kit%202011_Final.pdf

Cancer Care Ontario. (2010). "CCO Toolbox – Symptom Assessment and Management Tools." Retrieved from https://www.cancercare.on.ca/toolbox/symptools/

Capossela, C., & Warnock, S. (2004). *Share the care: How to organize a group to care for someone who Is seriously ill.* Touchstone Books.

Carr, F.M. (2013). "The role of sitters in delirium: An update." *Canadian Geriatrics Journal,* 16(1), 22–36. doi:10.5770/cgj.16.29

Carteret, M. (2011). "Cultural aspects of pain management." Retrieved from http://dimensionsofculture.com/2010/11/cultural-aspects-of-pain-management/

Causton, E. (2016). Personal communication.

CCPNR (Canadian Council for Practical Nurse Regulators). (2013). "Code of ethics for Licensed Practical Nurses in Canada." Retrieved from http://www.clpna.com/wp-content/uploads/2013/02/doc_CCPNR_CLPNA_Code_of_Ethics.pdf

Chapple, A., Ziebland, S., McPherson, A., & Herxheimer, A. (2006). "What people close to death say about euthanasia and assisted suicide: A qualitative study." *Journal of Medical Ethics,* 32, 706–710.

Cheatham, Carla. (2016). Personal communication.

Chochinov, H.M. (2010). "The Patient Dignity Question." Retrieved from http://dignityincare.ca/en/toolkit.html#The_Patient_Dignity_Question

Chochinov, H.M., Johnston, W., McClement, S.E., Hack, R.F., Dufault, B., Enns, M., ... Kredentser, M.S. (2016). "Dignity and distress towards the end of life across four non-cancer populations." *Public Library of Science Online,* 11(1). doi:10.1371/journal.pone.0147607

Chow, K., Cogan, D., & Mun, S. (2015). "Nausea and vomiting." In B.R. Ferrell, N. Coyle, & J.A. Paice (Eds.), *Oxford Textbook of Palliative Nursing* (4th ed.). New York, NY: Oxford University Press. doi:10.1093/med/9780199332342.003.0010

CHPCA (Canadian Hospice Palliative Care Association). (2012). "The palliative approach: Improving care for Canadians with life limiting illnesses." The Way Forward. Retrieved from http://www.hpcintegration.ca/resources/discussion-papers/palliative-approach-to-care.aspx

CHPCA. (2013). "A model to guide hospice palliative care." Retrieved from http://www.chpca.net/media/319547/norms-of-practice-eng-web.pdf.

CHPCA. (2015). "Fact sheet: Hospice palliative care in Canada." Retrieved from http://www.chpca.net/media/400075/fact_sheet_hpc_in_canada_march_2015_final.pdf

CHPCA. (2016). "How to do advance care planning." Retrieved from http://www.advancecareplanning.ca/making-your-plan/

CHPCA & QELCCC (Quality End-of-Life Care Coalition of Canada) (2015). "The Way Forward National Framework: A roadmap for an integrated palliative approach to care." Ottawa, Ontario: CHPCA.

Collier, R. (2011). "Bringing palliative care to the homeless." *Canadian Medical Association Journal,* 183(6). doi:10.1503/cmaj.109-3756

Columbia School of Social Work. (2016). "Complicated grief." Retrieved from http://www.complicatedgrief.org

Coyle, N. (2015). "Introduction to palliative nursing care." In B.R. Ferrell, N. Coyle, & J.A. Paice (Eds.), *Oxford Textbook of Palliative Nursing* (4th ed.). New York, NY: Oxford University Press. doi:10.1093/med/9780199332342.003.0010

Dahlin, C.M. (Ed.). (2013). *Clinical practice guidelines for quality palliative care. National Consensus Project for Quality Palliative Care.* Retrieved from http://www.nationalconsensusproject.org/guidelines_download2.aspx

Dahlin, C.M., & Cohen, A.K. (2015). "Dysphagia, xerostomia, and hiccups." In B.R. Ferrell, N. Coyle, & J.A. Paice (Eds.), *Oxford Textbook of Palliative Nursing* (4th ed.). New York, NY: Oxford University Press. doi:10.1093/med/9780199332342.003.0010

Daniels, N., James, E., & Sabin, J.E. (2002). *Setting limits fairly: Can we learn to share medical resources?* New York, NY: Oxford University Press.

Danis, M. (2015). "Stopping artificial nutrition and hydration at the end of life." Retrieved from http://www.uptodate.com/contents/stopping-artificial-nutrition-and-hydration-at-the-end-of-life

Davidson, K.M. (2011). "Evidence-based practice guideline: Family preparedness and end-of-life support before the death of a nursing home resident." *Journal of Gerontological Nursing, 37*(2), 11–16.

Davies, B., Steele, R., Krueger, G., Albersheim, S., Baird, J., Bifirie, M. ... Zhao, Y. (2016). "Best practice in provider/parent interaction." *Qualitative Health Research,* 1–15. doi: 10.1177/1049732316664712

Death with Dignity. (2016). "How to access and use death with dignity laws." Retrieved from https://www.deathwithdignity.org/learn/access/

Diamond, E.L., Russell, D., Kryza-Lacombe, M., Bowles, K.H., Applebaum, A.J., Dennis, J., DeAngelis, L.M., & Prigerson, H.G. (2016). "Rates and risks for late referral to hospice in patients with primary malignant brain tumors." *Journal of Neuro-Oncology, 18*(1), 78–86. doi:10.1093/neuonc/nov156

Doane, G.H., & Varcoe, C. (2016). *How to nurse: Relational inquiry with individuals and families in changing health and health care contexts.* Baltimore: Lippencott Williams and Wilkins.

Dodson, S., Baracos, V.E., Jatoi, A., Evans, W.J., Cella, D., Dalton, J.T., & Steiner, M.S. (2011). "Muscle wasting in cancer cachexia: clinical implications, diagnosis, and emerging treatment strategies." Annual Review of Medicine, 62, 265-79. doi:10.1146/annurev-med-061509-131248

Doka, K.J., & Martin, T.L. (2010). *Grieving beyond gender: Understanding the ways men and women mourn.* New York, NY: Routledge.

Downing, M., & Wainwright, W. (2006). *Medical care of the dying.* Victoria. B.C.: Victoria Hospice.

Dudgeon, D. (2015). "Dyspnea, terminal secretions, and cough." In B.R. Ferrell, N. Coyle, & J.A. Paice (Eds.), *Oxford Textbook of Palliative Nursing* (4th ed.). New York, NY: Oxford University Press. doi:10.1093/med/9780199332342.003.0010

Dwyer, P. (2016). *Conversations on dying.* Toronto: Dundurn Press.

Dy, S. (2006). "Enteral and parenteral nutrition in terminally ill cancer patients: A review of the literature." *American Journal of Hospice Palliative Care, 23*(5), 369–377.

Economou, D.C. (2015). "Bowel management: Constipation, diarrhea, obstruction, and ascites." In B.R. Ferrell, N. Coyle, & J.A. Paice (Eds.), *Oxford Textbook of Palliative Nursing* (4th ed.). New York, NY: Oxford University Press. doi:10.1093/med/9780199332342.003.0010

ELMMB. (2013). "Topical morphine for painful skin ulcers in palliative care: A treatment guideline." East Lancashire Medicines Management Board. Retrieved from http://www.elmmb.nhs.uk/EasySiteWeb/getresource.axd?AssetID=34123&type

ELNEC. (2015). "End-of-life Nursing Education Consortium (ELNEC) Project. Advanced Palliative Care." Retrieved from http://www.aacn.nche.edu/elnec

Ferrell, B., Connor, S.R., Cordes, A., Dahlin, C.M., Fine, P.G., Hutton, N. ... The National Consensus Project for Quality Palliative Care Task Force Members. (2007). "NHPCO Special Article: The National Agenda for Quality Palliative Care: The National Consensus Project and the National Quality Forum." *Journal of Pain and Symptom Managment, 33,* 737–744.

Fraser Health Authority. (2006). "Nausea and vomiting." Retrieved from https://www.fraserhealth.ca/media/14FHSymptomGuidelinesNausea.pdf

Fraser Health Authority. (2009). "Dyspnea." Retrieved from http://www.fraserhealth.ca/professionals/hospice-palliative-care/hospice-palliative-care-symptom-guidelines/hospice-palliative-care-symptom-guidelines

Fraser Health Authority. (2011). "Refractory symptoms and palliative sedation therapy guidelines." Retrieved from https://www.fraserhealth.ca/media/RefractorySymptomsandPalliativeSedationTherapyRevised_Sept%2009.pdf

Fraser Health Authority. (2016a). "Principles of opioid management." In *Hospice palliative care program: Symptom guidelines.* https://www.fraserhealth.ca/media/16FHSymptomGuidelinesOpioid.pdf

Fraser Health Authority. (2016b). "Symptom Assessment Acronym." Retrieved from http://www.fraserhealth.ca/media/SymptomAssesment.pdf

Fraser Health Authority. (2016c). "Bowel care." Retrieved from https://www.fraserhealth.ca/media/04FHSymptomGuidelinesBowelCare.pdf

Friedman, B.T., Harwood, M.K., & Shields, M. (2002). "Barriers and enablers to hospice referrals: An expert overview." *Journal of Palliative Medicine, 5*(1), 73–84. doi:10.1089/10966210252785033

Friesen, K.J., Woelk, C., & Bugden, S. (2016). "Safety of fentanyl initiation according to past opioid exposure among patients newly prescribed fentanyl patches." *Canadian Medical Association Journal.* doi:10.1503/cmaj.150961

Gawande, A. (2014). *Being mortal: Medicine and what matters in the end.* New York, NY: Henry Holt and Company.

Gibson, J.L., Martin, D.K., & Singer, P.A. (2005). "Evidence, economics and ethics: Resource allocation in health services organisations." *Healthcare Quarterly, 8*(2), 50–59.

Ginsburg, M., Silver, S., & Berman, H. (2009). "Prescribing opioids to older adults: A guide to choosing and switching among them." *Geriatrics and Aging*, 12(1), 48–52.

Goldman, L. (2012). "The four tasks of grieving." Life and Death Matters Podcast. Podcast retrieved from http://lifeanddeathmatters.ca/products/podcast-library /kids-and-grief-supporting-grieving-children-four-tasks-of -grieving/

Goldstein, N., Carlson, M., Livote, E., & Kutner, J.S. (2010). "Brief communication: Management of implantable cardioverter-defibrillators in hospice: A nationwide survey." *Annals of Internal Medicine*, 152, 296–299.

Government of Canada. (2016a). "Compassionate care benefits." Retrieved from http://www.esdc.gc.ca/en/reports /ei/compassionate_care.page

Government of Canada. (2016b). "Bill C14 Royal Assent." Retrieved from http://www.parl.gc.ca/HousePublications /Publication.aspx?Language=E&Mode=1&DocId=8384014

Green, L.M. (2015). "A Surprise Question can help predict which patients are near the end of life." Retrieved from http://nursing.onclive.com/web-exclusives /a-surprise-question-can-help-predict-which-patients-are -near-the-end-of-life

Grossman, D., Rootenberg, M., Perri, G.A., Yogaparan, T., DeLeon, M., Calabrese, S., ... Mazzotta, P. (2014). "Enhancing communication in end-of-life care: A clinical tool translating between the Clinical Frailty Scale and the Palliative Performance Scale." *Journal of the American Geriatrics Society,* 62(8), 1532–5415.

Gueant, J-L. Aimone-Gastin, I., Namour, F., Laroche, D., Bellou, A., & Lazenaire, M-C. (1998). "Diagnosis and pathogenesis of the anaphylactic and anaphylactoid reactions to anaesthetics." *Clinical and Experimental Allergy,* 28, Supplement 4, 65–70.

Hadad, M. (2009). *The ultimate challenge. Coping with death, dying and bereavement.* Toronto, Canada: Nelson Education.

Halifax, J. (2013). "Being with dying. Experiences in end of life care." In T., Bolz & M. Singer (Eds.), *Compassion: Bridging Practice and Science.* Retrieved from http://www.compassion-training.org/

Halifax, J. (2014). "G.R.A.C.E. for nurses: Cultivating compassion in nurse/patient interactions." *Journal of Nursing Education and Practice,* 4(1), 121–8.

Harris, D. (2016). "The sustaining capacity of compassion in the midst of loss and grief." Webinar retrieved from http://www.adec.org/adec/Main/Continuing_Education /Webinars/Webinar_Details/ADEC_Main/Continuing -Education/We/Webinar_Details_Folder /Webinar_Details.aspx?webinar=WEB0116

Heart Rhythm Society. (2014). "End of life and heart rhythm devices." Retrieved from http://www.hrsonline.org/content /download/21396/940307/file/End%20of%20Life%20 and%20Heart%20Rhythm%20Devices.pdf

Hebert, R.S., Schulz, R., Copeland, V., & Arnold, R.M. (2008). "What questions do family caregivers want to discuss with health care providers in order to prepare for the death of a loved one? An ethnographic study of caregivers of patients at end of life." *Journal of Palliative Medicine,* 11(3), 476–483.

Heidrich, D.E., & English, N.K. (2015). "Delirium, confusion, agitation, and restlessness." In B.R. Ferrell, N. Coyle, & J.A. Paice (Eds.), *Oxford Textbook of Palliative Nursing* (4th ed.). New York, NY: Oxford University Press. doi:10.1093/med /9780199332342.003.0010

Herr, K., Coyne, P.J., Manworren, R., McCaffery, M., & Pelosi-Kelly, J. (2006). "Pain assessment in the nonverbal patient: Position statement with clinical practice recommendations." *Pain Management Nursing,* 7(2), 44–52.

Heyland, D.K. (2016). "Cardio-Pulmonary Resuscitation (CPR): A decision aid for patients and their families." Retrieved from http://www.thecarenet.ca/docs/CPRDecision_Aid_formatted _20101110.pdf

Horgas, A.L., Yoon, S.L., & Grall, M. (2013). "Nursing Standard of Practice Protocol: Pain management in older adults." In *Evidence-Based Geriatric Nursing Protocols for Best Practice.* New York, NY: Springer Publishing Company.

Huang, J. (2016). "Overview of delirium and dementia." Merck Manual. Retrieved from http://www.merckmanuals.com /professional/neurologic-disorders/delirium-and-dementia /overview-of-delirium-and-dementia

Hughes, A. (2015). "Poor, homeless, and underserved populations." In B.R. Ferrell, N. Coyle, & J.A. Paice (Eds.), *Oxford Textbook of Palliative Nursing* (4th ed.). New York, NY: Oxford University Press. doi:10.1093/med /9780199332342.003.0010

Hyslop Christ, G. (2000). *Healing children's grief: Surviving a parent's death from cancer.* New York, NY: Oxford University Press.

Ingleton, C., & Larkin, P.J. (2015). *Palliative care nursing at a glance.* Oxford: John Wiley and Sons.

International Council of Nurses. (2012). "Code of Ethics." Retrieved from http://www.icn.ch/who-we-are/code-of -ethics-for-nurses/

iPANEL (Initiative for a Palliative Approach in Nursing: Leadership and Education). (2014). *Integration of a palliative approach in home, acute medical, and residential care settings: Findings from a province-wide survey.* Province of B.C.

iPANEL. (2016). "A port in a storm: A day of education and discussion about equitable access in palliative care for structurally vulnerable people in Victoria." Retrieved from http://www.ipanel.ca/news-events/news/354-a-port-in-the-storm

ISMP (Institute for Safe Medication Practices). (2011). "FDA and ISMP lists of look-alike drug names with recommended Tall Man letters." Retrieved from https://www.ismp.org/tools/tallmanletters.pdf

Johnson, C.E., Girgis, A., Paul, C.L., & Currow, D.C. (2011). "Palliative care referral practices and perceptions. The divide between metroplitian and non-metropolitan general practitioners." *Palliative and Supportive Care*, 9, 181–189.

Jonsen, A.R., Siegler, M., & Winslade, W.J. (2002). "Clinical ethics: A practical approach to ethical decisions in clinical medicine." New York, NY: McGraw-Hill.

Joseph, S. (2013). *What doesn't kill us: The new psychology of posttraumatic growth.* New York, NY: Basic Books.

Joseph, S. (2014). "Postraumatic growth." *Psychology Today.* Retrieved from https://www.psychologytoday.com/blog/what-doesnt-kill-us/201402/posttraumatic-growth

Kabat-Zinn, J. (1994). *Wherever you go, there you are: Mindfulness meditation in everyday life.* New York, NY: Hachette Books.

Kangas, M., Bovbjerg, D.H., & Montgomery, G.H. (2008). "Cancer-related fatigue: A systematic and meta-analytic review of non-pharmacological therapies for cancer patients." *Psychology Bulletin,* 134(5), 700–41. doi:10.1037/a0012825

Katz, A. (2016). "Sexuality at end of life" The Exchange, Virtual Hospice. Retrieved from http://virtualhospice.ca

Kaiser Commission on Medicaid and the Underinsured. (2009). "Health insurance coverage of America's children." Retrieved from http://kff.org/about-kaiser-commission-on-medicaid-and-the-uninsured/

Kellehear, A. (2005). *Compassionate cities: Public health and end of life care.* New York, NY: Routledge.

Kennedy, B. (2016). "Hospice palliative care program—Symptom guidelines—Principles of opioid management." Fraser Health Authority. Accessed March 7, 2016. http://www.fraserhealth.ca/media/HPC_SymptomGuidelines_Opioid.pdf.

Kirolos, I., Tamariz, L., Schultz, E.A., Diaz, Y., Wood, B.A., & Palacio, A. (2014). "Interventions to improve hospice and palliative care referral: A systematic review." *Journal of Palliative Medicine,* 17(8), 957–964.

Kitwood, T. (2003). "Dementia reconsidered: The persona comes first." In R.S. Morrison & D.E. Meier (Eds.), *Geriatric Palliative Care.* Oxford, UK: Oxford University Press.

Klass, D., Silverman, P.R., & Nickman, S.L. (Eds.). (1996). *Continuing bonds: New understandings of grief.* Philadelphia, PA: Taylor & Francis.

Larkin, P. (2016). Personal communication.

Larkin, P.J., Sykes, N.P., Centeno, C., Ellershaw, J.E., Eisner, F., Eugene, B. … Zyyrmond, W.W.A. (2008). "The management of constipation in palliative care: clinical practice recommendations." *Palliative Medicine,* 22, 796–807

Lawlor, P., & Bush, S. (2014). "Delirium diagnosis, screening and management." *Supportive and Palliative Care,* 8(3), 286–295. Retrieved from http://www.supportiveandpalliativecare.com

Lemieux, L., Kaiser, S., Pereira, J., & Meadows, L.M. (2004). "Sexuality in palliative care: Patient perspectives." *Palliative Medicine,* 18(7), 630–7.

Levine, Stephen. (1989). *Meetings at the edge: Dialogues with the grieving and the dying, the healing and the healed.* New York, NY: Anchor Press.

Living Well with COPD. (2008). "Managing your breathing and saving your energy." Retrieved from http://www.livingwellwithcopd.com/DATA/DOCUMENT/57_en~v~managing-your-breathing-and-saving-your-energy.pdf

Lynn, J. (2004). *Sick to death and not going to take it anymore! Reforming health care for the last years of life.* Berkeley: University of California Press.

Mathieu, F. (2012). *The Compassion Fatigue Workbook: Creative tools for transforming compassion fatigue and vicarious traumatization.* New York: Taylor & Francis Group.

Matzo, Marianne. (2015). "Sexuality." In B.R. Ferrell, N. Coyle, & J.A Paice (Eds.), *Oxford Textbook of Palliative Nursing* (4th ed.). New York: NY: Oxford University Press. doi:10.1093/med/9780199332342.003.0010

Mazanec, P., & Panke, J.T. (2015). "Cultural considerations in palliative care." In B.R. Ferrel, N. Coyle, & J.A, Paice (Eds.), *Oxford Textbook of Palliative Nursing* (4th ed.). New York, NY: Oxford University Press. doi:10.1093/med/9780199332342.003.0010

McCaffery, M. (1968). "Nursing practice theories related to cognition, bodily pain, and man-environment interactions." Los Angeles: UCLA Students' Store.

McDonald, J. (2013a). "Quality palliative care in long term care." Retrieved from http://www.palliativealliance.ca/communication

McDonald, J. (2013b). "Quality palliative care in long term care, peer led debriefing toolkit: Guidelines for promoting effective grief support among front line staff." Retrieved from http://www.palliativealliance.ca/assets/files/Alliance_Reources/Org_Change/Toolkit_Sept

McGee. P., & Johnson, M. (2014). "Developing cultural competence in palliative care." *British Journal of Community Nurses,* 19(2), 91–93.

McInerney, F. (2000). "Requested death": A new social movement." *Social Science and Medicine,* 50(1), 137–54.

Meisel, A. (1989). *The right to die: The law of end-of-life decision making.* New York: Wiley Law Publications.

Mertes, P.M., & Laxenaire, M-C. (2000). "Anaphylaxis during general anaesthesia: Prevention and management." *Central Nervous System Drugs,* 14(2), 115–133.

Morley, J.E., Thomas, D.R., & Wilson, M.G. (2006). "Cachexia: Pathophysiology and clinical relevance." *American Journal of Clinical Nutrition,* 83, 735–43.

Mulcahy, Jim. (2014). *A story about care.* Video produced by Canadian Virtual Hospice and Canadian Association of Schools of Nursing. Retrieved from http://www.casn.ca /2014/10/story-care

NCHS (National Center for Health Statistics). (2012). "Health, United States." *Department of Health and Human Services Publication,* 2013–1232.

NCHS. (2015). "Mortality in the US 2014 NCHS Data Brief 229." Center for Disease Control. Retrieved from http://www.cdc .gov/nchs/data/databriefs/db229.pdf

NHPCO (National Hospice and Palliative Care Organization). (2009). "Disabilities outreach guide." Retrieved from http://www.nhpco.org/sites/default/files/public/Access /Outreach_Disabilities.pdf

NHPCO. (2015). "Statistics and Research Facts and Figures 2015." Retrieved from http://www.nhpco.org/sites/default /files/public/Statistics_Research/2015_Facts_Figures.pdf

NHPCO. (2016a). "History of Hospice Care." Retrieved from http://www.nhpco.org/history-hospice-care

NHPCO. (2016b). "Palliative Care. An Explanation of Palliative Care." Reproduced with permission from John Mastrojohn, chief operating officer. Retrieved from http://www.nhpco .org/palliative-care-4

NHS (National Health Services) Lothian. (2016). "Home." *Supportive and Palliative Care Indicators Tool.* University of Edinburgh. Retrieved from http://www.spict.org.uk/

Nouwen, H., McNeill, D.P., & Morrison, D.A. (1981). *The way of the heart, desert sprituality and contemporary ministry.* New York: The Seabury Press.

Olsen, M.L., Swetz, K.M., & Mueller, P.S. (2010). Ethical decision making with end-of-life care: Palliative sedation and withholding or withdrawing life-sustaining treatments. Mayo Clinic Proceedings, 85(10), 949–954. http://doi.org/10.4065/mcp.2010.0201

Olsson, L., Östlund, G., Strang, P., Jeppsson Grassman, E., & Friedrichsen, M. (2010). "Maintaining hope when close to death: Insight from cancer patients in palliative home care." *International Journal of Palliative Nursing,* 16(1), 607–12.

O'Neil-Page, E., Anderson, P.R., & Dean, G.E. (2015). "Fatigue." In B.R. Ferrell, N. Coyle, & J.A. Paice (Eds.), *Oxford Textbook of Palliative Nursing* (4th ed.). New York, NY: Oxford University Press. doi:10.1093/med/9780199332342.003.0010

Oregon Public Health Division. (2016). "Oregon Death with Dignity Act: 2015 Data Summary." Retrieved from https://public.health.oregon.gov/ProviderPartnerResources /EvaluationResearch/DeathwithDignityAct/Documents /year18.pdf

Paice, J.A. (2015). "Pain at the end of life." In B.R. Ferrell, N. Coyle, & J.A. Paice (Eds.), *Oxford Textbook of Palliative Nursing* (4th ed.). New York, NY: Oxford University Press. doi:10.1093/med/9780199332342.003.0010

Palliative Care Australia. (2005). "A guide to palliative care service development: A population based approach." Retrieved from http://www.pallcare.org.au

Pallium Canada. (2013). *The Pallium Palliative Pocketbook: A Peer Reviewed Reference Resource.* Edmonton: Pallium Canada.

Parkes, C.M., & Prigerson, H.G. (2013). *Bereavement: Studies of grief in adult life* (4th ed.) New York: Routledge.

Pasacreta, J.V., Minarik, P.A., Nield-Anderson, L., & Paice, J.A. (2015). "Anxiety and depression." In B.R. Ferrell, N. Coyle, & J.A. Paice (Eds.), *Oxford Textbook of Palliative Nursing* (4th ed.) New York, NY: Oxford University Press. doi:10.1093/med/9780199332342.003.0010

Pasero, C. (1994). *Acute pain service: Policy and procedure manual.* Los Angeles, California: Academy Medical Systems.

Pasero, C. (2009). "Assessment of sedation during opioid administration for pain management." *Journal of Perianesthesia Nursing,* 24(3), 186–90. doi:10.1016/j.jopan .2009.03.005

Patient Global Platform. (2014). "Scored Patient-Generated Subjective Global Assessment (PG-SGA)." Retrieved from http://pt-global.org/?page_id=6098

Pharmacist's Letter. (2012). "Equianalgesic Dosing of Opioids for Pain Management." PL Detail-Document #280801. Retrieved from https://www.nhms.org/sites/default/files/Pdfs /Opioid-Comparison-Chart-Prescriber-Letter-2012.pdf

Podymow, T., Turnbull, J., & Coyle, D. (2006). "Shelter-based palliative care for the homeless terminally ill." *Palliative Medicine,* 20(2), 81–6.

Post, S.G. (2003). "The place of love in the care of persons with advanced dementia." In R.S. Morrison & D.E. Meier (Eds.), *Geriatric Palliative Care.* New York, NY: Oxford University Press.

Puchalski, C.M. (2008). "Spiritual issues as an essential element of quality palliative care: A commentary." *Journal of Clinical Ethics,* 19(2), 160–162. Retrieved from https://smhs.gwu.edu /gwish/global-network

Puchalski, C.M., & Romer, A.L. (2000). "Taking a spiritual history allows clinicians to understand patients more fully." *Journal of Palliative Medicine,* 3(1), 129–137.

Puchalski, C., Ferrell, B., Virani, R., Otis-Green, S., Baird, P., Bull, J. ... Sulmasy, D. (2009). "Improving the quality of spiritual care as a dimension of palliative care: The report of the Consensus Conference." *Journal of Palliative Medicine,* 12(10), 885–904. doi:10.1089/jpm.2009.0142

Rando, T.A. (1984). *Grief, dying, and death: Clinical interventions for caregivers.* Champaign, Illinois: Research Press Company.

Rawlings, D. (2012). "End-of-life care considerations for gay, lesbian, bisexual, and transgender individuals." *International Journal of Palliative Nursing,* 18(1), 29–34. doi.org/10.12968/ijpn.2012.18.1.29.

Remen, N. (1997). *Kitchen table wisdom: Stories that heal.* New York: Putnam Press.

Reuter, S.E., & Martin, J.H. (2016). "Pharmacokinetics of cannabis in cancer cachexia-anorexia syndrome." *Clinical Pharmacokinetics,* 55(7), 807–12. doi:10.1007/s40262-015 -0363-2.

Richardson, L.A., & Jones, G.W. (2009). "A review of the reliability and validity of the Edmonton Symptom Assessment System." *Current Oncology,* 16(1), 55.

Rockwood, K., Song, X., MacKnight, C., Bergman, C., Hogan, D.B., McDowell, I., & Mitnitski, A. (2005). "A global clinical measure of fitness and frailty in elderly people." *Canadian Medical Association Journal,* 173(5), 489–495.

Saunders, C. (2010). *Quotes from Cicely Saunders.* Retrieved from http://www.lifebeforedeath.com/thelastword /deathquotes.shtml

Sawatzky, R., Porterfield, P., Lee, J., Dixon, D., Lounsbury, K., Pesut, B. ... Stajduhar, K. (2016). "Conceptual foundations of a palliative approach: A knowledge synthesis." *Biomed Central: Palliative Care,* 15(5). doi:DOI 10.1186/s12904-016 -0076

Sherazi, S., Mcnitt, S., Aktas, M.K., Polonsky, B., Shah, A.H., Moss, A.J., Daubert, J.P., & Zareba, W. (2013). "End-of-life care in patients with implantable cardioverter defibrillators." *Pacing and Clinical Electrophysiology,* 36(10), 1273–1279.

Silverman, P.R. (2000). *Never too young to know: Death in children's lives.* New York, NY: Oxford University Press.

Smith, H., & Passik, S. (2008). *Pain and Chemical Dependency.* New York, NY: Oxford University Press.

Smith, A.K., Cenzer, I.S., Knight, S.J., Puntillo, K.A., Widera, E., Williams, B.A., Boscardin, W.J., & Covinsky, K.E. (2010). "The epidemiology of pain during the last two years of life." *Annals of Internal Medicine,* 153(9), 563–569.

Snow, A.L., Weber, J.B., O'Malley, K.J., Cody, M., Beck, C., Bruera, E., & Ashton, C. (2004). "NOPPAIN: A nursing assistant-administered pain assessment instrument for use in dementia." *Dementia and Geriatric Cognitive Disorders,* 17, 240–246.

Statistics Canada. (2011). *Population projections: Canada, the provinces and territories 2012-2036.* Retrieved from http://www.statcan.gc.ca/daily-quotidien/100526 /dq100526b-eng.htm

Stienstra, D., & Chochinov, H.M. (2006). "Vulnerability, disability, and palliative end-of-life care." *Journal of Palliative Care,* 22(3), 166–176.

Sweetman, S. (2005). *Martindale: The Complete Drug Reference.* (34th ed.). New York, NY: Pharmaceutical Press.

Synder, S., Hazelett, S., Allen, K., & Radwany, S. (2012). "Physician knowledge, attitude and experiences with advance care planning, palliative care and hospice: Results of a primary care study." *American Journal of Hospice and Palliative Medicine,* 30(5), 419–4.

Taylor, B., & Davis, S. (2007). "The extended PLISSIT model for addressing the sexual wellbeing of individuals with an acquired disability or chronic illness." *Sexuality and Disability,* 25(3), 135–139.

Tedeschi, R.G., & Calhoun, L.G. (2004). "Posttraumatic growth: Conceptual foundations and empirical evidence." *Psychological Inquiry,* 15, 1–18. doi:http://dx.doi.org/10.1207/s15327965pli1501_01

Temel, J.S., Abernethy, A.P., Currow, D.C., Friend, J., Duus, E.M., Yan, Y., & Fearon, K.C. (2016). "Anamorelin in patients with non-small-cell lung cancer and cachexia (ROMANA 1 and ROMANA 2): Results from two randomised, double-blind, phase 3 trials." *Lancet Oncology,* 15, S1470–2045. doi:10.1016/S1470-2045(15)00558-6

Temel, J.S., Greer, J.A., Muzikansky, A., Gallagher, E.R., Admane, S., Jackson, V.A., ... Lynch, T.J. (2010). "Early palliative care for patients with metastatic non-small-cell lung cancer." *New England Journal of Medicine,* 363(8), 733–742.

Tervalon, M., & Murray-Garcia, J. (1998). "Cultural humility versus cultural competence: A critical distinction in defining physician training outcomes in multicultural education." *Journal of Health Care for the Poor and Underserved,* 9(2), 117–127.

Thomas, K. (2011). "Gold Standards Framework Prognostic Indicator Guidance." Version 4. Gold Standards Framework. Retrieved from http://www.goldstandardsframework.org .uk/cd-content/uploads/files/General%20Files/Prognostic %20Indicator%20Guidance%20October%202011.pdf

Toronto Central Community Care Access Centre. (2008). "Community Ethics Toolkit." Retrieved from http://www.jointcentreforbioethics.ca/partners/documents/cen_toolkit2008.pdf

Truth and Reconciliation Commission of Canada. (2012). "Calls to Action." Retrieved from http://www.trc.ca/websites/trcinstitution/File/2015/Findings/Calls_to_Action_English2.pdf

Tuffrey-Wijne, I., Hogg, J., & Curfs, L. (2007). "End-of-life and palliative care for people with intellectual disabilities who have cancer or other life-limiting illness: A review of the literature and available resources." *Journal of Applied Research in Intellectual Disabilities, 20*, 331–344.

Twycross, R., & Wilcock, A. (2001). "Pain Relief." In R. Wilcock, A. Twycross, & C.S. Toller (Eds.), *Symptom Management in Advanced Cancer* (4th ed). Nottingham: UK: Palliative Drugs.

UC Berkeley. (2016). "What Is compassion?" Retrieved from http://greatergood.berkeley.edu/topic/compassion/definition

US Medicare. (2016). Medicare Part A: Hospice Care Coverage. Retrieved from https://www.medicare.gov/coverage/hospice-and-respite-care.html

UTHealth (University of Texas Health Sciences Center Medical School). (2016). "Chapter 8: Pain Modulation and Mechanisms." In Department of Neurobiology and Anatomy (Ed.), *Neuroscience Online*. Retrieved from http://www.neuroscience.uth.tmc.edu/s2/chapter08.html

van der Molen, T. (1999). "Clinical COPD Questionnaire Health Care Professionals." Retrieved from http://www.ccq.nl/.

Vick, J.B., Pertsch, N., Hutchings, M., Neville, B.A., Lipsitz, S., Gawande, A., Block, S., & Bernacki, R. (2015). "The utility of the Surprise Question in identifying patients most at risk of death." *Journal of Clinical Oncology, 33*(suppl; abstr 8).

Victoria Hospice Society. (2009). "Victoria Bowel Performance Scale (BPS)." Retrieved from http://www.victoriahospice.org/sites/default/files/vhs_bowel_performance_scale_handout_2016_sample.pdf

Victoria Hospice Society. (2011). "Palliative Performance Scale, PPS v2." Retrieved from http://www.victoriahospice.org/sites/default/files/pps_for_distribution_2015_-_with_watermark_sample.pdf

Victoria Hospice Society. (2014). "Bereavement Risk Assessment Tool." Retrieved from http://www.victoriahospice.org/health-professionals/clinical-tools

Victoria Hospice Society. (2016). "Psychosocial Assessment Tool." Retrieved from http://www.victoriahospice.org/sites/default/files/psychosocial_assessment_2010_01.pdf

Victoria Hospice Society, Wainwright, W., & Thompson, M. (2016). *Transitions in Dying and Bereavement. A Psychosocial Guide for Hospice and Palliative Care* (2nd ed.). Baltimore, MD: Health Professions Press.

VIHA (Vancouver Island Health Authority). (2014). "Confusion Assessment Method (CAM) for delirium." Retrieved from http://www.viha.ca/NR/rdonlyres/6121360B-B90F-4EF3-88F6-D50CC4825EE7/0/camshortform.pdf

VP-NET (Vulnerable Persons and End of Life New Emerging Team). (2006). "People with disabilities, vulnerability, and dignity conserving care." Retrieved from http://www.umanitoba.ca/outreach/vpnet/articles/DignityConservingCare%20Final.doc

Walter, L.C., Brand, R.J., Counsell, S.R., Palmer, R.M., Landefeld, C.S., Fortinsky, R.H., & Covinsky, K.E. (2001). "Development and validation of a prognostic index for 1-year mortality in older adults after hospitalization." *Journal of the American Medical Association, 285*(23), 2987–94.

Warden, V., Hurley, A.C., & Volicer, L. (2003). "Development and psychometric evaluation of the Pain Assessment in Advanced Dementia (PAINAD) Scale." *Journal of the American Medical Directors Association, 4*(1), 9–15.

Warnick, A. (2010). "The three C's children have about dying." Life and Death Matters podcast. Retrieved from http://lifeanddeathmatters.ca/products/podcast-library/kids-and-grief-the-3-cs-of-talking-with-children-about-dying/.

Warnick, A. (2015a). "When to tell the children: Preparing children for the death of someone close to them." Virtual Hospice podcast. Retrieved from http://www.virtualhospice.ca/en_US/Main+Site+Navigation/Home/Topics/Topics/Communication/When+to+Tell+the+Children_+Preparing+Children+for+the+Death+of+Someone+Close+to+Them.aspx

Warnick, A. (2015b). "The unvoiced questions of children experiencing an illness, dying, or death in their family." Podcast from This Changed My Practice. Retrieved from http://thischangedmypractice.com/unvoiced-questions-of-children-grief/

Weiner, D., Peterson, B., & Keefe, F. (1998). " Evaluating persistent pain in long term care residents: What role for pain maps?" *Pain, 76*(1–2), 249–257. doi:doi.org/10.1016/S0304-3959(98)00059-1

WHO. (2012). "Defining palliative care." Retrieved from http://www.who.int/cancer/palliative/definition/en/

Wholihan, D. (2015). "Anorexia and Cachexia." In B.R. Ferrell, N. Coyle, & J.A. Paice, (Eds.), *Oxford Textbook of Palliative Nursing* (4th ed.). New York, NY: Oxford University Press. doi:10.1093/med/9780199332342.001.0001

Wiseman, T. (1996). "A concept analysis of empathy." *Journal of Advanced Nursing, 23*(6), 1365–2648. doi:http://dx.doi.org/10.1046/j.1365-2648.1996.12213.x

Woods, A., Willison, K., Kington, C., & Gavin, A. (2008). "Palliative care for people with severe persistent mental illness: A review of the literature." *Canadian Journal of Psychiatry, 53*(11), 725–36.

Worden, J.W. (1991). *Grief counseling & grief therapy: A handbook for the mental health practiioner.* New York, NY: Springer Publishing Company Inc.

Wright, D.K., & Brajtman, S. (2011). "Relational and embodied knowing: Nursing ethics within the interprofessional team." *Nursing Ethics*, 18, 20–30.

Yennurajalingam, S. (2016). "Fatigue." In E. Bruera & S. Yennurajalingam (Eds.), *Oxford American Handbook of Hospice and Palliative Medicine and Supportive Care.* New York, NY: Oxford University Press.

You, J.J., & Fowler, R.A. (2014). "Just ask: Discussing goals of care with patients in hospital with serious illness." *Canadian Medical Association Journal,* 186(6), 425–432.

Zalonis, R., & Slota, M. (2014). "The use of palliative care to promote autonomy in decision making." *Clinical Journal of Oncology Nursing,* 18(6), 707–711.

Index

grieving style
  intuitive and instrumental 199–200
individual pathway 194
model 197
post-traumatic growth 202
stages—Kubler-Ross 194
sudden death 4
supportive care
  compassion 205
theories 194–195
types
  anticipatory 198–199
  complicated 199
  disenfranchised 198
whole body experience 195–196
grieving
  supportive care 202–204
growth hormone receptor agonists 125
growth, post-traumatic 202
GSF PIG
  Gold Standards Framework Prognostic Indicator Guidance 51

H

hallucination
  delirium 138
  supporting, during delirium 141
heart attack
  CPR in last days and hours 236
  sudden death trajectory 4
heart disease
  clinical indicators of decline 53
holistic care
  anorexia and cachexia 123
  palliative approach 23
hope
  supporting 202
hospice
  registration criteria 13
hospice and palliative care
  barriers to accessing 19–21. *See* **accessibility to hospice
    and palliative care**
  benefits 15
  expanding 13
  goals 12
  models 13
  moving upstream 15
  principles 13
Huffing/Coughing Technique 151
hydration, artificial
  last days and hours 241
hydromorphone 102
hypodermoclysis
  last days and hours 241

I

infection
  nausea and vomiting 163
information sharing
  assessing preferences 50
intake
  changes, last days and hours 240
  changes with progressive illness 123
  fiber and constipation 127
  screening with PPS 64
intimacy and sexuality 223–224
  addressing fears/concerns 223
  quality of life 223

J

journaling, reflective practice 44

K

Klass, Silverman, Nickman
  grief theory 195
Kubler-Ross, Elizabeth
  grief theory 194

L

last days and hours 231–253
  preparing person and family 231–234
    responding to questions 233
  preparing to care 235–239
    arranging support 24/7 237
    CPR 236
    developing a plan 235
    implantable cardioverter defibrillators 237
    medication changes 236
    rituals/care preferences 238
    strategies for caring with compassion 239
  providing care 240–246
  sharing information 231
  when death occurs 247–252
laxative 130, 131
life-limiting illness
  definition 3
  slow decline 7
  stuttering decline 6
liver disease
  delirium 135
  prognosticating 57
loss 192
  ambiguous losses 193
  basic truths 193
  coping with denial 201
  definition 192
  expected losses 193
  experienced by family 192–193
  post-traumatic growth 202

steady decline 4
  benefits 5
  disadvantages 5
stuttering decline 6
  challenges 6
  life-limiting illness 6
sudden death 4
transitions in dying 190–192

V

vestibular issues
  nausea and vomiting 163
Victoria Bowel Performance Scale (BPS) 128
visceral pain
  definition 175

W

World Health Organization (WHO)
  definition, palliative care 12